FRACTURES OF THE HIP

FRACTURES OF THE HIP

Marvin H. Meyers, M.D.

Clinical Professor
Orthopaedic Surgery and Rehabilitation
University of California, San Diego
School of Medicine
San Diego, California

YEAR BOOK MEDICAL PUBLISHERS, INC.
CHICAGO

0 9 8 7 6 5 4 3 2 1

Library of Congress Cataloging in Publication Data

Meyers, Marvin H.
  Fractures of the hip.

  Includes bibliographies and index.
  1. Hip joint—Fractures.   2.   Internal fixation in fractures.   I. Title.   [DNLM: 1.   Hip Fractures. WE 855 M613f]
  RD772.M46   1985   617'.158   84-25654
  ISBN 0-8151-5897-1

Sponsoring editor: James D. Ryan, Jr.
Editing supervisor: Frances M. Perveiler
Production project manager: Max Perez
Proofroom supervisor: Shirley E. Taylor

MEYERS, MARVIN H.

Fractures of the Hip

Contributors

TIMOTHY J. BRAY, M.D.
Assistant Professor of Orthopaedics
University of California, Davis, School of
  Medicine
Chief, Orthopaedic Trauma Service
University of California, Davis, Medical
  Center
Sacramento, California

ROBERT W. BUCHOLZ, M.D.
Associate Professor of Orthopaedic
  Surgery
University of Texas Southwestern Medical
  School
Parkland Memorial Hospital
Dallas, Texas

MICHAEL W. CHAPMAN, M.D.
Professor and Chairman
Department of Orthopaedics
University of California, Davis, School of
  Medicine
Sacramento, California

LORRAINE DAY, M.D.
Associate Professor of Orthopaedic
  Surgery
University of California, San Francisco
Acting Chief, Orthopaedic Surgery Service
San Francisco General Hospital
San Francisco, California

WILLIAM M. DEYERLE, M.D.
Fellow, American College of Surgeons
Clinical Professor of Orthopaedics
Medical College of Virginia
Senior Consultant
McGuire Veterans Administration Hospital
Richmond, Virginia

JOSEPH H. DIMON, III, M.D.
Associate, Peachtree Orthopaedic Clinic
Atlanta, Georgia

VICTOR H. FRANKEL, M.D., Ph.D.
Director, Department of Orthopaedic
  Surgery
Hospital for Joint Diseases Orthopaedic
  Institute
New York, New York

KEVIN D. HARRINGTON, M.D.
Clinical Associate Professor of Orthopaedic
  Surgery
University of California, San Francisco
Children's Hospital Medical Center
San Francisco, California

LESLIE J. HARRIS, M.D.
Assistant Clinical Professor
University of Southern California
Chairman, Department of Orthopedics
San Pedro Peninsula Hospital
San Pedro, Torrance, Los Angeles

EMMETT M. LUNCEFORD, Jr., M.D.
Professor, Orthopaedic Surgery
University of South Carolina School of
  Medicine
Orthopaedic Surgeon
Richland Memorial Hospital
Columbia, South Carolina

MARVIN H. MEYERS, M.D.
Clinical Professor
Orthopaedic Surgery and Rehabilitation
University of California, San Diego
School of Medicine
San Diego, California

ALONZO J. NEUFELD, M.D.
Former Chief Physician (Retired)
Los Angeles County USC Hospital
Emeritus Attending Physician
Los Angeles USC Medical Center
Los Angeles, California

MICHAEL J. PATZAKIS
Associate Professor
University of Southern California School of
  Medicine
University of Southern California Medical
  Center
Los Angeles, California

JAMES PUGH, Ph.D.
Department of Orthopaedics
State University of New York School of
  Medicine
Health Sciences Center
Stony Brook, New York

ERIC R. SIGMOND, M.D.
Staff Orthopedic Surgeon
Northwest Community Hospital
Arlington Heights, Illinois
Humana Hospital
Hoffman Estates, Illinois

FRANKLIN H. SIM, M.D.
Professor of Orthopedic Surgery
Mayo Medical School
Consultant, Department of Orthopedics
Mayo Clinic and Mayo Foundation
Rochester, Minnesota

EDWIN T. WYMAN, Jr., M.D.
Assistant Clinical Professor of Orthopaedic
  Surgery
Harvard Medical School
Visiting Orthopaedic Surgeon
Massachusetts General Hospital
Boston, Massachusetts

ROBERT E. ZICKEL, M.D.
Clinical Professor, Orthopedic Surgery
Columbia University
College of Physicians and Surgeons
Attending Orthopedic Surgeon
St. Luke's-Roosevelt Hospital Center
New York, New York

Preface

FRACTURES OF THE HIP are relatively common injuries that impose a severe medical and economic burden on health service providers as well as on patients. The treatment of hip fractures, in particular those that are displaced, is challenging. The voluminous literature on this subject and the plethora of innovative metallic devices that continue to be introduced attest to the vicissitudes of surgery for hip fractures.

As for displaced fractures of the femoral neck, Dickson in 1953 called this the "unsolved fracture"[1] and Barnes in 1967 reported that many of his colleagues regarded it as an "unsolvable fracture."[2]

Defeatism pervaded the medical community in regard to the treatment of hip fractures until the early 1900s. Later, with the advent of radiography and internal fixation techniques, the results of treatment improved, with greater success being achieved with extracapsular fractures than intracapsular fractures. As patient prognosis improved, and with the availability of new techniques, orthopedic surgeons began to express a more aggressive approach to the treatment of fractures of the upper end of the femur.

Present treatment methods are directed mainly at better reduction of hip fractures and fixation with stouter metallic devices. Recently, sliding nails that allow compression of fracture fragments and replacement arthroplasty for intracapsular fractures, especially in the elderly, have been gaining favor. Careful review of the literature on hip fracture reveals a striking disparity in results of treatment—many surgeons using innovative techniques report results superior to those achieved at teaching institutions. Differences in the rate of success in treating hip fractures in large institutions may in part be explained by the proportion of participating surgeons with limited experience. Some papers reflect a lack of appreciation for the principles of treatment expounded by the experts.

Whichever treatment method is selected, a thorough understanding of the anatomy, biomechanics, physiology, pathology, pathogenesis, and complications is essential before the surgery is undertaken. The principle on which each method is based is perhaps as important as the details of the method itself. Failure to understand principles inevitably will lead to selection of inappropriate treatment and will jeopardize results. An essential ingredient is the experienced orthopedic surgeon who has a thorough knowledge of the principles of treatment, instrumentation, and available metallic devices, as well as impeccable surgical technique. Too often, treatment of these difficult injuries is relegated to less experienced junior house officers in teaching institutions. The results are inferior and there is a higher incidence of complications.

The plethora of internal fixation devices that have been introduced suggests that none has achieved general acceptance as the ideal device for the treatment of any hip fracture. It is unlikely that a perfect internal fixation device will ever be devised. More likely, improved results will come from a clearer understanding of biomechanical and physiologic principles involved, and therefore better use of devices based on these principles. Chapters 14, 16, 18, and 20 provide detailed explanations of the proper surgical technique for the popular internal fixation devices used to treat common hip fractures. The authors base their techniques on solid principles of treatment. Chapter 17 discusses use of the muscle pedicle graft as a means of decreasing the incidence of late segmental collapse of the femoral head, a frustrating complication following treatment of displaced intracapsular hip fractures.

This book brings together the principles of treatment and the basic knowledge in support of these principles. The practical aspects of treating fractures of the proximal end of the femur are discussed in detail. It has been written with several objectives. The book is to serve as a resource for students, orthopedic residents, and orthopedic surgeons on the principles and methods of hip fracture treatment.

The contributing authors have described in great detail the steps to be taken to avoid pitfalls and complications. Their comments should aid the surgeon in treating the many complications that arise during the treatment of hip fractures.

MARVIN H. MEYERS, M.D.

REFERENCES

1. Dickson J.A.: The "unsolved fracture." A protest against defeatism. *J. Bone Joint Surg.* 35A:805–822, 1953.
2. Barnes R.: Fracture of the neck of the femur. *J. Bone Joint Surg.* 49B:607–617, 1967.

Contents

x
Contents

General Considerations: History, Epidemiology, Diagnosis, Principles of Treatment

Marvin H. Meyers, M.D.

Until the early 20th century, fractures of the hip were frustratingly difficult to treat. Although hip fractures were recognized for many years, it was not until 1823 that Astley Cooper[1] first distinguished between intracapsular and extracapsular fractures in terms of both type of union (or nonunion) and prognosis (poor for intracapsular fractures, good for extracapsular fractures). Cooper suggested that nonunion could be related to loss of blood supply to the proximal fragment and that fibrous union was likely in most cases, and specifically in cases of intracapsular fractures, in which osseous union did not occur. In addition, Cooper proposed the first plan of treatment that included early mobilization, having recognized that immobilized elderly patients often died.

There followed a series of observations pointing to improved diagnosis and treatment. Gross, a physician active in the mid-1800s, disagreed with Cooper, but had little influence on the profession. He believed that union was possible if contact of the fragments could be achieved and immobilization maintained for a sufficient period of time.[2] Robert Smith, a contemporary of Gross, reported that osseous union of intracapsular fractures was more likely to occur when the fractures were impacted.[3] Bigelow, in 1869, noted that a false joint was a frequent result of an unimpacted fracture.[4] Nonunion and an impaired blood supply to the proximal fragment following fracture were recognized as problems by these surgeons more than a century ago. Percival Pott, among others, had recognized quite early that traction was necessary to treat fractures of the upper end of the femur.[5]

Some improvement in the reduction and healing of hip fractures came about with the introduction of roentgenographic techniques to study injured bone. Royal Whitman believed that reduction could be accomplished by careful manipulation. He advocated maintenance of the reduction in a plaster spica cast with the fractured leg held in abduction and internal rotation,[6] a method known as Whitman's abduction treatment. Whitman claimed improvement in healing with the use of his technique but never formally reported his results. Leadbetter modified the abduction method of manipulation by using perpendicular manual traction of the flexed hip, followed by abduction and internal rotation.[7] He proposed the heel-and-palm test as a means of rapidly assessing whether reduction was successful and advocated a nonpadded spica cast after fracture reduction.

Others seeking to improve treatment and results suggested changes to the nonoperative treatment protocol. Kleinberg advised early weight-bearing in a plaster cast.[8] Cotton advocated impaction of the fragments by striking the trochanter with a mallet shielded by a leather or felt pad.[9] Wilkie described a system which utilized the well leg to maintain hip abduction and fixed rotation of the leg.[10] So-called Wilkie boots were cotton dressings, supported by plaster bandages on both legs with a metallic bar between them. In 1932 Roger Anderson reported using this system to apply countertraction against the well leg.[11] These methods permitted mobilization without the need for a cumbersome spica cast.

Interest in the internal fixation of hip fractures grew right along with interest in operative and nonoperative reduction methods. Again, methods pertinent to modern surgical techniques take us back to the early and mid-19th century. Stinson's *A Treatise on Fractures,* published in 1883, refers to internal fixation of fractures by Burton at Philadelphia in 1834.[12] Von Langenbeck, in 1878, is credited with initial attempts at internal fixation of a fractured hip with a silver pin.[13] The procedure failed because of infection. Others advocated the use of nails to treat human hip fractures in serious cases.[14, 15] However, internal fixation of fractures did not receive wide acceptance because of the profession's fear of open surgery. In the early 1880s Senn demonstrated that the rate of union of femoral neck fractures in dogs could be improved by the use of internal fixation.[16] He believed that accurate reduction and firm immobilization were necessary to achieve osseous union.

Many attempts were made at internal fixation of intracapsular fractures, although Whitman's conservative treatment, based on the principles of end-to-end apposition of the fracture fragments, pressure of the fragments on each other, and immobilization, was the accepted method for treating intracapsular hip fractures.[17-19] However, the development of a triflanged nail by Smith-Peterson in 1931 introduced the modern era of treatment of hip fractures.[20, 21] This event, coupled with improved patient management and anesthesia, led to a significant increase in the number of successfully treated patients. Nevertheless, the results were far from ideal. The frustration in achieving further improvement in the rates of nonunion and osteonecrosis following internal fixation of displaced femoral neck fractures is epitomized by the publication of two papers, "The unsolved fracture," by Speed, in 1935,[22] and "The unsolved fracture: A protest against defeatism," by Dickson, in 1953.[23] Barnes in 1967 noted that some surgeons still considered these fractures "unsolvable."[24]

Many innovative design changes for internal fixation of hip fractures have been described in the literature since 1931. Even though the various designers have claimed better results with the use of their individual devices, statistical analysis of comparative results has not demonstrated significant improvement in the overall success rate. Variables present in each study make comparison of results difficult. A detailed account of each of these devices would not be pertinent to a general historical review. Nevertheless, some devices led to changes in technique that simplified surgical treatment, and in some instances improved results as well.

Closed reduction and internal fixation with the triflanged nail under roentgenographic control was recommended by Smith-Peterson. He reemphasized the principles of internal fixation and impaction outlined earlier by Martin and King[19] and by Hey-Groves,[18] both in 1922. Although significant improvement in results occurred with this technique as compared to nonoperative treatment, dissatisfaction remained because of the high rates of nonunion and osteonecrosis with segmental collapse.

Technical improvements in the triflanged nail simplified treatment and in some instances improved the results slightly. The cannulated nail and the addition of side plates were proposed to improve technique and fixation.[25, 26]

Thornton in 1937 suggested that a side bar attached to a hip nail would be useful to treat intertrochanteric fractures.[26] Neufeld in 1940 devised a single nail plate, which Taylor, Neufeld, and Janzen used in the first large series of patients treated successfully with such a device.[27] Jewett in 1941 developed a single nail plate which also was used extensively.[28] Although these single nail plate devices proved to be good internal metallic fixation devices for stable intertrochanteric fractures, they left much to be desired insofar as intracapsular and unstable intertrochanteric fractures were concerned. Both absorption due to disuse and settling of the fracture fragments frequently resulted in penetration of the femoral head by the nail end. The introduction of telescoping nails and screws with a side plate decreased the incidence of femoral head penetration and improved the rate of union.[29, 30] Nonetheless, the incidence of osteonecrosis remained the same in healed intracapsular fractures.

Shortly after the introduction of the triflanged nail, Moore in 1934[31] and Knowles in 1936[32] reported that firmer fixation of the intracapsular fracture fragments could be obtained by the use of multiple threaded pins. This had been advocated earlier by Martin and King.[19] This technique with various modifications is presently the treatment of choice in most centers.

Cotton in 1911 had promoted accurate reduction and impaction as necessary preconditions to achieve a successful union.[9] He utilized a hammer to effect a blow over the greater trochanter in order to obtain fragment impaction. Smith-Peterson reemphasized the importance of impaction. Henry in 1931 utilized a flanged screw with a nut placed laterally to impact the fracture fragments.[33] Others added innovations which were designed to provide increased contact and thus continuous impaction.[34-37]

The addition of a plastic side plate by Harmon[38] in 1944 and of a metal one by Deyerle[39] in 1959 was suggested to provide stronger fixation and permit the pins to slide distally rather than proximally when bone absorption occurred at the fracture site.

Bone grafts have been suggested as a desirable method to promote healing of intracapsular fractures and to augment repair of severely comminuted intertrochanteric fractures. Albee in 1915 reported on a small series of intracapsular fractures treated with an autogenous tibial bone graft without internal fixation.[40] King advocated use of an autogenous fibula graft with internal fixation.[41] These methods did not become popular because of technical problems, increased time for surgery, and the lack of long-term reports to show that results were improved by this technique.

Judet et al. introduced the muscle pedicle graft utilizing the quadratus femoris muscle and internal fixation to improve the revascularization process in the head fragment in an attempt to reduce the incidence of osteonecrosis.[42] They did not report their results. My colleagues and I treated a large series of patients with a modified Judet technique; we noted significant improvement in the rate of union and a decrease in the incidence of late segmental collapse.[43]

Many authors had placed great emphasis on the posterior neck comminution as a major cause for failures in the treatment of displaced intracapsular fractures.[38, 44, 45] My colleagues and I suggested the addition of supplemental iliac bone to fill a large defect which was present in the posterior aspect of the neck in 70% of cases.

The failure to improve on the high rates of nonunion and late segmental collapse led to the development of hemiarthroplasty. Moore introduced a self-locking vitallium prosthesis in 1952.[46] Changes in the design of endoprostheses have been proposed by others. Hemiarthroplasty has been popular in the treatment of older, less active patients. Loosening, subsidence, and postoperative pain have been late complications. Many advocate the adjunctive use of methylmethacrylate cement to prevent loosening and subsidence of the prosthesis.

Kuntscher in 1970 introduced intramedullary fixation for peritrochanteric fractures.[47] This method was developed to reduce blood loss, anesthetic time, and infection. Ender developed a simpler technique utilizing multiple nails which are more flexible than the rigid, single Kuntscher nail.[48] The Ender nails are easier to insert and provide rotational stability not provided by the single stiff nail. At the same time, they have the same advantages for the patient that are provided by the Kuntscher procedure.

EPIDEMIOLOGY

Fractures of the hip are most frequent in patients over the age of 40 and the incidence increases with each decade of life thereafter. These fractures are rare in children and infrequent in adults under the age of 40. Fractures of the hip in the elderly account for a large number of invalids.

Females sustain the injury three times as often as males, and caucasians more often than blacks.

Osteoporosis and osteomalacia are significant factors responsible for the high incidence of hip fractures in the elderly. Elderly patients often have debilitating medical diseases, which makes them more vulnerable to injury. In elderly patients the fracture most often results from a minor fall, twisting injury, or a stress fracture in osteoporotic hips, whereas in patients below the age of 40 and in children, severe trauma invariably is the cause.

There has been much speculation concerning the etiology of hip fractures. Some have theorized that a fall precedes the fracture; others believe the fracture occurs prior to the fall because of strain caused by disordered weight-bearing in osteoporotic bone. The biomechanics responsible for the fracture are discussed in chapter 3.

The socioeconomic problems caused by fractures in elderly patients are enormous. A large number of beds in a general hospital are occupied by this group of patients, placing a burden on health resource allocations.

In one study, two thirds of patients with hip fractures were admitted from their home and one third from institutions. The mean hospital stay was 3–4 weeks. Only 62% of those admitted from their home returned directly home.[49, 50]

It has been estimated that 200,000 hip fractures occur each year in the United States, at a cost of $750,000,000 for treatment. Approximately 19% of these patients die as a result of the fracture.[51] The incidence of recurrence, whether ipsilateral, at the same site, or contralateral, has been estimated at 20%–29%.[52, 53]

Rehabilitation requires larger resources and great effort on the part of ancillary rehabilitation personnel. In one report, the prognosis in terms of survival, mobility, and ability to carry on activities of daily living was better for patients admitted from the home rather than from institutions. However, many required walking aids, and more than half were unable to shop for themselves.[49]

DIAGNOSIS

The diagnosis of a fractured hip usually is not difficult to make. This fracture occurs most often in the aged patient following a single twisting injury or fall. It is far less frequent in children and patients under the age of 40. In young patients it usually follows a violent injury. There is a higher incidence in women than men and a lower incidence in blacks than in caucasians.

Symptoms and Signs

PAIN.—The pain accompanying intertrochanteric fractures is more severe than the pain accompanying intracapsular fractures. Movement of the limb markedly increases the pain. Intracapsular fractures are more likely to cause groin pain, while intertrochanteric and subtrochanteric fractures cause lateral hip and thigh pain. Patients with stress fractures and undisplaced intracapsular fractures frequently complain of knee rather than hip pain.

TENDERNESS.—Tenderness in the hip region is almost always present.

ECCHYMOSIS.—Ecchymosis does not occur with intracapsular fractures. In 48 hours there may be large areas of skin ecchymosis below Poupart's ligament. Ecchymosis is frequent in the thigh and posterior buttock following intertrochanteric and subtrochanteric fractures.

LIMB ATTITUDE.—The patient holds his leg in external rotation when the fracture is displaced, but usually it is held in the normal attitude when the fracture is undisplaced or impacted.

WEIGHT-BEARING.—The patient is unable to bear weight. Walking with a limp may be possible with impacted or incomplete fractures such as a stress fracture.

SWELLING.—Swelling occurs but may not be discernible because of the large volume of tissue clothing the hip joint.

LIMB SHORTENING.—Limb length is equal in undisplaced fractures. Shortening is present in the displaced fracture due to overriding of the fragments. In intracapsular fractures leg-length shortening follows varus displacement.

FALSE MOTION AND CREPITUS.—These are cardinal signs of a fracture but no attempt should be made to elicit these signs because manipulation causes severe pain. These signs are not essential to the diagnosis.

Diagnostic Tests
X-Ray

Routine x-ray studies will yield the diagnosis in most cases. Occasionally, undisplaced intracapsular and stress fractures cannot be visualized on x-ray films made in the first few days after fracture. The fracture line may not be discernible for several days, and may never be discernible in stress fractures. In order to obtain a true anteroposterior (AP) view, the limb should be held in internal rotation to eliminate the obliquity of anteversion (Fig 1–1). Usually this view will provide the diagnosis. An AP view of the pelvis is the crucial x-ray view. Often a lateral view will provide essential information concerning the degree of comminution. This view may be difficult to obtain because positioning the limb causes increased pain in most patients. It is essential to obtain a lateral view in patients with impacted femoral neck fractures since the AP view may not reveal the fracture or the degree of displacement, if any. If a lateral view is desired, a cross-table view can be obtained after first putting manual traction in line with the extended limb for several minutes. A "frogleg" view cannot be obtained because of the increased pain when the limb is moved.

Radioisotope Scanning

Technetium 99m scans are helpful in the assessment of viability of the femoral head. Technetium 99m methyldiphosphonate (MDP) scans are not useful

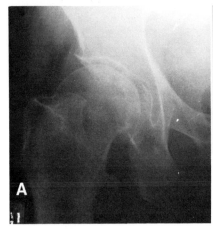
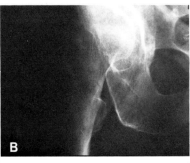

*Fig 1–1—**A,** AP x-ray film showing externally rotated leg. Fracture of neck cannot be visualized. **B,** AP x-ray film with leg internally rotated 20°. Fracture is visible.*

until 48 hours after injury. The phosphorous portion to which the radioisotope is attached is used in bone formation, and because bone production is increased in fracture healing and bone turnover, the scan will demonstrate increased activity. If circulation is absent in the head fragment, the radioisotope cannot accumulate in the head. Bone turnover does not occur in an avascular environment.

A technetium 99m MDP scan is particularly useful in the early diagnosis of stress fractures. A fracture line may not be visible on routine x-ray films, but the increased activity at the fracture line will be reflected in an increased uptake of radioisotope (see Chapter 12).

Technetium 99m sulfur colloid (SC) scans, on the other hand, can provide information concerning the vascularity of the head fragment soon after the fracture. The sulfur colloid portion is phagocytosed by reticuloendothelial cells in the marrow. Approximately 15% of this radioisotope is picked up by the bone. The remainder is picked up mainly in the liver and spleen. An early assessment of vascularity is possible since circulation to the head fragment is impaired at the time of the fracture. The technetium 99m SC scan is not valid if the uninjured hip shows no activity. Very often there is diminished hematopoietic marrow in the femoral head of the elderly patient. This accounts for the absent or minimal phagocytic activity and negative scan in viable femoral heads in many aged patients with femoral neck fractures.

Gallium scans may be helpful if an infection of the hip following surgery is suspected. However, the surgeon must keep in mind that false positive and false negative readings are frequent.

Computerized Tomography

CT scans are useful in some cases of pathologic fracture when it is necessary to assess the extent of the lesion. They also have a role in determining the position of the fragment in fracture dislocation of the femoral head.

Bone Conduction Test

Undisplaced femoral neck fractures may be extremely difficult to discern. In other cases, the physician may not be able to ascertain whether the fracture is new or healed. Since a fresh fracture will interrupt the transmission of sound across the fracture site, a simple test frequently can aid in determining whether a fracture is present or whether a sclerotic line is due to an impacted fresh fracture or a healed fracture. The test is performed by placing a stethoscope over the pubic bone and striking each patella smartly with the tip of the middle and index fingers. A muffled sound will be audible when the patella on the side of the fracture is struck, compared to a more distinct sound when the test is carried out on the intact side. The change in sound is related to "the mechanical properties of the tissue and the absorption of impact by the fractured hip as compared with that of the control" (see chapter 3). As healing of the fracture progresses, less energy is absorbed at the fracture site and the sound becomes more audible.

CLASSIFICATION

Basically, hip fractures can be classified on an anatomical basis. There are two main divisions, intracapsular fractures and extracapsular fractures. Intracapsular fractures comprise fractures of the femoral head, the subcapital area, and the transcervical area. Extracapsular fractures comprise fractures of the basal neck (partially intracapsular, anteriorly); intertrochanteric, peritrochanteric, and subtrochanteric fractures; and fractures of the greater and lesser trochanter. More detailed classifications are discussed in later chapters.

PRINCIPLES OF TREATMENT

Factors that influence the choice of treatment may be categorized into three groups: patient factors, factors pertaining to the fracture itself, and factors pertaining to operation and operating room personnel. Patient factors include age, the patient's physical and mental condition, and the bone structure. Factors pertaining to the fracture itself include the level of the fracture, the degree of displacement, and whether any complicating joint disease is present. Factors pertaining to the operation and operating room personnel include the surgeon's degree of technical skill and past experience with the operation, the availability of appropriate instruments and a good selection of internal fixation devices, the availability of good-quality x-ray equipment and image intensification, and use of a fracture table.

Most patients with hip fractures are elderly and may be debilitated, dehydrated, in electrolyte imbalance, undernourished, or have other serious medical ailments. Some surgeons have suggested that these patients be treated on an emergency basis as a life-saving measure. However, it was noted in a recent study that mortality was highest in patients who had open reduction and internal fixation of the hip in the first few days after surgery compared to those patients who were not operated on until a complete evaluation had been done and all medical problems were stabilized.[54]

Prolonged bed rest of the elderly patient is accompanied by a higher incidence of thromboembolic disease, pneumonia, and decubitus ulcers. The elderly do not respond well to treatment methods that confine them to bed rest. Organ systems function at a more efficient level in an active, ambulatory person. Bed rest produces substantial and adverse changes in the physiology of various organ systems, changes which are then superimposed on preexisting illness or debilitation. Mortality is high in elderly patients with hip fractures who are treated with prolonged bed rest.

Effects of Bed Rest on Organ Systems

CARDIAC SYSTEM.—The supine position increases the workload of the heart. Cardiac output, heart rate, and stroke volume are all increased. After a few days, the response to a change to the upright position is marked increase in heart rate and a significant drop in blood pressure.

BLOOD VESSELS.—Venous stasis due to recumbency, lack of muscular contractions, and increased venous pressure due to a reduction in circulation favor thrombus formation.

RESPIRATORY SYSTEM.—There is decreased respiratory movement, which leads to a disturbance of the oxygen and carbon dioxide balance as well as diminished movement of pulmonary secretions. Narcotics, sedatives, and anesthetic agents depress the CNS respiratory centers, which contributes to the limitation of chest expansion, further decreasing respiratory function. The additive effect of bed rest and drugs that depress respiration account for the increase in the incidence of pulmonary complications.

URINARY SYSTEM.—Stasis, incontinence, infection, and calculi as a consequence of increased calcium output are the results of bed rest in many elderly patients. Consequently there is an increased incidence of urinary complications.

GASTROINTESTINAL SYSTEM.—Gastrointestinal function is impaired in the supine position. Ingestion and digestion are impeded. Peristalsis decreases and muscles that participate in elimination become less efficient, resulting in constipation and fecal impaction.

MUSCULOSKELETAL SYSTEM.—Disuse atrophy and loss of muscle strength result from a decrease in muscular contraction. Prolonged bed rest reduces the need for joint motion, and without full range of motion after several days the muscle fibers shorten, causing contractures.

Osteoporosis is accelerated when patients are confined to bed rest. The equilibrium of bone mineralization is adversely affected when the stress of activity and weight-bearing is removed.

OTHER EFFECTS.—Decubitus ulcers and psychological disturbances are frequent. However, the surgical assault may be more hazardous for the patient with significant medical problems since he may not be capable of adjusting physiologically and biochemically until his medical status is stabilized. A delay of 24–48 hours to allow assessment of the physical status of the patient and control of serious medical problems is a prudent course. With careful preoperative assessment, death from anesthetic and medical complications may be prevented. In my experience, mortality is significantly higher in the first few days following hip fracture if surgery is performed before adequate measures have been taken to stabilize the general medical condition of the patient.

Alleviation of the pain of hip fracture is of utmost importance. Unless pain is reduced in the course of medical stabilization prior to surgery the patient's physical and mental condition may deteriorate substantially. Thus, the patient may become a greater surgical risk. If surgery is delayed by 2–3 days and pain is not eliminated in the interim, the patient may die.

In general, fractures of the hip should be considered semiemergencies in order to prevent deterioration of the patient's condition, bed sores, and pulmonary or thromboembolic complications.

Postoperatively, early mobilization as well as breathing and calf exercises should be instituted. These measures require meticulous attention on the part of nursing and allied health professionals. Diet, adequate fluid intake, and electrolyte balance deserve the physician's utmost interest. Pulmonary embolism is a life-threatening complication, and in some centers prophylactic anticoagulation therapy is routine. This question is addressed in chapter 25.

Early surgery has been advocated for intracapsular fractures as a means of decreasing the incidence of femoral head osteonecrosis. In one report of a large series of cases, surgery delayed for several days did not result in an increase in the number of patients that subsequently developed osteonecrosis.[18]

Several authors have advocated aspiration of the hip joint following intracapsular fracture in order to prevent osteonecrosis of the femoral head.[38] This procedure is unnecessary and is not supported by clinical experience or physiologic principles (see chapter 4).

The choice of an appropriate treatment method is based on a thorough understanding of hip anatomy, the biomechanics of hip fractures, the physiology of the hip joint, and the pathophysiology of hip fractures. These issues are addressed in the following chapters.

Rehabilitation

Rehabilitation after internal fixation of hip fractures is extremely important for the aged patient. A good rehabilitation program too frequently is overlooked by the treating surgeon, whose interest in rehabilitation frequently ends when the patient is discharged from the hospital. The patient may go to a convalescent home, a private residence, or a nursing care facility, where rehabilitation ends.

The importance of carrying out a program to reach rehabilitation goals to restore hip motion, muscle strength, body tone, and eventually normal gait cannot be emphasized enough. The elderly patient must be encouraged and motivated to achieve these goals. Unless a rigorous program is planned and carried out, the patient will languish and quickly deteriorate mentally as well as physically. Gentle, passive range-of-motion exercises should be started at the end of 24 hours after surgery, with progression to active assistance and active range-of-motion exercises as soon as they are tolerated.

Simultaneously with range of motion exercises, strengthening of the quadriceps and hamstring muscles is begun. Muscle strengthening measures commence with isometric muscle setting and progress to isokinetic exercise. Hip adductor strengthening is started by placing a pillow between the knees as resistance to isometric contraction.

Abduction exercises are begun as tolerated, commencing with active abduction in the supine position and progressing to abduction in the contralateral decubitus position as the patient gets stronger. The patient usually cannot begin abduction exercises for several days after starting other muscle strengthening procedures. As soon as the patient can begin ambulation between parallel bars or with a walker, hip elevation exercises are encouraged.

Whole body fitness can be maintained by ambulation and stationary bicycle riding in the physical therapy department.

Proper gait training under the guidance of a trained therapist is essential. Alert patients progress rapidly to a walker or crutches. Other patients need instruction, encouragement, and careful supervision. Many patients have a tendency to shift the trunk laterally during the stance phase or to walk with a Trendelenburg gait. These deviations are due to hip abductor weakness, contractures, or pain. It is therefore important to eliminate the pain with appropriate medication or have the physician check the patient to be sure that there has been no change in the position of the fracture fragments or fixation. The therapist must be certain that sufficient muscle strength has returned to permit progressive gait training exercises.

REFERENCES

1. Cooper A.R.: *A Treatise on Dislocations and on Fractures of the Joints,* ed. 2, London, Longman Hurst, 1823, p. 570.

2. Gross S.O.: *System of Surgery.* Philadelphia, Blanchard & Lea, 1859, vol. 2, pp. 252-240.

3. Smith R.W.: *A Treatise on Fractures in the Vicinity of Joints.* New York, Samuel S. and William Wood, 1845, p. 111.

4. Bigelow H.J.: *The Mechanism of Dislocation and Fracture of the Hip.* Philadelphia, Henry C. Lea, 1869, p. 137.

5. Pott P.: *Chirurgical Works.* London, 1783.

6. Whitman R.: A new method of treatment for fractures of the neck of the femur, together with remarks on coxa vara. *Ann. Surg.* 36:746, 1902.

7. Leadbetter G.W.: Treatment for fracture of the neck of the femur. *J. Bone Joint Surg.* 15:931, 1933.

8. Kleinberg S.: The value of early weight bearing in the treatment of the neck of the femur. *J. Bone Joint Surg.* 19:964, 1937.

9. Cotton F.J.: Artificial impaction in hip fracture. *Am. J. Orthop. Surg.* 8:680, 1911.

10. Wilkie D.P.D.: A new treatment for fracture of the neck of the femur. *Surg. Gynecol. Obstet.* 44:529, 1927.

11. Anderson R.: New methods for treating fractures utilizing the well-leg for countertraction. *Surg. Gynecol. Obstet.* 54:207, 1932.

12. Stinson L.A.: *A Treatise on Fractures.* Philadelphia, C. Lea's Son & Co., 1883, p. 598.

13. Von Langenbeck B.: *Verhandl. d. deutsch. Gesellsch. f Chir.* 1878, p. 92.

14. König S.: Congress Irith Sitzeing, 1875, p. 12.

15. Nicolaysen J.: Lidt om Diagnosen ag Behandligen af Fractura colli femoris. *Nord. Med. Arkiro.* 8:1, 1897.

16. Senn N.: Fractures of the neck of the femur with special reference to bony union after intracapsular fracture. *Trans. Am. Surg. Assoc.* 1:333, 1881-1883.

17. Delbet P.: Resultat elorgne d'un visage pour fracture transcervicale du femur. *Bull. Soc. Clin. Paris* 45:305, 1919.

18. Hey-Groves E.: *Modern Methods of Treating Fractures.* Bristol, England, John Wright and Sons, Ltd, 1916.

19. Martin E., King A.: A new method of treating fractures of the neck of the femur. *New Orleans Med. Surg. J.* 75:710, 1923.

20. Smith-Peterson M.N., Cave E.F., von Gorden W.: Intracapsular fracture of the neck of the femur. *Arch. Surg.* 23:715-759, 1931.

21. Smith-Peterson M.N., Cave E.F., von Gordon W.: Treatment of fractures of the femur by internal fixation. *Surg. Gynecol. Obstet.* 64:287-295, 1937.

22. Speed K.: The unsolved fracture. *Surg. Gynecol. Obstet.* 60:341, 1935.

23. Dickson J.A.: The "unsolved fracture": A protest against defeatism. *J. Bone Joint Surg.* 35A:805-822, 1953.

24. Barnes R.: Fracture of the neck of the femur. *J. Bone Joint Surg.* 49B:607-617, 1967.

25. Johannson S.: On the operative treatment of medial fractures of the femoral neck. *Acta Orthop. Scand.* 3:362-385, 1932.

26. Thornton L.: The treatment of trochanteric fracture: Two new methods. *Piedmont Hosp. Bull.* 10:21, 1937.

27. Taylor G.M., Neufeld A.J., Janzen J.: Internal fixation for intertrochanteric fractures. *J. Bone Joint Surg.* 26:707-712, 1944.

28. Jewett E.L.: One piece angle nail for trochanteric fractures. *J. Bone Joint Surg.* 23:803-810, 1941.

29. Massie W.K.: Functional fixation of femoral neck fractures: Telescoping nail technique. *Clin. Orthop.* 12:230-255, 1958.

30. Pugh W.L.: A self-adjusting nail-plate for fractures about the hip joint. *J. Bone Joint Surg.* 37A:1085-1093, 1955.

31. Moore A.T.: Fractures of the hip joint (intracapsular): A new method of skeletal fixation. *J. South Carolina Med. Assoc.* 30:199-205, 1934.

32. Knowles F.C.: Fractures of the neck of the femur. *Wisconsin Med. J.* 35:106-109, 1936.

33. Henry M.D.: Intracapsular fracture of the hip. *J. Bone Joint Surg.* 13:530, 1931.

34. Charnley J.: Treatment of fractures of neck of femur by compression. *J. Bone Joint Surg.* 38B:772, 1956.
35. Godoy-Moreira F.E.: A special studbolt screw for fixation of fractures of the neck. *Zentralbl. Chir.* 77:316, 1952.
36. Lippmann R.K.: A new device for securing and maintaining compression in femoral neck fractures. *J. Mt. Sinai Hosp.* 3:65, 1936.
37. Lorenzo F.A.: Molybdenum steel lag screw in internal fixation in fractured neck of the femur. *Surg. Gynecol. Obstet.* 73:98, 1941.
38. Harmon P.H.: Treatment of trochanteric, subtrochanteric, and transcervical fractures of the upper femur by fixation with plastic plate and stainless steel screws. *South. Clin. Bull.* 14:10, 1944.
39. Deyerle W.M.: Absolute fixation with contact compression in hip fractures. *Clin. Orthop.* 13:279-297, 1959.
40. Albee F.H.: The bone graft peg in treatment of fractures of the neck of the femur. *Ann. Surg.* 62:85-91, 1915.
41. King T.: The closed operation for intracapsular fracture of the neck of the femur. *Br. J. Surg.* 26:721-748, 1939.
42. Judet R., Judet J., Lord G., et al.: Treatment of fractures of the femoral neck by pedicled graft. *Presse Med.* 69:2452-2453, 1961.
43. Meyers M.H., Harvey J.P. Jr., Moore T.M.: Treatment of displaced subcapital and transcervical fractures of the femoral neck by muscle-pedicle bone graft and internal fixation. *J. Bone Joint Surg.* 55A:257-274, 1973.
44. Garden R.S.: Stability and union in subcapital fractures of the femur. *J. Bone Joint Surg.* 46B:630-647, 1964.
45. Hargadon E.J., Pearson J.R.: Treatment of intracapsular fractures of the femoral neck with the Charnley compression screw. *J. Bone Joint Surg.* 45B:305-311, 1963.
46. Moore A.T.: A new self-locking vitallium prosthesis. *South. Med. J.* 45:1015-1019, 1952.
47. Kuntscher T.G.: A new method of Rx of peritrochanteric fractures. *Proc. R. Soc. Med.* 63:1120, 1970.
48. Ender J., Simon-Weidner R.: Die Fixierung der trochenteren Bruche mit rundem elastischen Condylennageln. *Acta Chirurg. Aust.* 1:40, 1970.
49. Ceder L., Ekelund L., Inerot S., et al.: Rehabilitation after hip fracture in the elderly. *Acta Orthop. Scand.* 50:681, 1979.
50. Ceder L., Lindbergh L., Odberg E.: Differential care of hip fracture in the elderly. *Acta Orthop. Scand.* 51:157-162, 1980.
51. Lewinnek F.G., Kelsey J., White A.A., et al.: The significance and a comparative analysis of the epidemiology of hip fractures. *Clin. Orthop.* 152:35-43, 1980.
52. Melton J.L., Ilstrup D.M., Bechenbaugh R.D., et al.: Hip fracture recurrence. *Clin. Orthop.* 167:131-138, 1982.
53. Stewart I.M.: Fracture of the neck of the femur: Survival and contralateral fracture. *Br. Med. J.* 2:922, 1957.
54. Kenzora J.E., McCarthy R.E., Lowell J.D., et al.: Hip fracture mortality: Relation to age, treatment, preoperative illness, time of surgery and complications. *Clin. Orthop.* 186:45, 1984.

Chapter 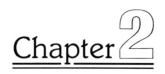2

Anatomy of the Hip

Marvin H. Meyers, M.D.

GROSS ANATOMY

The hip joint is a synovial joint and the most striking example of the ball-and-socket configuration. Its various parts provide a high degree of stability as well as a good range of movement.

The acetabulum is a cup-shaped, deep socket on the lateral aspect of the pelvis. The inner aspect is a horseshoe-shaped articular surface lined with hyaline cartilage (Fig 2–1,A). The anteroinferior rim is deficient and termed the acetabular notch (Fig 2–1,A). The floor of the acetabulum or fossa contains a fat pad covered by synovial membrane (Fig 2–1,B). Weight-bearing occurs in the upper part of the acetabulum where the cartilaginous strip is widest.

A fibrocartilaginous rim, the acetabular labrum (Fig 2–1,B), is attached to the bony rim, deepening the acetabulum and also narrowing the opening. The acetabular notch is crossed by the transverse ligament, which is attached to the labrum.

The head of the femur is completely covered by hyaline cartilage and forms slightly more than half a sphere (see Fig 2–1,B). It is gripped by the bony cavity of the acetabulum, which is deepened by the fibrocartilaginous labrum. The labrum grips the femoral head beyond its greatest diameter, increasing the stability of the joint. Inferior and behind the center of the head is a small depression to which the ligamentum teres is attached (see Fig 2–1,B). It is not covered by cartilage.

The capsular ligament of the joint encloses the hip joint as in a sleeve. It is attached to the acetabular labrum and bone behind the acetabulum, the trochanteric line of the front of the femur, and the posterior aspect of the femoral neck, with about half the posterior base of the neck remaining extracapsular.

Thickened bands called ligaments strengthen the capsular ligament and resist tensile strain. The anterior aspect of the capsular ligament is reinforced by the strong, dense, iliofemoral ligament which is attached to the anteroinferior iliac spine below the origin of the straight head of the rectus femoris. It is triangular in shape and divides into two bands as it passes downward to insert into each end of the trochanteric line. It has the appearance of an inverted Y. The inferomedial aspect of the hip joint is supported by the pubofemoral ligament, which runs from the iliopectineal eminence and blends with the lower and anterior part of the capsular ligament. The posterior aspect of the joint is strengthened by the ischiofemoral ligament, which blends with the capsular ligament from the ischium below the acetabulum.

The iliofemoral and ischiofemoral ligaments resist hyperextension of the hip. The pubofemoral ligament resists hyperextension and excessive abduction of the hip.

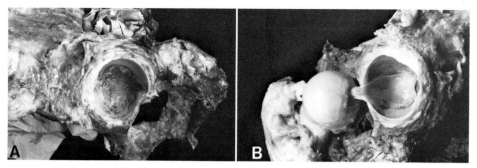

Fig 2–1—**A,** *horseshoe-shaped articular surface of acetabulum, acetabular notch, and fat pad in acetabular fossa.* **B,** *acetabular labrum deepening the socket. Ligamentum teres inserts into the fovea of the femoral head.*

The ligamentum teres lies within the joint and is covered by a tube of synovial membrane (see Fig 2–1,B). It runs from the fovea (the pit) on the head of the femur to the transverse ligament and margins of the acetabular notch.

The synovial membrane lines the capsular ligament and is reflected at its femoral attachment to cover the intracapsular portions of the femoral neck. As it lines the transverse ligament the membrane enters the joint to cover the fat in the acetabular fossa and the ligamentum teres. The ligamentum teres is a weak ligament. Probably, its sole function is to support the artery in its course to the fovea of the femoral head.

The superomedial part of the quadratus femoris, together with its nerve and vessels, the obturator internus tendon, and the gemelli, are in immediate relationship with the posterior capsule separating the sciatic nerve from the joint. The piriformis and gluteus minimus muscles near the insertion of the quadratus femoris lie on the superior aspect of the joint.

HIP MUSCLES

The muscles surrounding the hip joint are responsible for movement strength and provide additional stability by assisting the ligaments.

The *sartorius* muscle arises from the anterosuperior iliac spine and descends over the anterior aspect of the thigh to insert into the medial surface of the tibia just below the knee joint. It makes up the anterior portion of the pes anserinus.

The *pectineus* muscle arises from the superior ramus of the pubis and crosses in front of the medial part of the capsular ligament of the hip joint to insert just lateral to the lesser trochanter on the posterior aspect of the femur.

The *iliopsoas* tendon is a conjoined tendon made up of the psoas and iliacus muscles. The psoas muscle arises from the sides of the 12th thoracic to 5th lumbar vertebral bodies and intervening disks, as well as from the transverse processes. The tendon passes behind the inguinal ligament, after joining with the tendon of the iliacus muscle across the medial anterior aspect of the capsular ligament, to insert into the lesser trochanter.

The *iliacus* muscle arises from the fossa of the ilium. The medial fibers join with the psoas to form the iliopsoas tendon, and the lateral fibers attach to the femur below the lesser trochanter.

The *rectus femoris* muscle is one of the four parts of the quadriceps muscle. It has two heads. The straight head originates in the upper portion of the anterior inferior iliac spine. The reflected head originates in an area of the ilium just above the acetabulum. It runs downward between the sartorius and tensor fasciae latae superficial to the other three parts of the muscle.

The femoral vessels are separated from the anterior aspect of the capsular ligaments by the lateral edge of the pectineus, the iliopsoas muscles, and the straight head of the rectus muscle.

The *adductor longus* muscle arises from the body of the pubis between the crest and symphysis. It becomes wider as it descends and inserts into the medial lip of the linea aspera.

The *adductor brevis* muscle arises below the origin of the adductor longus. It runs posterior to the latter and inserts into the posterior aspect of the femur from the lesser trochanter to the linea aspera.

The *adductor magnus* muscle lies posterior to the adductor brevis. It arises from the pubic arch, under cover of the adductor brevis, and from the ischial tuberosity. It inserts into the gluteal tuberosity, linea aspera, and medial supracondylar line.

The *gracilis* muscle arises in the margin of the upper part of the pubic arch and the adjoining part of the body of the pubis. It inserts into the upper medial surface of the tibia.

The *obturator externus* muscle originates in the outer surface of the obturator membrane and the bony margins of the obturator foramen. It inserts into the trochanteric fossa after crossing the posterior aspect of the capsular ligament.

The *gluteus maximus* muscle is a large powerful muscle that arises over a large area encompassing the posterior part of the gluteal surface of the ilium, the dorsal aspects of the sacrum and coccyx, and the sacrotuberous ligament. It inserts into the gluteal tuberosity of the femur and the iliotibial tract in the upper posterior part of the fascia lata.

The *piriformis* muscle arises in the front of the sacrum and inserts into the upper border of the greater trochanter.

The *obturatorius internus* muscle arises in the margins of the obturator foramen on the internal surface of the pelvis and the inner surface of the obturator membrane. Part of its origin is the pelvic surface of the coxal bone. It inserts into the upper border of the greater trochanter under cover of the trochanteric crest.

The *superior gemellus* muscle originates in the posterior surface of the ischial spine and inserts into the upper border of the greater trochanter, forming a common tendon with the obturatorius internus, which lies inferior, and the inferior gemellus, which is inferior to the obturatorius internus. The latter arises on the upper border of the ischial tuberosity.

The *quadratus femoris* muscle arises from the lateral ischial tuberosity and inserts into the inferior aspect of the trochanteric crest.

The *gluteus medius* muscle originates on the gluteal surface of the ilium from the iliac crest to the middle gluteal line and behind to the posterior gluteal line. It inserts into the lateral aspect of the greater trochanter.

The *gluteus minimus* muscle arises from the gluteal surface of the ilium between the middle and inferior gluteal line and inserts into the anterior surface of the greater trochanter.

The *tensor fascia lata* arises from the anterior portion of the outer lip of the iliac crest and inserts into the iliotibial tract.

The *semimembranosus* muscle originates on the upper lateral aspect of the ischial tuberosity by means of a strong tendon and inserts into the posteromedial aspect of the medial condyle of the tibia.

The *semitendinosus* muscle arises from the lower medial impression on the ischial tuberosity in common with the long head of the biceps and inserts into the upper part of the medial surface of the tibia just below the gracilis muscle.

The long head of the *biceps femoris* arises from the posteromedial aspect of the ischial tuberosity and the lower part of the sacrotuberous ligament. The biceps femoris also has a short head, which arises from the lateral lip and the linea aspera and the lateral supracondylar line and lateral intermuscular system. It inserts into the head of the fibula.

The function of each muscle in the region of the hip as well as the nerve innervation is listed in Table 2–1.

TABLE 2–1.—Muscles, Functions, and Nerve Innervations in the Hip

Location	Muscle	Function	Nerve Innervation
Front of thigh	Sartorius	Flexion	Femoral
	Pectineus	Flexion and Adduction	Femoral
	Iliopsoas tendon		
	Iliacus	Flexion	Femoral
	Psoas	Flexion	L1–4 nerve roots
	Rectus	Flexion	Femoral
Medial side of thigh	Adductor longus	Adduction, flexion, lateral rotation	Obturator
	Adductor brevis	Adduction, flexion, lateral rotation	Obturator
	Adductor magnus	Adduction, flexion, lateral rotation, extension	Obturator and sciatic
	Gracilis	Adduction, flexion, lateral rotation	Obturator
	Obturatorius externus	Lateral rotation	Posterior division of obturator nerve
Gluteal region	Gluteus maximus	Lateral rotation, extensor	Inferior gluteal
	Piriformis	Lateral rotation	Anterior primary rami, S1–2
	Obturatorius internus	Lateral rotation Abduction when hip is flexed	Nerve to obturatorius internus
	Superior gemellus	Lateral rotation	Nerve to obturatorius internus
	Inferior gemellus	Lateral rotation	Nerve to quadratus femoris (L4–5, S1)
	Quadratus femoris	Lateral rotation	Nerve to quadratus femoris (L4–5, S1)

Continued.

TABLE 2–1.—Continued

Location	Muscle	Function	Nerve Innervation
Gluteal region—cont'd	Gluteus medius	Medial rotation/abduction	Superior gluteal
	Gluteus minimus	Medial rotation/abduction	Superior gluteal
	Tensor fascia lata	Medial rotation	Superior gluteal
Posterior aspect of thigh	Semimembra-nosus	Extension	Sciatic
	Semitendinosus	Extension	Sciatic
	Biceps femoris	Extension	Sciatic

THE PROXIMAL END OF THE FEMUR

The rounded head of the femur is securely gripped by the acetabular labrum beyond its maximum diameter. The head forms a separate epiphysis, and the epiphyseal cartilage separates it from the femoral neck. The epiphysis ossifies at the end of the first year of life and joins the shaft at about age 18 or 19. It is entirely intracapsular. The femoral head forms two thirds of a sphere. The axes of the head and neck are parallel. In the lateral plane both axes usually form a continuous straight line. The globular head is covered by articular cartilage which varies in thickness. The superior weight-bearing surface has the thickest cartilage. The fovea to which the ligamentum is attached is devoid of cartilage (see Fig 2–1,B).

The neck projects superiorly, anteriorly, and medially from the upper femoral shaft medial to the origin of the greater trochanter, forming an average angle of 135° with the long axis of the femoral shaft. The femoral neck is broader at its base and narrower at the subcapital junction (Fig 2–2). It is somewhat flattened anteriorly. The

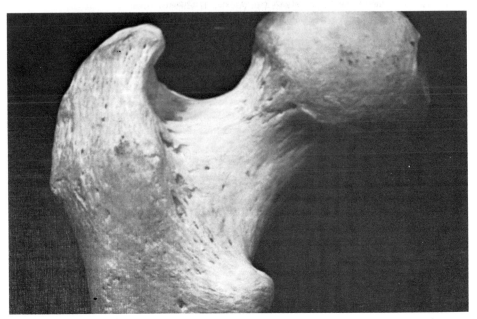

Fig 2–2—Posterior view of upper end of femur. Note broad base of neck and narrower subcapital end. The trochanteric crest decreases in height from the tip of the trochanter to its cephalad end at the upper edge of the lesser trochanter.

anterior surface of the neck lies entirely within the capsular surface of the hip joint. On the posterior aspect, the capsular ligament and the synovial membrane cover the neck in its medial part but never extend so far as the trochanteric crest. This aspect, therefore, is partly intracapsular and partly extracapsular. The periosteum covering the neck is devoid of the cambium layer, which accounts for the absence of periosteal callus in the healing process of a fracture.[1]

The greater trochanter, the most prominent projection of the hip, can be felt subcutaneously one handbreadth below the iliac crest. It has a separate center of ossification and its epiphysis includes the attachments of the gluteus minimus in front, gluteus medius on the lateral side, piriformis and obturatorius internus on its free border, and obturatorius externus in the trochanteric fossa.

The lesser trochanter cannot be palpated in the living subject. It gives attachment to the tendon of the psoas major and forms a scale-like epiphysis between ages 14 and 18. The trochanteric line crosses the front of the upper end of the shaft. It gives attachment to the capsular ligament and upper and lower parts of the ilio-femoral ligament of the hip joint. Below and medially it runs into the spiral line that passes below the lesser trochanter, and reaches the lip of the linea aspera. The origin of the vastus medialis follows the lower part of the trochanteric line and the spiral line to the linea aspera. The trochanteric crest crosses the posterior aspect of the bone and runs into the lesser trochanter below (see Fig 2–2). Its middle is the point of insertion of the quadratus femoris muscle.

The trabecular structure of the proximal femur enables it to withstand the considerable tensile and compressive forces to which it is normally subjected. There are two main trabecular systems in the upper end of the femur, a compression system and a tension system (Fig 2–3). The compression system arises from the medial portion of the shaft and extends upward into the head. The tensile group arises from the lateral portion of the neck and the inferior portion of the head. A mainly intertrochanteric system connects the two major groups, forming a triangle. The area of lessened density in the triangle delineated by the major trabecular systems is known as Ward's triangle (see Fig 2–3).

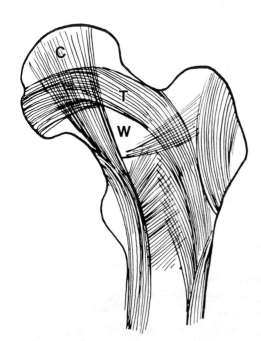

Fig 2–3—Coronal section of upper end of the femur demonstrating tension (t) and compression (c) trabeculae and Ward's triangle (w)

The calcar femorale is a dense vertical plate of bone within the femur.[2,3] It originates in the posteromedial portion of the femoral shaft under the lesser trochanter and radiates laterally through the cancellous tissue toward the greater trochanter (Fig 2–4,A). Superiorly the calcar femorale fuses firmly with the cortex of the posterior aspect of the femoral neck; distally it extends for about 2 inches anterior to the lesser trochanter (Fig 2–4,B) and then fuses into the posteromedial aspect of the diaphysis (Fig 2–4,C). The calcar femorale appears to act as a reinforcement to the posteromedial angle of the intertrochanteric portion of the femur.[3] When this structure fails, unstable intertrochanteric fracture is the result. The thickened inferior neck of the femur is referred to erroneously as the calcar in many publications on hip fractures and total hip replacements.

The neck projects medially from the shaft, forming an average angle of 135° in the adult (the neck shaft angle). The femoral neck also projects anterior to the coronal plane of the shaft. This is referred to as anteversion. The average measure-

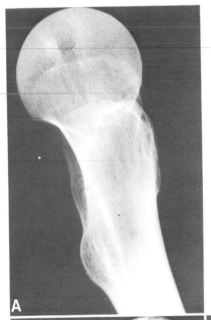

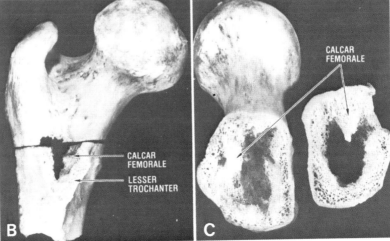

Fig 2–4—Calcar femorale. The calcar femorale is located in the intramedullary portion of the femoral neck and is not part of the inferior femoral neck. **A,** lateral x-ray view of upper end of the femur. The dense line running from the posterior neck to the lesser trochanter is the dense bone of the calcar femorale. **B,** posterior view of upper end of the femur. The femoral cortex is denuded, revealing the calcar femorale. **C,** calcar femorale. Note its location anterior to the lesser trochanter and in an intramedullary position. (**B** and **C** from Griffin.[2] Reproduced by permission.)

CALCAR
FEMORALE

LESSER
TROCHANTER

CALCAR
FEMORALE

ment of anteversion is 7° in the male and 10° in the female caucasian. There may be differences in the normal average anteversion of the femoral neck in different ethnic groups, based on the work of Hoaglund and Low.[4]

CIRCULATION

Bone is a vascular tissue. The hyaline cartilage covering the femoral head is avascular. The blood supply to the upper end of the femur is extensive. The arteries supplying the femoral head are particularly vulnerable to injury.

There is a ring of arteries surrounding the femoral neck at its base (Fig 2–5). Posteriorly a branch of the medial femoral circumflex artery and anteriorly a branch of the lateral circumflex artery, both arising from the medial or posterior aspect of the femoral artery, or the profunda, which is a branch of the femoral artery, form most of the circle.

The superior gluteal artery, derived from the internal iliac artery, and the first perforating artery, derived from the profunda, anastomose with the circle, thereby forming the crucial anastomosis.

Branches from the arterial ring of the femoral neck are given off periodically. They pierce the capsule and are covered by retinacula of synovial membrane. These branches pass upward along the femoral neck to enter the superoposterior aspect of the femoral neck near its junction with the femoral head articular cartilage (Fig 2–6). The description of the vasculature of the femoral head is based on the work of Trueta and Harrison (Fig 2–7).[5] Excellent descriptions of the arteries supplying the upper end of the femur can be found in articles by Chung[6] and Crock.[7]

These vessels are divided into epiphyseal and metaphyseal arteries. The lateral epiphyseal arteries (four or more in number) probably are the major source of blood to the femoral head (Fig 2–8). They gain access to the femoral head at the junction of the articular cartilage and the superoposterior aspect of the femoral neck

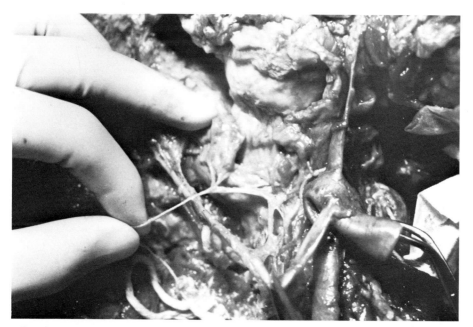

Fig 2–5—Anatomical dissection showing ring formed by anastomosis of the medial and lateral circumflex arteries from the profunda femoris artery.

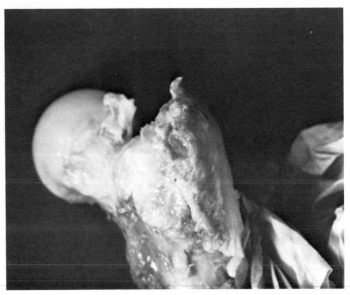

Fig 2–6—*Anatomical dissection showing lateral epiphyseal vessels entering the superoposterior aspect of the femoral neck near its junction with the articular cartilage of the femoral head. The superior retinaculum has been dissected off the femoral neck.*

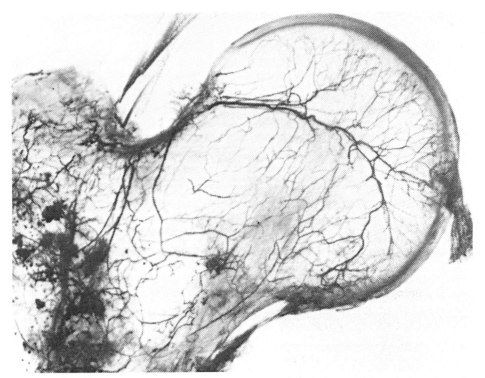

Fig 2–7—*Micropaque-infiltrated preparation of the femoral head showing the major arterial supply to the femoral head. Lateral epiphyseal vessels form an arcade that supplies most of the femoral head. (From Sevitt and Thompson.[8] Reproduced by permission.)*

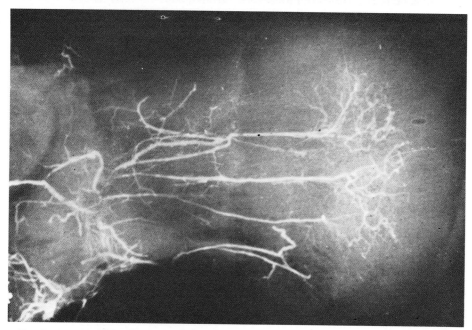

Fig 2–8—Lateral roentgenogram of decalcified, barium-infiltrated femoral head and neck. Note four lateral epiphyseal vessels entering the superoposterior aspect of the femoral head and forming a network of vessels. (From Wertheimer, L.J., et al.: Arterial supply of the femoral head. J. Bone Joint Surg. 53A:549, 1971. Reproduced by permission.)

in a superior retinaculum. The superior metaphyseal vessels enter separately or after joining the lateral epiphyseal arteries prior to entering the femoral neck. They supply the superior metaphysis of the femoral neck. The lateral epiphyseal vessels are ruptured or may be crushed at the fracture site as they enter the bone (see chapter 4) in displaced femoral neck fractures.

The posteroinferior capsular arteries gain access to the femoral neck in the inferior retinaculum and supply the inferior metaphysis and a small area of the inferior portion of the femoral head.[8] In 20% of specimens the collateral circulation can adequately supply the femoral head if the main circulation from the lateral epiphyseal vessels is disrupted.[8]

There are several small arteries which penetrate the bone inferior to the femoral head articular cartilage, anteriorly.

Branches from the obturator artery traverse the ligamentum teres to enter the fovea of the head and supply a small portion of the femoral head in the region of the fovea. In approximately 4% of adults these vessels have sufficient collateral circulation to adequately supply blood to the entire femoral head.[1,8]

The vascular pattern of the femoral head during growth has been described by Trueta.[9] The pattern changes several times until puberty, when the adult pattern is established. At birth, vessels of the ligamentum teres do not penetrate the epiphysis. From age 18 months to age 7 years, the metaphyseal vessels decrease in number and the lateral epiphyseal vessels become more important as the supply of blood to the epiphysis.

Vessels from the ligamentum teres do not penetrate the epiphysis until approximately age 6.

Most of the blood flow to the epiphysis is derived from the lateral epiphyseal vessels. Penetration of the epiphysis by vessels in the ligamentum teres occurs after age 6 in caucasians but is usually present at birth in African children. The arteries of the ligamentum teres and lateral epiphyseal vessels anastomose 7–11 years after the former penetrate the epiphysis.

The vasculature of the proximal metaphysis increases markedly from the 11th year until the growth plate disappears. The anastomosis of vessels from the epiphysis and metaphysis proceeds gradually as the growth plate disappears.

REFERENCES

1. Schmorl G.: Die pathologische Anatomie der Schenkelholsbrakturen. *München. Med. Wochenschr.* 71:1381-1385, 1924.
2. Griffin J.B.: The calcar femorale redefined. *Clin. Orthop.* 164:211-214, 1982.
3. Harty M.: The calcar femorale and the femoral neck. *J. Bone Joint Surg.* 39A:625-630, 1957.
4. Hoaglund F.W., Low W.D.: Anatomy of the femoral neck and head with comparative data from caucasians and Hong Kong Chinese. *Clin. Orthop.* 152:10-16, 1980.
5. Trueta J., Harrison M.H.M.: The normal vascular anatomy of the femoral head in an adult man. *J. Bone Joint Surg.* 35B:442, 1953.
6. Chung S.M.K.: The arterial supply of the developing proximal end of human femur. *J. Bone Joint Surg.* 58A:961, 1976.
7. Crock H.V.: A revision of the anatomy of the arteries supplying the upper end of the human femur. *J. Anat.* 99:77-88, 1965.
8. Sevitt S., Thompson R.G.: The distribution and anastomosis of arteries supplying the head and neck of the femur. *J. Bone Joint Surg.* 47B:560-573, 1965.
9. Trueta J.: The normal vascular anatomy of the human femoral head during growth. *J. Bone Joint Surg.* 39B:3, 1957.

Chapter 3

Biomechanics of Hip Fractures

James Pugh, Ph.D.
Victor H. Frankel, M.D.

For the purpose of biomechanical characterization, fractures of the femur can be classified into distinct categories according to the tissues involved and the type of loading. The tissue categories are (1) intra-articular, (2) extra-articular. The loading categories include (1) fractures due to static forces, and (2) fractures due to dynamic forces. Consideration of the mechanisms of fracture and fracture healing must take into account these four categories, as well as the mechanical properties of the ancillary tissues involved in fracture type.

Intra-articular fractures and extra-articular fractures are both produced through similar loading mechanisms. However, intra-articular fractures involve to a much greater extent tissues that show a significant rate dependence of the mechanical properties, such as articular cartilage, ligaments, capsule, and synovium. Extra-articular fractures have a more significant static component than intra-articular fractures. Because of their location and the potential for disruption of vascularity, intra-articular fractures often pose significant challenges in treatment. Intra-articular fractures must necessarily involve the mechanics of cancellous bone to a greater extent than fractures farther away from the joint, since the proportion of cortical bone to cancellous bone increases greatly in the direction away from the joint.

Muscle force, on the other hand, must play a greater role in the production and treatment of extra-articular fractures, again because of their location distal to the joint. Minimization of muscle force is often a prerequisite to successful healing of these fractures. Intra-articular fracture healing is often assisted by the application of dynamic loads. The trend in fracture treatment is toward early weight-bearing and often passive range-of-motion exercise during the early stages. This trend implies that a consideration of the static and dynamic components of the tissues during fracture healing is germane.

STATICS

Statics is that aspect of mechanics dealing with systems in force and moment equilibrium. The two criteria for static equilibrium are the following: (1) the sum of the forces in any and all directions must equal zero, and (2) the sum of the moments about any and every point must be zero. The first criterion ensures that there are no net forces on the system and that the system is not linearly accelerating. The second criterion ensures that there are no net moments and that the system is not angularly accelerating. Examples of static systems include passive weight-bearing, as well as activities occurring over protracted periods of time, such as very slow walking, slow leg-raising, and similar exercises. Even when there is motion, implying *nonzero* net force and net moment, and therefore *net* linear and angular accelerations, each increment of time can be broken down into quasi-static increments for individual analysis and final summation into the observed action.

The usefulness of static analysis, such as the freebody technique,[1] lies in its potential for predicting the nominal forces, and hence the stresses, on and in the components involved in a fracture. It is not the purpose of this chapter to develop the principles of freebody analysis. For this the reader is referred to a number of authoritative sources.[2, 3]

The response of a material to static loading is best illustrated by its force-deformation response, as shown in Figure 3–1. This test is usually performed in tension or compression and entails measurement of the force sustained by a specimen as a function of deformation at a constant rate of loading. In a static test such as this, the loading rate is usually specified as being no greater than 1 inch of deformation in 10 minutes.

The information bearing on fractures and healing that results from a static test concerns the following: stiffness, yield strength, fracture strength, deformability, and toughness. Stiffness is simply the relationship between force and deformation in the initial linear portion of the force-deformation relationship. Stiffness is quantitated by the slope of the force-deformation curve in the initial linear region of the curve. Stiffness is the so-called Hookean parameter, given by:

$$S = F/D \qquad \text{(Eq. 1)}$$

where S is the stiffness, F the applied force, and D the deformation. The compliance of a material is herein denoted C and is simply the inverse of the stiffness. It is given by:

$$C = D/F \qquad \text{(Eq. 2)}$$

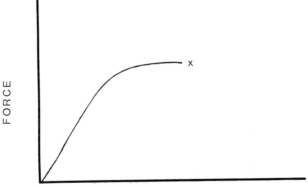

DEFORMATION

Fig 3–1—Force versus deformation relationship for a typical material. This is the output from a machine that applies a constant rate of compression or tension to the specimen. The load or force is monitored by a load cell. The deformation is monitored by a displacement gage. X is the fracture point, at which the material breaks into two pieces. The stiffness S is given by force divided by deformation (F/D) in the initial linear portion of the curve.

The energy stored in an elastic deformation is shown in Figure 3–2 and is given by:

$$E = \frac{1}{2} S D^2 \qquad \text{(Eq. 3)}$$

This energy, in purely elastic materials, is released when the force F is removed.

The strength properties of interest of these materials are the yield strength and the fracture strength. The yield strength is simply that force at which the test specimen takes on a permanent deformation (see Fig 3–2). The fracture strength is the force necessary to break the specimen into two pieces. Deformability is the amount of deformation that the specimen can sustain prior to breaking.

All of the foregoing properties determine the toughness, which is the energy required to break the specimen into two pieces. This is quantitated by the area under the curve shown in Figure 3–3. The toughest materials have an optimum combination of high yield strength, high fracture strength, and high deformability.

Materials are said to be purely elastic if their mechanical response is independent of time or duration of loading. If the mechanical properties of a material change with rate of loading, as shown in Figure 3–4, the material is said to be viscoelastic. This means that the material has part elastic (Hookean), and part fluid (Newtonian) properties. Notice that at a high rate of loading, all of the mechanical properties are enhanced. The stiffness, yield strength, fracture strength, deformability, and toughness all increase with increases in loading rate. This rate sensitivity of the mechanical properties of materials, especially those involved in hip fractures and healing, are especially dominant in rates of loading consistent with dynamics.

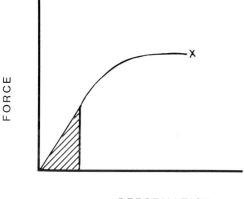

DEFORMATION

Fig 3–2—Same curve as Figure 3–1 with the elastic portion of the curve shaded to show the energy stored in an elastic deformation. Since energy and work are equivalent, the area under the elastic portion of the curve is basically the product of force and deformation. The yield strength is the force at the end of the shaded elastic region. Any force in excess of the yield strength will cause plastic deformation and permanent injury to the tissue.

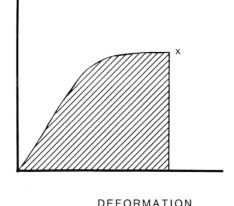

DEFORMATION

Fig 3–3—Same curve as Figure 3–1 with the energy required to cause fracture indicated by the entire area under the curve. This is termed the toughness of the material, or the resistance to fracture. The area depicted here is the sum of the elastic energy stored in a deformation and the energy required to plastically or permanently deform the specimen. The latter is equivalent to the hysteresis depicted in Figure 3–8, except that Figure 3–8 refers to sub-yield strength forces applied to a viscoelastic material.

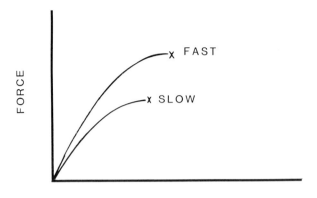

DEFORMATION

Fig 3–4—Two force versus deformation curves for similar-sized pieces of the same material. One was tested at a low rate of loading. The other was tested at a high rate of loading. A material that shows significant enhancement of properties with increases in rate of loading is described as viscoelastic.

DYNAMICS

Dynamics differs from statics in that there *are* net forces and moments. Dynamics is the study of systems in static equilibrium. There are net linear accelerations and net angular accelerations. Thus, dynamics is more applicable to analysis of activities of daily living, because those activities involve the production of useful work and of necessity require energy input. Considerations of energy and work are more germane to the analysis of dynamic systems than to the analysis of static systems.

Dynamics also encompasses systems in which forces are rapidly applied. In contrast to the analysis of static systems, in which loads are applied over periods of approximately 10 minutes, in the analysis of dynamic systems loads are applied over periods of approximately 1 second or less. Thus, any activity involving rapidly applied loads is a problem in dynamics. Audiofrequency steady-state forces (such as those applied during swept sine tests) as well as impact forces (such as those applied to the foot during heel strike in walking) are considered dynamic.

Fatigue situations also fall in the realm of dynamics. Fatigue failures are produced by repeated applications of the same load that would not fracture the specimen were it to be applied only once. These cyclic loading–induced fractures are discussed in detail in chapter 12. The reader is also referred to Morris and Blickenstaff.[4] The reader is reminded that any repeatedly applied load is capable of inducing fatigue effects.

Polymeric materials, of which collagenous materials comprise a subgroup, can be generally characterized by their degree of viscoelasticity or degree of rate dependence of their mechanical properties. As a rule, materials with a more fluid content and lower stiffness exhibit a greater rate dependence of their mechanical properties.

It is perhaps appropriate in this regard to refer to the work of Noyes, DeLucas, and Torvik,[5] who showed that ligaments exhibit less of a strain rate hardening than bone. Theoretically, we would expect the opposite. In fact, Noyes' experiments showed that at moderate strain rates, ligament-bone preparations failed at the bony section. At rates 100 times higher, the ligaments predominantly failed. This, of course, implies a higher strain rate dependence of the mechanical properties of bone relative to that of ligaments. The bone, in fact, became stronger relative to the ligaments at the higher strain rates. Another germane rationalization lies in the intrinsic structure of the ligaments relative to the structure of bone. In bone, the collagen is already organized in a direction roughly parallel to the direction of loading. In the relaxed ligament, the collagen fibers are slightly kinked. On application of a load, the collagen fibers will tend to align. Noyes' experiments showed, perhaps, that the collagen of the ligaments does not align as well at high strain rates as at low rates, which compromises its mechanical properties and its resistance to failure at the highest strain rates.

One of the fundamental modes of testing for viscoelastic response is the swept sine test (Fig 3–5). In this test, a sinusoidal force is applied to a specimen, and the resulting sinusoidal deformation is measured. The form of the applied force is the following:

$$F(t) = F_o \sin \omega t \qquad \text{(Eq. 4)}$$

where F_o is the amplitude of the applied force, ω is the angular frequency, and t is time. The resulting deformation as a function of time, for a purely elastic material, is:

$$D(t) = D_o \sin \omega t \qquad \text{(Eq. 5)}$$

where D_o is the amplitude of the deformation. Notice that for a purely elastic material, $F(t)$ and $D(t)$ are exactly in phase. The maximum in force coincides temporally with the maximum in deformation. There is no lag between the applied force and the resulting deformation. Of course, the stiffness is given by F_o/D_o, which is exactly the same as the stiffness as measured by the static test shown in Figure 3–1.*

---

*Except for the subscripts denoting maximum values of F and D, F_o and D_o are the same as force and deformation, respectively.

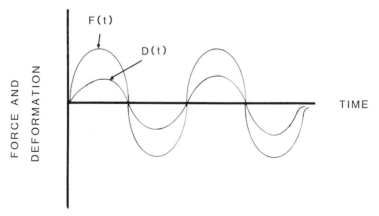

Fig 3–5—Force, F(t), and deformation, D(t), represented as functions of time in a swept sine test. Such a test involves the application of a sinusoidal force F(t) and the monitoring of the force level as a function of time along with monitoring of the deformation D(t) as a function of time. Notice in this purely elastic material that the force and deformation are exactly in phase. The forces applied here are beneath the yield point of the material depicted in Figure 3–1. In a swept sine test, the amplitudes of F(t) and D(t) are recorded as a function of increasing frequency of application of the sinusoidal force F(t).

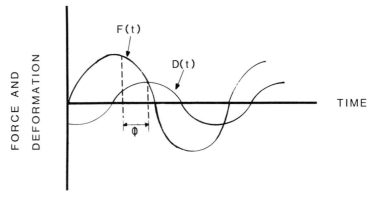

Fig 3–6—A similar depiction of a swept sine test showing force and deformation as functions of time. Notice here that the maximum in deformation D(t) *occurs at a time* φ *later than the maximum in* F(t). *This phase lag is consistent with significant viscoelastic behavior of the material and indicates that the material is capable of a much greater enhancement in properties with rate of loading than the material tested in Figure 3–5.*

A viscoelastic material, on the other hand, shows time dependence in its deformation relative to the applied force. Figure 3–6 shows the results of a corresponding swept sine test for a viscoelastic material, such as bone, cartilage, or ligament. The force applied to the specimen is again given by:

$$F(t) = F_o \sin \omega t \qquad \text{(Eq. 6)}$$

The deformation as a function of time, in this case, is given by:

$$D(t) = D_o \sin (\omega t - \phi) \qquad \text{(Eq. 7)}$$

where ϕ is the phase angle representing the lag between force and deformation. It is clear that for materials exhibiting significant viscoelastic behavior, the maximum of deformation occurs later in time than the maximum in the applied force. It is this fundamental feature of viscoelastic materials that leads to rate dependence of their mechanical properties.

The formula for deformation as a function of time (equation 7) can be rewritten trigonometrically, as follows:

$$D(t) = D_o \cos \phi \sin \omega t - D_o \sin \phi \cos \omega t \qquad \text{(Eq. 8)}$$

If we assign the symbols D' and D'' to the quantities $D_o \cos \phi$ and $D_o \sin \phi$, respectively, equation 8 becomes

$$D(t) = D' \sin \omega t - D'' \cos \omega t \qquad \text{(Eq. 9)}$$

The compliance of the material, which is the reciprocal of the stiffness, is now given by two quantities,

$$C' = D'/F_o \qquad \text{(Eq. 10)}$$

and

$$C'' = D''/F_o \qquad \text{(Eq. 11)}$$

Thus, compliance, in this case, is a complex quantity, given by:

$$C^* = C' + iC'', \tag{Eq. 12}$$

where i is $\sqrt{-1}$. A similar relationship can be derived for the stiffness and results in

$$C^* = S' + iS'' \tag{Eq. 13}$$

Thus, in dynamic function of materials, the maximum in deformation lags behind the maximum in force by a phase angle ϕ. This means that the material will show hysteresis, or energy loss per cycle of applied load. A purely elastic material will have the force-deformation response shown by Figure 3–7. Notice that force and deformation are in phase, as evidenced by the absence of hysteresis in this cycle of loading and unloading. In contrast, a viscoelastic material shown in Figure 3–8 shows significant hysteresis, or energy loss per cycle. The amount of purely elastic response of a material is given by S'. The amount of hysteresis is given by S''. In both cases the phase lag is related to stiffness and compliance by:

$$\tan \phi = S''/S' = C''/C' \tag{Eq. 14}$$

In dynamic loading conditions, the energy that must be dissipated into the surrounding tissue is reflected by the phase lag ϕ. The greater the phase lag, the greater the amount of hysteresis shown in Figure 3–8 relative to the elastic energy shown in Figure 3–2 in a typical cycle of deformation.

---

*Except for the subscripts denoting maximum values of F and D, F_o and D_o are the same as force and deformation, respectively.

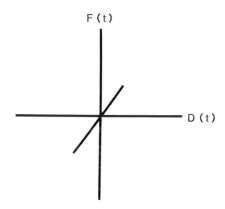

Fig 3–7—Force as a function of time and deformation as a function of time as plotted relative to each other rather than as in Figure 3–5. Notice that there is no hysteresis, or area within the linear relationship shown here.

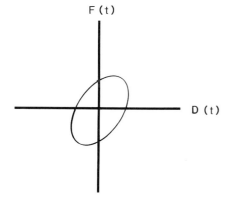

Fig 3–8—Force as a function of time and deformation as a function of time plotted relative to each other, as in Figure 3–7. This is a plot of F(t) versus D(t) for the curves shown in Figure 3–6. Notice the significant hysteresis or area within the loop for this viscoelastic material relative to the purely elastic material depicted in Figure 3–7. This is consistent with the curves shown in Figure 3–6, showing a large phase angle between F(t) and D(t).

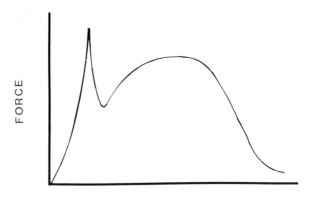

FORCE

TIME

Fig 3–9—Force versus time as measured on the heel of a person walking. Note the sharp spike at heel strike and the broad peak during weight-bearing. The sharp heel strike spike contains much higher frequency components than the broad weight-bearing peak.

The mode of functioning of tissues in the body is not truly swept sine. The profile for force versus time for walking is shown schematically in Figure 3–9. Notice that there is a sharp peak at heel strike, followed by a weight-bearing peak of relatively long duration. Such a force-time profile, with its inherent frequency components,* impinges on the foot of a normal person during each step of walking. McMahon and Greene[6] have shown convincingly that comfort can be considerably improved by eliminating the sharp peak occurring at heel strike and producing a force-time profile similar to that in Figure 3–10. This can be accomplished by providing a sole material or a walking surface of a relatively compliant, high phase lag, viscoelastic material.

It is left to the reader to infer that materials of which the hip is composed, as well as those materials produced at various stages of healing, have different viscoelastic behaviors, different phase lags, and different propensities to absorb and dissipate energy. The roll-off of the high frequencies shown in Figure 3–9 and 3–10 is accomplished, during normal biomechanical functioning, by the eccentric contractions of the muscle groups that span each joint. (Eccentric contraction is defined as forced stretching of tensed muscle.) This is the fundamental mechanism of shock absorption in the musculoskeletal system. Thus, muscle tone is a potential key in producing a mode of force transmission that can serve to prevent fracture of a bone by attenuating the peak force level.

Figure 3–11 shows two force-time profiles. One is the force applied across the joint without active eccentric muscle contraction. The broader peak shows the attenuation that is produced by active muscle intervention. In the former, the tissues in the joint (bone and cartilage) alone serve to attenuate the applied force through elastic and viscoelastic modes of response. Relative to tensed muscle, this is a poor mode of shock absorption. In the latter, the muscle is serving as a variable stiffness spring capable of storing large amounts of elastic energy, as per Figure 3–2, as well

---

*The frequency components in such a plot as shown in Figure 3–9 are the basis for frequencies chosen in a swept sine test of Figure 3–5.

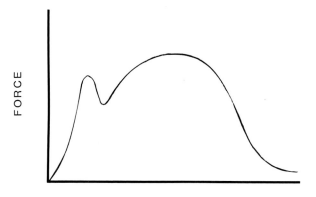

TIME

Fig 3–10—Force versus time as measured on the heel of a person walking on a much more compliant or softer surface than in Figure 3–9. Note that the broad weight-bearing peak remains unchanged relative to that depicted in Figure 3–9. The sharp heel strike peak is significantly reduced in height. This results from interaction of the heel of the test subject with a surface showing significant shock absorption. Materials that are candidates for shock absorption show high compliance and significant viscoelasticity. Such materials have high hysteresis and are therefore capable of absorbing impact energy rather than transmitting this energy through the heel to the body.

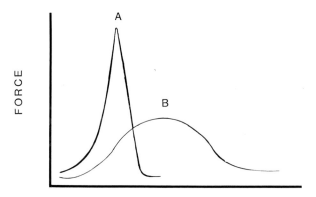

TIME

Fig 3–11—Force across a joint versus time for the following: A, fully extended joint without active muscle function. This response is indicative of deficient shock absorption supplied only by the cartilage and bone adjacent to the joint. B, flexed joint with significant eccentric muscle action. The forced stretching of tensed muscle allows significant energy storage and greatly increased shock absorption. This spreading out of the force over time results in a decrease in the levels of peak force in an activity such as walking or running. These two plots should be compared and contrasted with those depicted in Figures 3–9 and 3–10. Notice that active eccentric muscle action can accomplish the same effect as a change in floor surface or a change in shoe material.

as possessing significant hysteresis due to its inherent viscoelastic functioning and large phase angle, thus sparing the joint from the potentially damaging force levels experienced when the muscle is inactive.

The positive feature of hysteresis of tissue under dynamic loading is that a synchronous roll-off in peak force occurs. The negative feature of this hysteresis is that of energy dissipation in the tissue itself. This energy dissipation, in the form of heat or permanent deformation of the tissue, is a key feature of injury.

The components of the musculoskeletal system act in concert to produce force-time profiles potentially sparing of injury to the involved tissues. It should be evident that, in cases of muscle atrophy, the energy storage or dissipation must be parceled out to the involved tissues in a different manner, or to different tissues. This fundamental mode of functioning can be used to advantage or disadvantage in the treatment of hip fractures.

Impact such as that occurring at heel strike during walking also produces a rebounding of the bones in the leg against the relatively compliant end points consisting of the articular cartilage of the joints spanned by the ligaments and muscles, as shown by the $D(t)$ plot in Figure 3–12. (This rebounding can be seen by expanding the force-time plot of Figure 3–9 and removing the weight-bearing segment.) Similar rebounds are set up by clinical test methods such as impact, percussion, or osteophony. A healing fracture will sequentially show changes from the $D(t)$ response shown in Figure 3–13 to the response illustrated in Figure 3–12. This variation in impact response is intrinsically related to the viscoelastic mechanical properties of the tissue involved in the healing process.

During fracture healing, the application of dynamic loads such as those produced during walking will result in a greater energy dissipation in the initial osteoid

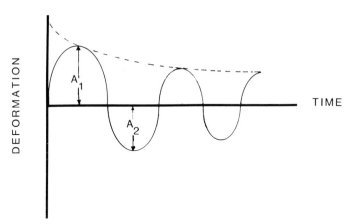

Fig 3–12—Deformation as a function of time for an impact test. The time axis here is greatly expanded ($\times 4$) relative to that in Figures 3–9, 3–10, and 3–11. Such decaying sinusoids are set up during walking and running and represent a rebounding of the bones against the elastic end points. The frequency of this rebounding is roughly the same as that of the sharp heel strike peak shown in Figure 3–9. Figure 3–12 is quantitated by the damping, defined as A_1/A_2. If A_2 is attenuated relative to A_1, the damping is high. If A_2 is roughly the same as A_1, the damping is low. The dotted line shows the exponentially decaying successive rebounds. The coefficients of the exponential function describing the decay in amplitudes is also a quantitative means of describing the damping.

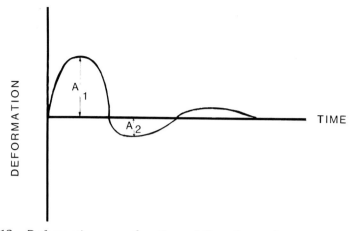

Fig 3–13—Deformation as a function of time for an impact test resulting in significantly greater damping than in Figure 3–12. Note that A_2 is much smaller than in Figure 3–12, resulting in a much larger value of A_1/A_2. This increased damping is typical of compliant tissues having large phase lags, as shown in Figures 3–6 and 3–8. The exponential decay envelope drops off to zero much more quickly than that in Figure 3–12.

present at the site of the healing fracture. Therefore, the application of dynamic loads during this first stage of healing potentially delays the healing process, because that initial tissue is of necessity involved in heat absorption as well as plastic damage consistent with the relatively enhanced tendency to absorb impact energy. During the progressive tissue changes occurring during fracture healing, the tissue, becoming less and less compliant, will absorb less and less energy. This renders the healing fracture more and more suitable for supporting impact loads as time progresses.

These observations are consistent with the "sound" heard in a stethoscope during impaction of a fractured hip when compared with the "sound" produced by impaction of the contralateral control: the fractured hip sounds "dull," compared with the contralateral control. Percussion resulting in a response of the type shown in Figure 3–12 is characteristically described as "sharp and ringing," while that of the type shown in Figure 3–13 is described as "dull." The audible change in sound is fundamentally related to the mechanical properties of the tissue and the absorption of impact by the fractured hip as compared with that of the normal control. When both sides sound identical, the fracture process can be assumed to be mechanically completed.

TISSUE PROPERTIES

Figures 3–14 and 3–15 show schematically the relative mechanical properties of the tissues involved in intra-articular and extra-articular hip fractures, as well as those of the tissues involved in the healing of those fractures. Tendon, ligament, and muscle are relatively the weakest of the tissues involved, but potentially the most susceptible to enhancement of properties by rate of loading. They are also the most effective as shock absorbers, showing a response similar to that depicted in Figures 3–6, 3–8, and 3–13.

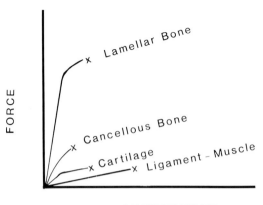

Fig 3–14—Force versus deformation curves for similar-sized pieces of tissue involved in the fracture process. Note the differences in stiffness, yield strength, fracture strength, toughness, and deformability for the various tissues. The most compliant of the tissues are the ligament, tendon, and muscle types of tissues, which contribute the most to shock absorption and to the attenuation of potentially disruptive peak forces.

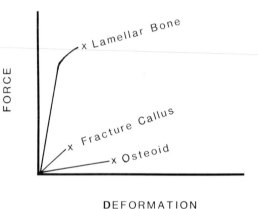

Fig 3–15—Force versus deformation curves for similar-sized pieces of tissue of interest in the fracture healing process. The material initially involved in the healing process, osteoid, is potentially most capable of storing energy in a manner consistent with that shown in Figures 3–6 and 3–8. As healing progresses, the properties of the healing tissue change as shown toward lamellar bone, which has dynamic properties with lower phase angles and less hysteresis than that shown in Figures 3–6 and 3–8.

The progression of strength is in the order upwards to cortical bone. The progression of shock absorption is downward in the same order. The response of cortical bone is more consistent with that shown in Figures 3–5, 3–7, and 3–12.

Intra-articular fractures must involve cancellous bone and cartilage, two tissues with inherent shock absorption capacity. Since these tissues are viscoelastic, they are capable of significant enhancement in their mechanical properties with increases in the rate of loading. It should be mentioned that extremely high peak forces, of very short duration, can be tolerated well by the joint, because of the enhancement in properties consistent with the increase in loading rate, as shown in Figure 3–4. Thus, intra-articular fractures would tend to be produced more frequently by lower loading rates or high rates of longer duration than extra-articular fractures, which do not involve the articular cartilage, and involve less cancellous bone.

Articular cartilage is not as resistant to shear forces applied perpendicularly to the surface as it is to compression and tension applied parallel to the surface. Thus intra-articular fractures are associated with significant shear developed across the surface of the articular cartilage. There will always be shear to some extent present in articular cartilage, since it rests on a bed of heterogeneous bone. This bed of variable stiffness amplifies the shear forces already present as loading rates and the loads themselves increase. Rupture of the articular cartilage necessarily involves rupture of the underlying subchondral cancellous bone. Thus, subchondral cancellous defects predispose joints to intra-articular fractures.[7] (Any subchondral heterogeneity of any significance will dramatically raise the shear stresses in the cartilage.) Weight-man has also shown a tendency for articular cartilage to fatigue fail.[8]

The extra-articular fractures of the femoral neck and the intertrochanteric and subtrochanteric regions involve compact cortical bone and cancellous bone. Because of the complex stress state in this region, fractures are invariably produced consistent with a mechanical path of least resistance through the numerous stress concentrators present in the cortical-cancellous complex. Computer simulations[9] of the bone in this region have shed light on the force transmission problem. This, however, is beyond the scope of the present discussion.

The tissues involved in the fracture healing process are largely osteoid, fracture callus, and fully remodeled lamellar bone. The progression of properties of these tissues is illustrated schematically in Figure 3–15. Again, the most compliant tissues show the greatest tendency toward strain rate–induced enhancement of mechanical properties and the greatest shock absorption. The static force-deformation curves shown are consistent with the observations of impact tests performed on healing fractures, as well as the swept sine tests on healing fractures. Osteoid shows the greatest shock absorption (see Figs 3–6 and 3–8). Lamellar bone shows the least shock absorption (see Figs 3–5 and 3–7).

It is possible that the inherent shock absorption mechanisms in the body accommodate a fracture by reacting accordingly to effect a prescribed level of shock absorption, as suggested by Voloshin and Wosk.[10] If this is the case, greater shock absorption at a fracture site would be consistent with less muscular shock absorption, which may place the healing fracture at risk, by mechanisms previously discussed.

DYNAMICS AND STATICS OF HEALING FRACTURES

Experiments were performed on white male New Zealand rabbits to assess the dynamics and statics of healing fractures. Transverse osteotomies were performed on the right tibias of nine rabbits. One rabbit served as a control. The rabbits were subsequently treated with a cast and/or an intramedullary rod for up to 94 days after operation. The rabbits were sequentially sacrificed at various intervals in the fracture healing period. The tibias were removed and x-rayed. Indices 1 through 5 were assigned to each fracture based on its radiographic appearance. Index 1 was assigned to a fresh fracture. Index 2 was assigned to those showing periosteal callus. Index 3 was indicative of tibias showing bridging callus. Index 4 was assigned to fractures showing trabeculations, and index 5 to completely healed fractures.

A small pendulum was constructed to impact the tibias longitudinally, to simulate the mode of transmission during normal walking. The profile of the impact peak is similar to that depicted in Figure 3–13. The ends of the tibias were machined flat with a precision slicing apparatus. The end opposite the impaction site was affixed with a piezoelectric accelerometer. The whole assembly was affixed to an elastic mount that allowed longitudinal translations only of low frequency. The impact response was quantitated by a damping ratio, as depicted in Figure 3–13.

Subsequent to this procedure of nondestructive testing, the tibias were tested to failure in three-point bending in an MTS electrohydraulic tester, at a rate consistent with static loading. This provided a link between static and dynamic properties. Fractures were produced consistently at the position of the osteotomy sites.

The results of these tests were as follows:

1. As the fractures healed, the impact response was sinusoidal, with a progressively less pronounced decay envelope. The fractures with greater healing showed consistently less shock absorption.

2. The fracture strengths were correlated with the index of x-ray assessment ($P < 0.01$).

3. The fracture strengths and shock absorption were inversely correlated ($P < 0.05$).

4. Interestingly, no significant correlation was found between x-ray assessment and damping ratio.

These results are largely consistent with our theoretical understanding of the mechanisms of healing fractures and the mechanical properties of the tissues involved in the healing process. The observation of decreased shock absorption with progression of healing is consistent with the clinical finding that sounds produced by percussion become more ringing and less dull as healing progresses.[11]

The inconsistent findings in the correlations of fracture strength with x-ray index and shock absorption with x-ray index are consistent with the notable unreliability of x-ray techniques to assess the integrity of healed fractures. It has been convincingly shown that fractures often require considerably longer to fully adapt mechanically than they do to become invisible on x-ray.[2]

SUMMARY

The basic biomechanical principles of statics and dynamics have been applied to the tissues involved in intra-articular and extra-articular fractures of the hip. Mechanisms have been proposed and results presented in the light of known clinical findings. It is hoped that the reader will regard the production of hip fractures and their subsequent treatment with increased consideration of the static and dynamic principles germane to those specific tissues involved in each type of fracture, coupled with the biomechanical environment of the fracture and the likely biomechanical environment of the healing tissues.

REFERENCES

1. Pugh J.: Biomechanics of the hip: Part I. *Orthop. Surg. Update Series* 2:1-8, 1982.
2. Frankel V.H., Burstein A.H.: *Orthopaedic Biomechanics.* Philadelphia, Lea & Febiger, 1970.
3. Frankel V.H., Nordin M.: *Basic Biomechanics of the Skeletal System.* Philadelphia, Lea & Febiger, 1980.
4. Morris J.M., Blickenstaff L.D.: *Fatigue Fractures: A Clinical Study.* Springfield, Ill., Charles C Thomas, Publisher, 1967.
5. Noyes R.R., DeLucas J.L., Torvik P.J.: Biomechanics of anterior cruciate ligament failure: An analysis of strain-rate sensitivity and mechanisms of failure in primates. *J. Bone Joint Surg.* 56-A:236-253, 1974.
6. McMahon T.A., Greene P.R.: The influence of track compliance on running. *J. Biomechanics* 12:893-904, 1979.
7. Pugh J.W., Rose R.M., Radin E.L.: A structural model for the mechanical behavior of trabecular bone. *J. Biomechanics* 6:657-670, 1973.
8. Weightman B.: Tensile fatigue of human articular cartilage, *J. Biomechanics* 9:193-200, 1976.
9. Mirabello, J.: *Finite element analyses of the proximal end of the human femur and its application to design of total hip prostheses,* thesis. Cooper Union School of Engineering, May 1974.

10. Voloshin A., Wosk J.: An *in vivo* study of low back pain and shock absorption in the human locomotor system. *J. Biomechanics* 15:21-27, 1982.
11. Weiss C., Pugh J., Gruber J., et al.: The application of structure-borne sound to the structural analysis of bone and fracture healing. *Bull. Hosp. Jt. Dis.* 38:26-28, 1977.

Chapter 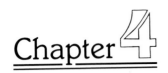4

Pathology and Pathophysiology

Marvin H. Meyers, M.D.

The extensive literature on the surgical treatment of hip fractures reveals an overwhelming concern with internal fixation and a relative neglect of the pathology and pathophysiology of these fractures. The continuing efforts to improve mechanical devices have overshadowed the importance of pathologic and pathophysiologic factors. The importance of appropriate stout metal fixatives inserted into the correct anatomical area is not to be downgraded. On the other hand, overlooking the basic vascular, anatomical, biomechanical, pathologic, and pathophysiologic relations that bear on surgical treatment can only lead to unsatisfactory results. A thorough understanding of the factors that may lead to complications and unsatisfactory results is as important to the success of the procedure as are proper fracture reduction and placement of internal fixation devices.

VASCULAR FACTORS

The vascularity of the femoral head is severely compromised in intracapsular fractures, but there is little if any damage to the circulation of the major fragments in extracapsular fractures. The fracture line in most subcapital and transcervical fractures includes the superior and posterior femoral neck at its confluence with the hyaline articular cartilage of the femoral head. It is here that the important lateral epiphyseal arteries, the major source of blood supply to the femoral head, enter the femur. (Fig 4–1).[1] One group of workers believes that the inferior rather than the superior retinacular vessels is the more important source of blood supply to the femoral head.[2]

The lateral epiphyseal vessels are subjected to tearing or crushing by fracture fragments, which interrupts the blood supply. Since the head fragment rotates posteriorly as it displaces it can entrap the superior retinaculum, crushing the vessels within between the two major fragments. I have documented this mechanism on numerous occasions (Fig 4–2).

The importance of the lateral epiphyseal vessels as the major source of blood supply to the femoral head has been strongly supported by an elegant experiment performed by Sevitt and Thompson.[1] They infused micropaque material into the common femoral artery of fresh cadavers. The vessels supplying the femoral head were interrupted by cutting the femoral neck in various ways. Sevitt and Thompson showed that the superior retinacular arteries were the most important arterial supply to the femoral head. The arteries in the ligamentum teres were an unimportant arterial supply, and the inferior retinacular vessels were of only subsidiary importance.

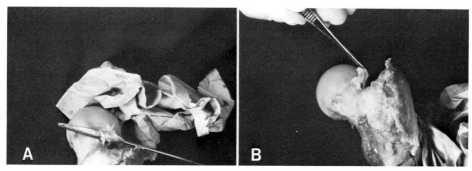

Fig 4–1—**A** and **B,** *lateral epiphyseal arteries entering the superoposterior neck through the superior retinaculum.*

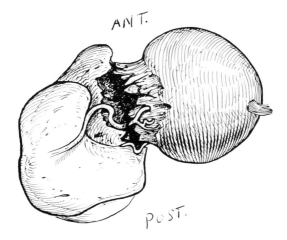

Fig 4–2—*As the head fragment rotates posteriorly it traps and crushes the lateral epiphyseal arteries.*

Because the lateral epiphyseal arteries, as they enter the head, are located in the fracture line, they are vulnerable to injury. Therefore, the head fragment in two thirds or more of displaced fractures is completely or subtotally avascular.[3,4] Some 15% of intracapsular fractures occur at the transcervical and cervicotrochanteric levels and usually do not involve the superior retinaculum; the incidence of avascularity and avascular necrosis with late segmental collapse is low at these levels. The subsequent development of late segmental collapse is discussed in chapter 25.

Approximately 10% of impacted femoral neck fractures will go on to late segmental collapse, compared to 30% of displaced fractures that unite. Figure 4–3 illustrates a typical impacted femoral neck fracture with crushing of fragments at the posterior superior segment where the lateral epiphyseal vessels enter the femoral head. The vulnerability of these arteries in impacted fractures is evident.

Segmental avascular necrosis may follow when large nails are inserted into the superoposterior half of the head fragment near the subchondral level of the femoral head (Fig 4–4). The intraosseous arcade from which the major portion of the femoral head receives its blood supply is vulnerable to injury at this point. The risk of interrupting the major intraosseous vascular pattern can be decreased by placing internal fixation devices in the inferoposterior half of the femoral head and by not using bulky nails.

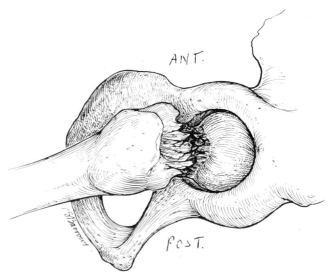

Fig 4–3—Impacted fracture with comminution and crushing of fragments at the posterosuperior aspect of the head-neck junction.

INTRACAPSULAR HEMORRHAGE AND AVASCULAR NECROSIS

Several authors have suggested that intracapsular hemorrhage following intracapsular fracture causes tamponade of the major blood vessels supplying the femoral head due to increased intracapsular pressure. Aspiration of the injured hip joint has been advocated to decrease the incidence of avascular necrosis.[2, 5, 6] In a recent study by Drake and Meyers, only 3 cc of blood or less could be aspirated from the hip joint of displaced femoral neck fractures within 48 hours of injury, and the average pressure measured by a transducer attached to a needle in the joint was 31 mm Hg, well below the normal average venous pressure.[8] There was an increase in pressure when the limb was held in extension and rotated internally. The conclusion reached in this study was that aspiration of the hip was not indicated following intracapsular fractures and that splinting or traction on the leg should be applied in the presenting position of external rotation with mild flexion of the hip until definitive treatment can be undertaken. The small volume of intracapsular hemorrhage does not extend the capsule significantly, and therefore the minor increase in the intracapsular pressure could not occlude the capsular vessels.

The arguments against intracapsular hemorrhage as a causative factor in avascular necrosis are many. The volume capacity for the hip is approximately 40 cc. It should be apparent that much more than 3 cc of blood would be required to appreciably increase intracapsular pressure in the hip joint. In 10%–15% of intracapsular hip fractures the capsule is torn.[2, 6, 8] It is unlikely that tamponade can be a factor when the capsule is torn. Finally, in undisplaced and impacted fractures the fracture surfaces are compressed together. The extraosseous vessels probably are not ruptured and hemarthrosis does not occur. Nevertheless, there is a 10%–15% incidence of late segmental collapse in the latter situation.

COMMINUTION OF THE POSTERIOR FEMORAL NECK

Major comminution of the posterior wall of the femoral neck is present in 70% of displaced femoral neck fractures (Figs 4–5 and 4–6).[9, 10] It has been con-

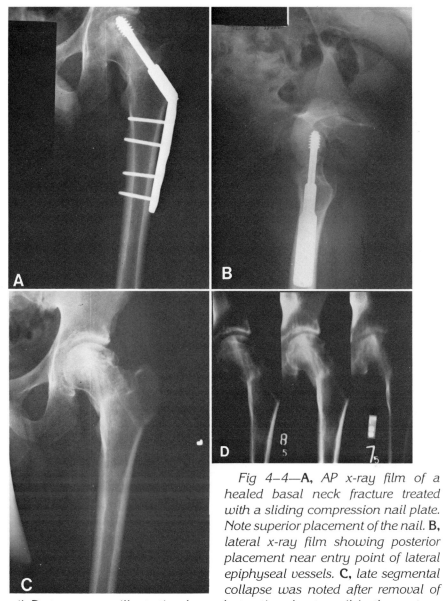

*Fig 4–4—**A,** AP x-ray film of a healed basal neck fracture treated with a sliding compression nail plate. Note superior placement of the nail. **B,** lateral x-ray film showing posterior placement near entry point of lateral epiphyseal vessels. **C,** late segmental collapse was noted after removal of the nail. **D,** tomograms illustrating bone destruction due to nail in the postero-superior aspect of the femoral neck where major vessels enter the head.*

sidered a poor prognostic sign because of loss of the buttressing effect of the posterior and inferior aspects of the femoral neck after fracture reduction.[10, 11] Additionally, displacement of the comminuted fragments frequently leaves a large gap that can only result in an increased incidence of delayed union or nonunion since fracture healing is by endosteal rather than periosteal callous formation in intracapsular hip fractures (see Fig 4–5).[12] The absence of a cambium layer in the periosteum of the femoral neck is the proximate cause for absence of periosteal callus. The gap is too large to expect osseous bridging by marrow callus.

Posterior comminution is caused by posterior and inferior displacement of the head fragment from the force of the fracture. The extreme compressive force on the thin cortex of the posterior aspect of the neck near the junction with the head

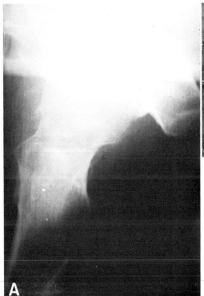

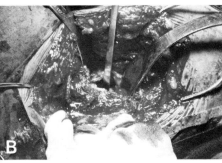

Fig 4–5—**A,** *lateral x-ray film showing severe comminution of the posterior aspect of the femoral neck.* **B,** *appearance at surgery. The osteotome is in the large defect created by the fracture; the femoral head fragment is above it.*

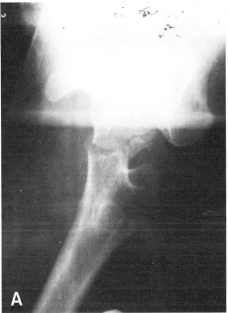

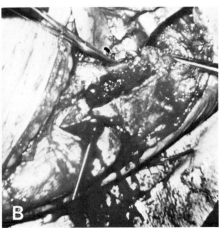

Fig 4–6—**A,** *lateral x-ray film showing posterior neck comminution.* **B,** *appearance at surgery. The hemostat is in the comminuted defect.*

accounts for the comminution. After reduction and fixation of the fracture in an anatomical position, the fracture often collapses because of the gap resulting from the posterior comminution.[10] This is due to loss of the buttressing effect of an intact posterior neck and the osteoporosis of the head fragment with a paucity of trabeculae. Rigid fixation is not possible in many cases because of osteoporosis. Closed reduction with internal fixation does not prevent the head fragment from again rotating posteriorly if the posterior wall of the neck is disorganized. Closure of the gap in the posterior neck with a bone graft can prevent further posterior rotational displacement of the femoral head.

OSTEOPOROSIS AND OSTEOMALACIA

Intracapsular fractures of the hip are most frequent in elderly women. There is a very high incidence of osteoporosis in this group of patients. Osteoporotic bones have a lower energy-absorbing capacity. Thus, failure of the bone can be expected with a moderately increased stress on the bone. Pins, nails, and screws are unlikely to gain a firm hold on the head fragment when the bone is osteoporotic (Figs 4–7 and 4–8). One can surmise that any force on the head fragment in an osteoporotic

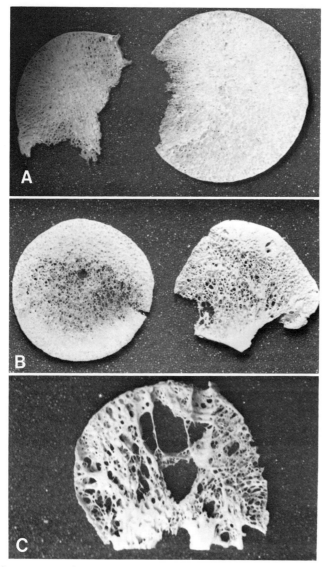

*Fig 4–7—***A,** *macerated coronal section of the femoral head from a 38-year-old woman. Note the normal concentration of trabeculae.* **B,** *macerated coronal and sagittal sections of the femoral head from a 55-year-old woman. Note the decreased concentration of trabeculae in the center but a normal concentration in the subchondral area.* **C,** *macerated sagittal section of the femoral head from a 75-year-old woman. There is a decrease in the number of trabeculae in all areas, including the subchondral region.*

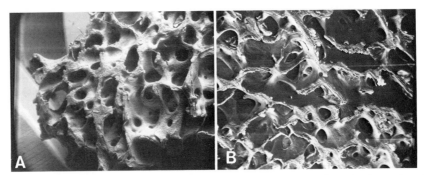

*Fig 4–8—**A,** scanning electron micrograph of macerated sagittal section from a 45-year-old woman. The trabeculae are of normal thickness and the spaces of normal size. **B,** scanning electron micrograph of macerated sagittal section from a 60-year-old woman. The trabeculae are very thin and the spaces are very wide.*

patient will tend to displace it posteriorly after internal fixation in the presence of posterior neck comminution unless the fixative can gain a firm hold in the sub-chondral bone. Migration ceases when the gap in the posterior neck closes and cortical contact is obtained. Malunion is a consequence if osseous union follows fragment displacement.

The incidence of femoral neck fractures has been shown to be closely related to the degree of osteoporosis.[13, 14] Enlargement of the medullary space due to greater endosteal rather than periosteal or cortical bone resorption is a feature of osteo-porosis. There is decreased trabecular volume. The cortical bone volume is also decreased geometrically and therefore the cortices are thin (see Fig 4–7,C). This results in larger intraosseous marrow spaces and thin trabeculae. The fragility of the femoral head trabeculae is supported by the studies of Stevens et al.[13, 14]

Singh and associates have used changes that occur in the trabecular pattern on roentgenograms to diagnose and grade osteoporosis.[15] Kranendonk and asso-ciates have disputed the accuracy of Singh's method to diagnose the severity of femoral head and neck osteoporosis.[16] Nevertheless, many surgeons have found Singh's method to be a useful clinical tool to roughly evaluate the degree of osteo-porosis present in bone.

In Singh's method, an anteroposterior x-ray film of the pelvis is made with the legs internally rotated. The findings are then graded as follows (Fig 4–9):

Grade 6: The normal trabeculae pattern, composed of principal and sec-ondary compressive and tensile groups as well as the greater tro-chanteric group, is readily seen. Ward's triangle is visible.

Grade 5: The principal compression and tensile trabeculae are accentuated, whereas the secondary compression group is barely or no longer seen. Ward's triangle is less prominent.

Grade 4: Grade 5 changes and tensile trabeculae are markedly reduced in number.

Grade 3: A break in continuity of the principal tensile group near the greater trochanter is now evident.

Grade 2: The principal compressive trabeculae are the only prominent ones.

Grade 1: There is a marked reduction in the number of the principal com-pressive trabeculae.

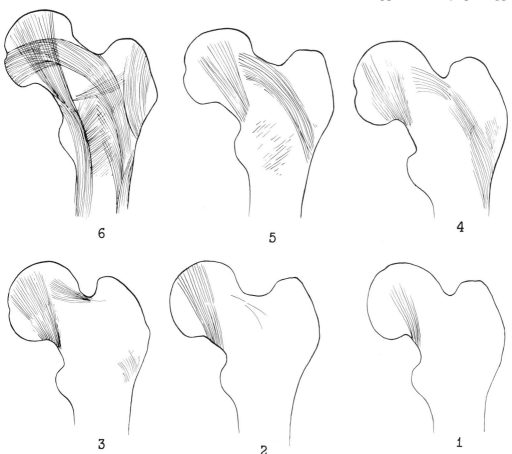

Fig 4–9—Osteoporosis grades, Singh's index. 6 is normal trabecular pattern at the upper end of the femur.

Occult osteomalacia was found in 25% of the fractured femoral heads biopsied during Austin Moore replacement arthroplasty in Caucasians.[7] This suggests soft bone. Osteomalacia results in impaired mineralization of the organic matrix. The etiology is a disturbance in vitamin D metabolism caused by adult nutritional deficiency, malabsorption syndromes, liver and renal disease, inadequate sunlight, alcoholism, and steroid therapy. Drugs such as dilantin and excessive ingestion of phosphate-binding antacids such as aluminum hydroxide may produce osteomalacia. Genetic and environmental factors play a significant role in the development of osteoporosis and osteomalacia.

Osteomalacia superimposed on osteoporotic bone makes it difficult to obtain firm fixation of the head fragment following femoral neck fracture. The incidence of fracture will be higher in these soft bones.

UNSTABLE FRACTURES

Unstable fractures (posterior comminution in intracapsular and basal neck fractures, posterior medial wall comminution in intertrochanteric fractures, and medial wall comminution in subtrochanteric fractures) must be recognized before surgery. Most stable fractures can be fixed adequately with the many metal devices currently available. However, unstable fractures can be stabilized successfully only with specific devices. These will be discussed in later chapters as each fracture type is considered individually.

Adequate roentgenographic evaluation is required to determine which fractures are unstable. Very often a true lateral x-ray film of the hip and upper shaft of the femur is obligatory to delineate fracture stability.

Other measures in addition to internal fixation may be required to treat instability. Bone grafts, additional fixation with interfragmentary screws, cerclage wires, and the like may be necessary to secure the fixation and ensure reconstitution of the medial buttress.

Failure to achieve cortical contact of displaced femoral neck fractures by means of impaction or bone graft and failure to obtain a firm hold in the osteoporotic femoral head by means of metal fixation devices allows the subsequent posterior rotation of the femoral head. This is followed by nonunion or malunion.

Cortical contact is imperative in unstable intertrochanteric fractures. Some surgeons opt for osteotomy and "pushover" techniques to obtain stability. Bone grafting and careful restoration of the bony anatomy with adequate fixation can also produce stability. Medial wall comminution in subtrochanteric fractures makes for an unstable fracture pattern. Tremendous forces are applied to the medial cortex in this fracture. Metal fatigue and subsequent failure of the fixation is frequent in the latter situation if stability is not restored. Stout fixation is necessary. The Zickel nail has been developed for unstable subtrochanteric fractures (see chapter 20).

TISSUE RESPONSE FOLLOWING HIP FRACTURES

Unlike other long bone fractures, intracapsular fractures do not develop an external callus because of absence of a cambium layer in the periosteum surrounding the femoral neck. When healing occurs in the femoral neck it is by formation of marrow callus. Subtrochanteric, intertrochanteric, and basal neck fractures do exhibit external callus. The basal neck fracture is extracapsular in the posterior aspect of the neck.

Banks has described the tissue response at the fracture site of intracapsular fractures.[12] Hemorrhage, fibrin, dead bone fragments, and debris characterize the fracture site. This is followed by a stromal response and new bone formation at the juxtaposed proximal femoral head and distal neck fracture surfaces. There is no stromal response on the proximal fracture surface if the head fragment is nonviable. However, osseous healing from the fracture surface of the distal fragment can occur if the fracture is anatomically reduced and rigidly fixed. Osseous union can be expected to take longer when the head fragment is not viable.

BONE NECROSIS FOLLOWING FEMORAL NECK FRACTURES

The pathology of bone necrosis following intracapsular fracture of the femoral neck has been thoroughly described by Catto.[3] Although there is a very high incidence of avascular necrosis (accounting for 85% of cases of total or subtotal avascularity[4]) following displaced femoral neck fractures, osseous union can be expected in 70%–90% of fractures that have been anatomically reduced and firmly fixed. Catto reported a 30% incidence of femoral head viability in a series of femoral heads removed at necropsy or at the time of primary arthroplasty. A nonviable head does not preclude fracture healing. However, 30% of healed displaced femoral neck fractures will go on to late segmental collapse of the femoral head. Ununited fractures with nonviable head fragments do not develop segmental collapse since the forces are dissipated at the nonunion site and do not result in sufficient force on the head fragment to cause collapse.

New vessels may grow into the dead marrow following fracture from the foveal vessels in the ligamentum teres or across the fracture from the viable distal fragment. Creeping apposition and creeping substitution along with the ingrowth of new vessels produces viable bone. In many cases fibrosis of the marrow interferes, causing cessation of the revascularization process. In any event, revascularization proceeds at a slow pace. This is the result of micromovement of the fracture fragments (which disrupts the new blood vessels crossing the fracture line), fibrosis at the fracture site following organization of the hematoma, fracture debris, and poor stability of the fracture fragments due to inadequate fixation. Revascularization frequently ceases and return of viability of the femoral head is incomplete for unknown reasons.

Histologic examination of femoral heads removed at arthroplasty revealed that only a third were viable according to the criteria of Catto. This was supported by tissue culture study of femoral head and neck biopsy specimens following fracture.[17]

Further discussion of avascular necrosis is found in chapter 25.

REFERENCES

1. Sevitt S., Thompson R.G.: The distribution and anastomosis of arteries supplying the head and neck of the femur. *J. Bone Joint Surg.* 47B:560-573, 1965.
2. Soto-Hall R., Johnson L.H., Johnson R.A.: Variations in the intra-articular pressure of the hip joint in injury and disease. *J. Bone Joint Surg.* 46A:509-516, 1964.
3. Catto M.: A histological study of avascular necrosis of the femoral head after transcervical fracture. *J. Bone Joint Surg.* 47B:749-776, 1965.
4. Sevitt S.: Avascular necrosis and revascularization of the femoral head after intracapsular fractures. *J. Bone Joint Surg.* 46:270-296, 1964.
5. Deyerle W.M.: Impacted fixation over resilient multiple pins. *Clin. Orthop.* 152:102-122, 1980.
6. Nagy E., Manninger J., Zalczer L., et al.: Data for the importance of intra-articular pressure and the tear of the capsule in fractures of the neck of the femur. *Aktuel. Traumatol.* 5:15-19, 1975.
7. Sokoloff L.: Occult osteomalacia in American (U.S.A.) patients with fracture of the hip. *Am. J. Surg. Pathol.* 2:21-30, 1978.
8. Drake J.K., Meyers M.H.: Intracapsular pressure and hemarthrosis following femoral neck fractures. *Clin. Orthop.* 182:172-176, 1984.
9. Meyers M.H., Harvey J.P. Jr., Moore T.M.: The muscle pedicle bone graft in the treatment of displaced fractures of the femoral neck: Indications, operative techniques and results. *Orthop. Clin. North Am.* 5:779, 1974.
10. Scheck M.: The significance of posterior comminution in femoral neck fractures. *Clin. Orthop.* 152:138-142, 1981.
11. Garden R.S.: Stability and union in subcapital fractures of the femur. *J. Bone Joint Surg.* 46B:630, 1964.
12. Banks H.H.: Tissue response at the fracture site in femoral neck fractures. *Clin. Orthop.* 61:116-128, 1968.
13. Stevens J., Freeman P.A., Nordin B.E.C., et al.: The incidence of osteoporosis in patients with femoral neck fracture. *J. Bone Joint Surg.* 44B:520-527, 1962.
14. Stevens J., Abrami G.: Osteoporosis in patients with femoral neck fractures. *J. Bone Joint Surg.* 46B:24-27, 1964.
15. Singh M., Hograth A.R., Maini P.S.: Changes in trabecular pattern of the upper end of the femur as an index of osteoporosis. *J. Bone Joint Surg.* 52A:457-467, 1970.
16. Kranendonk D.H., Jurist J.M., Lee H.G.: Femoral trabecular patterns and bone mineral content. *J. Bone Joint Surg.* 54A:1472-1478, 1972.
17. Richters V., Meyers M.H., Sherwin R.P.: Tissue cultures of bone from the fractured hip. *Clin. Orthop.* 101:268, 1974.

Chapter 5

Fracture of the Femoral Head

Marvin H. Meyers, M.D.

Fracture of the femoral head is a rare injury that is most often a complication of hip dislocation. It has been reported to occur in 5%–10% of traumatic hip dislocations.[1,2] There is no universally accepted treatment, perhaps because of the small number of cases in any series and the lack of statistically significant long-term follow-up. However, some surgeons have had sufficient experience to offer suggestions on effective forms of therapy, based on trends in results with small numbers of patients.

The fracture occurs when a portion of the head impinges on the lip of the acetabulum at the instant of dislocation. It is often associated with violent injuries and is seen in multiply injured patients. On some occasions comminuted fractures follow severe trauma.

Frequently diagnosis is delayed because small fragments fractured off the head are not recognized. Tomography and, more recently computerized tomography (CT) have been utilized to aid in the diagnosis (Fig 5–1). The position of the fragment can be localized by CT.

Fractures of the femoral head are classified according to the method of Pipkin,[3] as follows: type 1, dislocation with fracture of the femoral head caudad to the fovea capitis femoris (Fig 5–2); type 2, dislocation with fracture of the femoral head cephalad to the fovea capitis femoris (Fig 5–3); type 3, types 1 or 2 associated with fracture of the femoral neck (Fig 5–4); and type 4, types 1 or 2 associated with fracture of the acetabular rim. There may be overlapping of types as seen in Figure 5–5, which shows a combination of types 1 and 2, and in Figure 5–6, which shows a combination of type 3 and a fracture of the acetabular rim.

MECHANISM OF INJURY

The injury is usually produced by a severe force applied to the knee with the hip flexed. The shearing force produces the fracture as the femoral head impinges on the lip of the acetabulum. The size and location of the fracture probably depend on the degree of hip flexion at the time of impact. Rarely, fracture of the head has been reported with anterior hip dislocation.

Vigorous manipulation in attempting to relocate a dislocated hip could fracture the head. Often the fracture is seen after manipulation. One can only speculate whether or not the fracture occurred at the time of injury or as a result of manipulation.

Blunt injuries to the anterior aspect of the hip and direct gunshot wounds are extremely rare mechanisms of femoral head fracture.

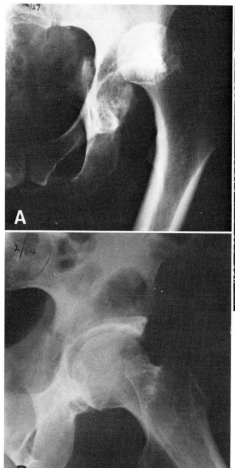

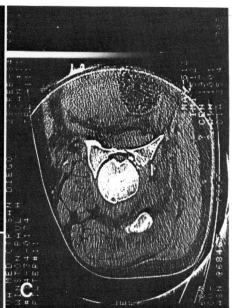

Fig 5–1—**A,** *fracture dislocation of the hip with fracture of the posterior lip of one acetabulum. Small fragments from the head are not discerned.* **B,** *dislocation reduced.* **C,** *CT scan shows fracture of the acetabulum and several small fragments from the femoral head lying in the joint.*

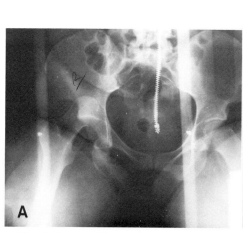

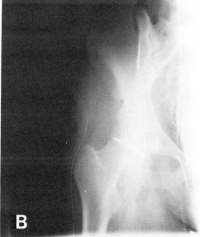

Fig 5–2—**A,** *AP x-ray film of pelvis showing a Pipkin type I injury with a large single fragment caudal to the fovea lying in the acetabulum.* **B,** *AP film of the hip after open reduction and screw fixation of the fragment.*

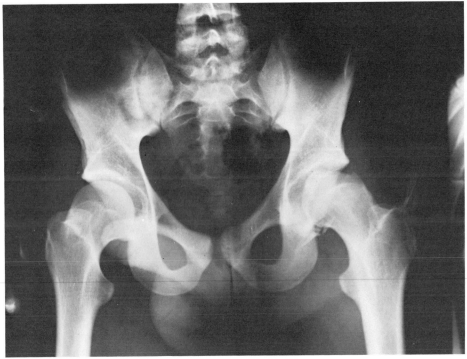

Fig 5–3—Pipkin type 2 injury with comminuted head fragments in the inferior aspect of the joint.

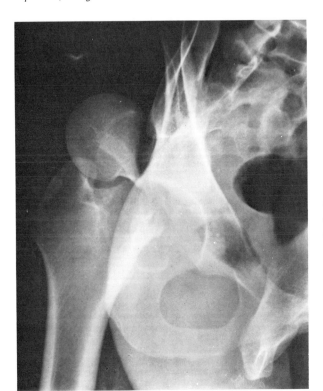

Fig 5–4—Pipkin type 3 injury with a large fragment of the femoral head caudal to the fovea.

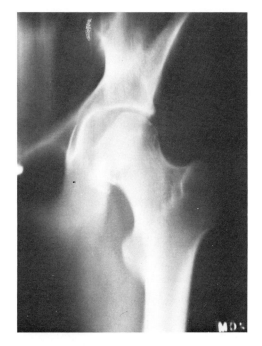

Fig 5–5—Combination of Pipkin types 1 and 2 fractures. There is a large femoral head fragment involving areas cephalad and caudal to the fovea (two thirds of the superior weight-bearing portion of the head is intact).

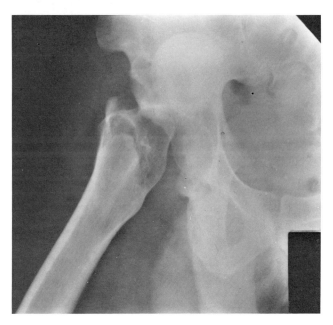

Fig 5–6—Pipkin type 4 fracture with a fracture of the superior acetabular rim.

TREATMENT

The method of treatment is largely dependent on the extent and location of the injury. In general, most authors agree that fracture dislocations should be reduced closed. Anatomical reduction of major fragments is achieved by open reduction and internal fixation if it cannot be achieved by closed manipulation. Small comminuted or inferior head fragments may be excised.

Pipkin Type 1

This injury is treated by closed reduction, usually under general anesthesia. If the fragment is large and cannot be reduced anatomically, treatment is by open reduction and internal fixation with countersunk screws (see Fig 5–2b). Small fragments may be excised since they are from a non-weight-bearing area of the femoral head. Occasionally a large fragment may be excised with impunity. However, it is probably wiser to fix internally larger fragments in an anatomical position to ensure congruity of the hip.

There is no agreement on what constitutes a large or a small fragment. The hip joint may become mechanically unstable if a large fragment is removed in type 1 injuries, and the stage is set for the development of traumatic arthritis. This is less likely to occur following removal of small fragments caudal to the fovea, since this area of the head is rarely involved in weight-bearing.

Large fragments must be anatomically reduced; otherwise they may obstruct hip function. Incongruity would result in hyaline cartilage dysfunction and traumatic abrasion of the cartilage with subsequent traumatic arthritis.

A hip spica cast is applied for 4–6 weeks following anatomical reduction. Rehabilitation with gradual resumption of weight-bearing is begun following removal of the cast.

Open reduction is required if the fragments are not anatomically reduced and thus act as a mechanical obstruction to congruity. A single large fragment is fixed with countersunk screws. A single small fragment or comminuted fragments are removed.

Pipkin Type 2

This fracture involves the major weight-bearing portion of the femoral head, and therefore single large fragments must be replaced to preserve congruity of the hip joint. Fixation is accomplished with one or two countersunk AO screws. When the fragment is comminuted so that internal fixation is not possible, removal of the fragments will lead to incongruity and inevitably to traumatic degenerative arthritis of the hip. If a significant area of the superior weight-bearing portion of the head is spared, comminuted fragments can be excised and the prognosis will be good. I have replaced the comminuted fracture segment with a fresh osteochondral allograft.[4] This is an experimental procedure and preliminary results have been promising. The technique is described in a recent publication.[4]

Pipkin Type 3

This fracture is a devastating injury. In all likelihood the circulation to the femoral head will be interrupted, resulting in osteonecrosis. Reduction and surgical repair of the injury are technically demanding. Small fragments caudal to the fovea should be excised, whereas fragments cephalad to the fovea require replacement and screw fixation. Internal fixation of the femoral neck fracture is then necessary. I prefer internal fixation and the quadratus femoris muscle pedicle graft as the treatment of choice. This procedure is designed to hasten union of the femoral neck fracture and prevent late segmental collapse of the femoral head (see chapter 17).

Pipkin Type 4

In addition to treating the type 1 or 2 components of the injury, as described above, the surgeon must internally fix the acetabular fragment if there is a large fragment of the posterior lip. If the hip is stable, small fragments may be left in situ without internal fixation.

PERSONAL PREFERENCE FOR SURGICAL MANAGEMENT

Satisfactory exposure can be obtained by a posterolateral approach to the hip. Usually it is necessary to section the ligamentum teres in order to anatomically replace the fragment and fix it. Large fragments are fixed with countersunk cancellous screws. The hip is relocated after the internal fixation has been secured and the wound is closed and all soft tissue layers, including the synovium and capsule, are replaced. The hip is maintained in balanced suspension for 2 weeks. Motion is started as soon as the pain subsides to a tolerable level. Non-weight-bearing ambulation is then permitted for 3–6 months. Weight-bearing can be resumed when there is radiologic confirmation of osseous union.

I prefer to use suction drainage of the hip for 24–48 hours after all hip surgery, and prophylactic antibiotics. A broad-spectrum antibiotic is given intravenously 30 minutes before surgery and is continued for 24 hours after surgery.

REFERENCES
1. Armstrong J.R.: Traumatic dislocation of the hip joint. *J. Bone Joint Surg.* 30B:430, 1948.
2. Epstein H.C.: Posterior fracture-dislocations of the hip: Long term follow-up. *J. Bone Joint Surg.* 56A:1103-1127, 1974.
3. Pipkin G.: The treatment of the grade IV fracture-dislocation of the hip: A review. *J. Bone Joint Surg.* 39A:1027-1042, 1957.
4. Meyers M.H., Jones R.E., Bucholz R.W., et al.: Fresh autogenous grafts and osteochondral allografts for the treatment of segmental collapse in osteonecrosis of the hip. *Clin. Orthop.* 174:107-112, 1983.

Chapter 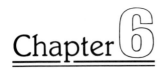6

Intracapsular Fractures of the Femoral Neck

Marvin H. Meyers, M.D.

Intracapsular fractures include fractures through the femoral neck and at the junction of the femoral head and neck. Basal neck fractures are partially intracapsular and partially extracapsular and are more appropriately considered in a discussion of intertrochanteric fractures (chapter 7).

The history of the treatment of intracapsular femoral neck fractures is long and controversial. No one treatment method has been accepted by orthopedic surgeons as superior because of the continuing high incidence of nonunion and avascular necrosis of the femoral head with late segmental collapse following treatment. The femoral neck fracture has been labeled the "unsolved fracture" because of failure to improve the poor results following operative as well as nonoperative treatment. Some surgeons have resorted to decapitation and prosthetic replacement as the treatment of choice because of dissatisfaction with results achieved by available treatment methods. Nevertheless, most orthopedic surgeons agree that the goal of treatment of intracapsular fractures is osseous union with a viable femoral head.

The highest incidence of nonunion and avascular necrosis with late segmental collapse occurs in displaced fractures as compared to undisplaced fractures. The difficulty in achieving anatomical reduction, rigid fixation, and good impaction of the fracture fragments makes this a difficult fracture to treat surgically. The extent of damage to the blood supply of the head fragment following fracture is an additional factor influencing results.

BIOMECHANICS OF FRACTURE

Most elderly patients have osteoporosis and osteomalacia, which cause structural weakness, a decrease in muscle mass and tone, and a gradual delay in reaction time by the neuromuscular system. These structural and physiologic changes contribute to the decreased capacity of the hip and its surrounding structures to dissipate energy. The decrease in energy-absorbing capacity causes an overload situation and mechanical failure.

Cyclic loading produces microfractures of the trabeculae which eventually lead to macrofracture. These changes precede a minor torsional injury which completes the fracture and causes a fall in a standing or walking person. In some instances turning in bed or catching the foot in the bedcovers provides the torsional force, the final event leading to complete fracture.

CLASSIFICATION

Far too much emphasis has been placed on classification of femoral neck fractures. Earlier writers emphasized that the more horizontal the fracture, the less the shearing force and therefore the better the prognosis. However, attention to the principles of fixation and the use of stout fixatives can provide adequate stability of the fracture fragments and neutralize shearing forces.

Historically the most popular classification systems for intracapsular fractures have been those of Pauwel[1] and of Garden.[2]

The key to Pauwel's system is the angle of inclination of the fracture line to the horizontal as seen on the anteroposterior (AP) roentgenogram (Fig 6–1). This angle is difficult to determine until the fracture is reduced. Therefore, presurgical diagnostic x-ray studies can be misleading. Pauwel stated that type 2 fractures resulted in a 50% incidence of nonunion and type 3 in an over 90% incidence of nonunion. In my experience the rate of nonunion is the same following type 2 and type 3 injuries. Other factors are more significant in causing nonunion and will be discussed later. This classification system has lost favor because type 1 is a stable fracture and when the obliquity and direction of the fracture line is 50% or more, it is unstable. The rate of nonunion is not significantly different in type 2 and 3 injuries.

Garden subdivided fractures into four stages, as follows: stage 1, incomplete fracture (Fig 6–2,A); stage 2, complete fracture without displacement (Fig 6–2,B); stage 3, complete fracture with partial displacement (Fig 6–2,C); and stage 4, complete fracture with full displacement (Fig 6–2,D).

Stage 1 is incorrectly classified as an incomplete fracture since the trabeculae and cortices are interrupted but maintain contact, although the complete fracture may not be visible on roentgenographic examination.

In stage 2 the fracture may be undisplaced, but frequently the head fragment rotates posteriorly a few degrees. The head fragment can rotate posteriorly as much

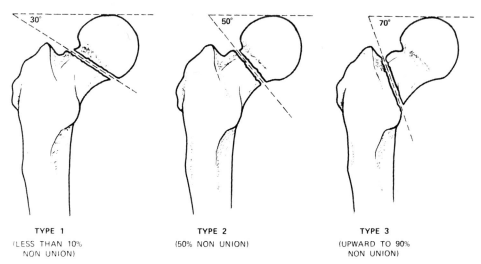

TYPE 1	TYPE 2	TYPE 3
(LESS THAN 10% NON UNION)	(50% NON UNION)	(UPWARD TO 90% NON UNION)

Fig 6–1—Pauwels' classification of fractures of the femur according to angle of inclination. In type 1, due to impaction and compression, there is a less than 10% incidence of nonunion; in type 2, due to sliding, tipping, and twisting, there is a 50% incidence of nonunion; and in type 3, due to shearing, sliding, tipping, pushing, pulling, and twisting, the incidence of nonunion may be as high as 90%. (Courtesy of Irwin S. Leinbach, M.D., St. Petersburg, Fla.)

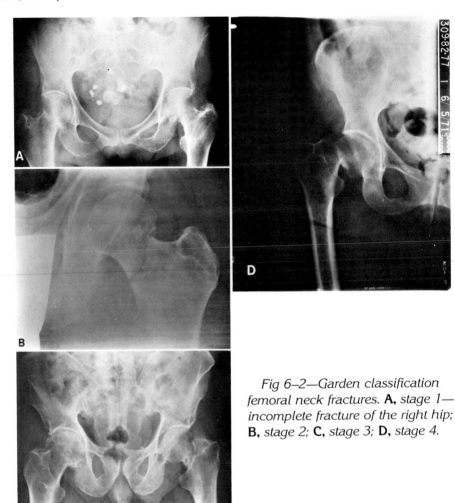

*Fig 6–2—Garden classification femoral neck fractures. **A**, stage 1— incomplete fracture of the right hip; **B**, stage 2; **C**, stage 3; **D**, stage 4.*

as 25° (as seen on a lateral roentgenogram) but gives the appearance of impaction on the AP roentgenogram (Fig 6–3). In essence, fractures in both stages are complete and in most cases minimally displaced, an acceptable position which does not require reduction. If posterior rotation between the head and distal fragments, as seen on the lateral roentgenogram, produces an angle of more than 15°, reduction of the fracture is required.

Stage 3 and 4 fractures are displaced and require reduction. It is more difficult to manipulate and accurately reduce a stage 4 fracture. However, the prognosis is the same for either stage once the fracture is accurately reduced and securely fixed. Therefore, it is my opinion that a practical classification for intracapsular fractures has only two stages: in stage 1, the stable fracture is undisplaced or minimally displaced with some valgus angulation and less than 15° of posterior rotation of the head fragment on the distal fragment as seen on the lateral x-ray film; in stage 2, the fractures are unstable and more than minimally displaced.

Appropriate radiologic studies are necessary in the preoperative period to assess the stage of the fracture and the presence or absence of posterior neck comminution. This information will help in deciding on treatment. An AP view is

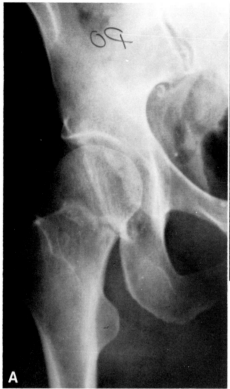
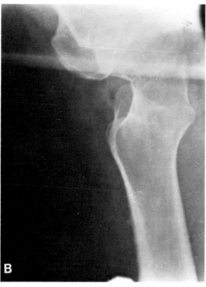

*Fig 6–3—**A,** AP roentgenogram of Garden stage 2 fracture. **B,** lateral roentgenogram of fracture with posterior angulation of 25°.*

obtained by gently pulling on the leg and gradually rotating it inwardly 20°. This maneuver will provide a true AP view of the femoral neck. Most patients will tolerate the mild traction necessary to get this view. A true lateral view is difficult to obtain because the "frogleg" maneuver is very painful. A cross-table lateral view requires the assistance of an experienced x-ray technician. If pain is too severe, these x-ray films can be obtained in surgery after the patient is anesthetized.

CHOICE OF TREATMENT

The choice of treatment depends on several factors, as described below.

Patient's Physical and Mental Status

The patient's physical and mental status has a great influence on the surgeon's decision. Nursing considerations, relief of pain, and prevention of complications caused by bed rest in the elderly debilitated patient with a fractured hip are strongly weighted toward a surgical approach that is simple. The patient must be able to tolerate an anesthetic. Simple reduction of the fracture and pinning it percutaneously or through a small incision will allow mobilization of the patient and provide relief of pain. Hemiarthroplasty is a slightly more difficult procedure but can be an effective alternative to in situ pinning. Other sophisticated alternative surgical methods such as open reduction with internal fixation, bone grafts, and total hip replacement may not be wise selections for the debilitated patient.

Patients bedridden prior to fracturing the hip are not expected to regain ambulatory status following successful surgery. In this situation medication with mild

Buck traction for 10 days to 2 weeks will alleviate pain. Thereafter, pain is minimal and the resulting nonunion is of no significance.

The mentally disturbed or disoriented patient is not expected to participate in a rehabilitation program and therefore is not a candidate for a sophisticated surgical procedure. The choice of treatment for these patients is very difficult. Hemiarthroplasty, which permits the patient to resume his preinjury ambulatory status, should be the surgeon's choice in most cases.

Semiactive patients, the so-called community ambulators, are usually unable to participate in non-weight-bearing postoperative regimens. Surgical procedures that permit early postoperative ambulation are the most reasonable choices for this group. Hemiarthroplasty and total hip replacement deserve serious consideration as treatment options for this group of patients.

Surgical options for the active patient with a reasonable life expectancy are many. The goal of surgery should be osseous union and a viable femoral head. Closed or open reduction with internal fixation augmented by a muscle pedicle graft of the quadratus femoris muscle is my treatment of choice.

The active patient with a short life expectancy is an appropriate candidate for a hemiarthroplasty and in some cases a total hip replacement.

Type of Fracture

The type of fracture influences the choice of treatment. Undisplaced or minimally displaced fractures can be treated nonoperatively or by pinning the fracture in situ. The incidence of disimpaction is 10% following nonoperative treatment of undisplaced or minimally displaced fractures.[3,4] Some authors have reported no disimpaction after internal fixation of this fracture.[5,6] Therefore, if the patient's physical condition will tolerate a surgical procedure, simple pinning of the fracture in situ should be the treatment of choice. The operation is relatively minor if the patient can tolerate an anesthetic, and the threat of disimpaction is minimized.

The treatment options for displaced fractures in active patients are open reduction and internal fixation, the muscle pedicle graft and internal fixation, hemiarthroplasty, and total hip replacement. Nonoperative treatment has no place in the treatment of displaced femoral neck fractures when the patient is healthy and active, as nonunion and disability would result in practically all cases.

Intraosseous Circulation

Avascular necrosis of the femoral head has been reported in 7%–20% of undisplaced femoral neck fractures whether or not the fracture has been pinned in situ.[3-6]

In 85% of displaced femoral neck fractures the femoral head is totally or subtotally avascular, and approximately 30% of those that unite go on to late segmental collapse of the femoral head. The absence of circulation is the primary reason for the quadratus muscle pedicle operation in displaced femoral neck fractures. I have successfully reduced the rate of late segmental collapse to 5% with the addition of the pedicle graft, in contrast to a 25% rate without the graft.

Comminution of Posterior Neck

Garden stated that comminution of the posterior cortex of the neck of the femur (Fig 6–4; see also Figs 4–5 and 4–6)[4-6] resulted in the loss of the buttressing effect against lateral rotation of the head fragment and was the main cause of

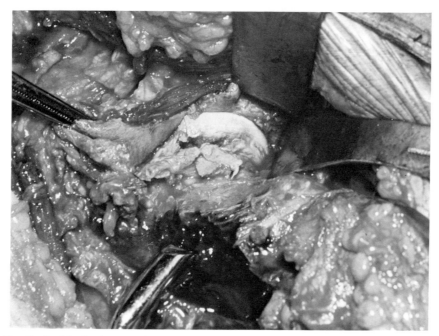

Fig 6–4—Marked comminution of posterior aspect of femoral neck after cap-sule had been incised and retracted.

instability even after internal fixation.[7] Others have reported comminution of the posterior neck visible on lateral roentgenograms in up to 65% of neck fractures.[8-10] It is probably a major reason for delayed union, nonunion, and malunion.

There frequently is a gap remaining in the posterior neck after manipulation and reduction (see Fig 4–5). This cavity, which is due to the severe comminution, must be filled with autogeneous iliac bone chips to provide a scaffold for the ingrowth of blood vessels. There is experimental evidence that iliac bone graft stimulates bone healing. The bone graft restores the stability lost by the comminution of the posterior aspect of the femoral neck. Otherwise, loss of the buttress effect provided by an intact posterior neck will result in rotation of the head fragment and subsequent nonunion or malunion.

Osteoporosis and Osteomalacia

The soft bone resulting from osteoporosis and osteomalacia influences the choice of treatment. These conditions are common in the elderly patient and result in demineralized bone with reduced, thinned trabeculae which are not suited for metallic fixation (see chapter 4). Postoperative shifting of the fracture fragments, and penetration or disengagement of the metallic fixation device is common in severe osteoporosis. Other options must be given serious consideration in these patients. Many surgeons utilize the Singh index to determine the degree of osteoporosis and base their selection of treatment on the stage of osteoporosis.

Concurrent Disease

A fracture in the hip joint with advanced osteoarthritis or rheumatoid arthritis limits the choice of treatment. This situation is an absolute indication for a total hip arthroplasty.

The treatment of pathologic fractures is discussed in chapter 27.

Advanced Parkinson's disease limits the choice of treatment for fractures of the femoral neck. Open reduction and internal fixation frequently fail because the patient is unable to comply with ambulation and non-weight-bearing on the fractured extremity.[9] Bed rest is not satisfactory for patients so afflicted.

PRINCIPLES OF SURGICAL TREATMENT

The techniques for various surgical options are discussed in detail in later chapters.

Most orthopedic surgeons agree that in order to achieve osseous union of femoral neck fractures, anatomical reduction, firm fixation, and impaction must be achieved. Even if these requirements are met the incidence of nonunion is about 20% on the average, as reported in the voluminous literature on this subject. Late segmental collapse of the femoral head occurs within 3 years in 30% of all displaced fractures that go on to osseous union after surgical pinning of the fracture fragments. These results are unacceptable in the healthy active patient.

The addition of the quadratus femoris muscle pedicle graft, augmented with autogenous bone to fill defects in the posterior femoral neck when they occur, has been reported to improve the rate of late segmental collapse significantly.[9] I prefer this method of treatment.

Anatomical Reduction

An anatomical reduction is difficult to achieve by manipulation. Comminution of the posterior wall of the femoral neck or the inferior neck will make an anatomical reduction unobtainable, even though incomplete coaptation of the fragments can be obtained. Distraction due to excessive traction on the leg and failure to derotate the distal fragment are other factors interfering with anatomical reduction. Usually, careful manipulation will produce near-anatomical coaptation of the fragments, which is required for osseous union of the fracture.

The adequacy of reduction can be determined by the angles formed by trabecular alignment described by Garden.[2] Figure 6–5 illustrates ideal reduction of the fracture. The AP x-ray film of the hip with the limb internally rotated will give a true AP view of the neck and femoral head. The axis through the head and neck should form a straight line. An angle up to 165° is acceptable. The lateral view should also project a straight line through the axis of the head and neck. An angle of 165° is acceptable.

Another method of gauging reduction accuracy is to draw a line down the central axis of the femoral head and neck. This line should form an angle of 130° with a line drawn down the central axis of the femoral shaft. The anatomical angle formed by the two axes may vary in some patients. An AP x-ray film of the pelvis will reveal the normal angle on the contralateral side.

Under anesthesia, reduction is accomplished by the Leadbetter maneuver[11] or by manual traction on the leg in a longitudinal direction followed by internal rotation of 20°. The latter method is usually successful and is less damaging to the fracture site. The Leadbetter maneuver is more vigorous, increasing the force across the fracture site, and theoretically it could cause additional comminution of the fracture.

The Leadbetter technique is performed in the following manner. An assistant fixes the pelvis by placing his hands over the anterosuperior iliac spines of the pelvis and maintains constant pressure on the pelvis. The surgeon places traction on the

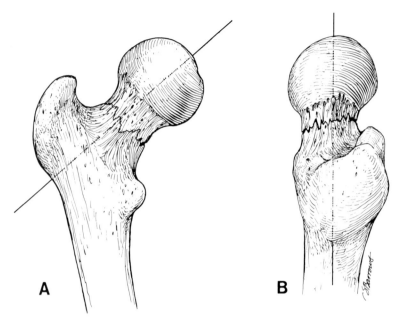

A   **B**

*Fig 6–5—**A,** AP view of ideal reduction. The axis of the head fragment and the distal neck axis form a straight line at an angle of 130° to the axis of the femoral shaft. **B,** lateral view. The axis of the head fragment and distal neck fragment forms a straight line.*

lower extremity. The knee and hip are flexed gradually to 90°, which relaxes the soft tissues. The thigh is adducted and internally rotated to 45° to engage the fragments. Finally, the hip is brought into abduction and extension while the thigh is maintained in internal rotation. Reduction has been achieved if full abduction can be maintained, the leg lengths are equal, and the leg doesn't fall into external rotation when traction on the extremity is discontinued.

Occasionally, more than one attempt at reduction is required. Open reduction is sometimes necessary. The fracture site is always exposed in the muscle pedicle graft procedure. Thus, the best reduction possible can be gained under direct vision.

Firm Fixation

Firm fixation requires placing metallic fixation devices in dense bone. They should be inserted into the areas of the head and neck that are least likely to permit penetration of the cortex.

The subchondral surface of the head fragment is an area of compact trabeculae where the denseness is greatest. The bone is dense enough to permit the device to gain a firm hold. The sparse trabeculation in the intramedullary portions of the head and neck fragments in the elderly patient is not conducive to firm fixation of nails. Compression and sliding nails may permit rotation of the head fragment on the distal fragment since the forces applied to the head fragment tend to rotate the fragment posteriorly as well as inferiorly and the decreased density offers little resistance to the rotary forces.

The recommended site for placing metal fixation devices is in the posterior and inferior halves of the femoral head and neck or in the exact center (Figs 6–6 and 6–7). If the head rotates posteriorly or inferiorly, bone will be compacted ahead

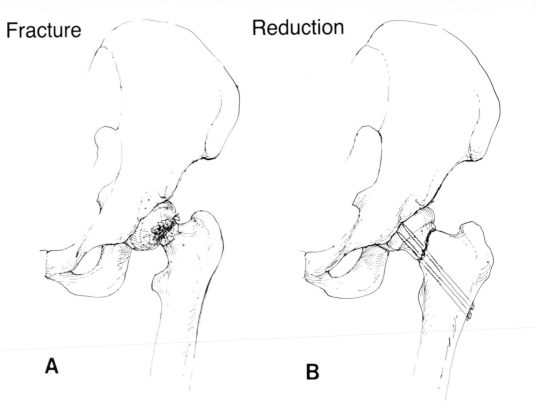

*Fig 6–6—**A,** anterior view of fracture. **B,** reduction and inferior placement of pins.*

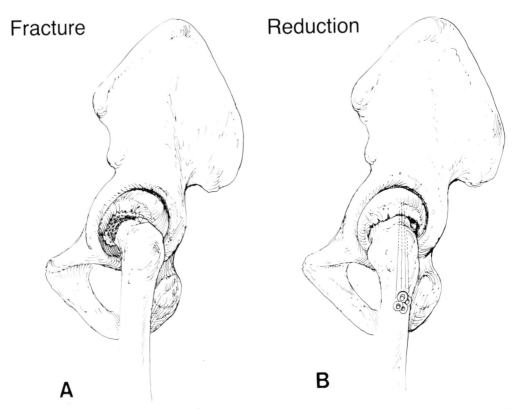

*Fig 6–7—**A,** lateral view of fracture. **B,** reduction and posterior placement of pins.*

of the metal and penetration will not take place before the head fragment comes to rest. There is a great risk that pins will penetrate the head if they are placed in the superior or anterior quadrants of the femoral head. The ends of the fixation device should come to rest in the subchondral surface of the femoral head within 5 mm of the cortical surface since the direction of the compression force on the femoral head will cause rotation of the head fragment posteriorly and inferiorly. A nail placed in this recommended position acts as a neutralization force.

Impaction

Impaction of the fragment can be produced by force or by the use of compression devices such as the compression nail plate, cancellous screws and washers, etc. Deyerly advocates striking the upper end of the distal fragment with a hammer to achieve fragment impaction.

PERSONAL PREFERENCE FOR TREATMENT
Undisplaced or Minimally Displaced Fractures

My preference is to pin the fracture in situ and to augment internal fixation with a muscle pedicle graft if circulation to the femoral head has been seriously impaired by the fracture (Fig 6–8).[12] A bone scan with technetium 99m sulfur colloid prior to surgery is a reliable indicator of the vascular status of the femoral head.[13] I require a technetium 99m sulfur colloid scan preoperatively in all undisplaced or minimally displaced femoral neck fractures to assess the circulatory status of the femoral head. Absence of radioisotope uptake in the femoral head is indicative of severe damage to the circulation.

In a small series of 31 cases of undisplaced or minimally displaced femoral neck fractures, three had internal fixation of the fracture augmented by a muscle pedicle graft because of a negative technetium 99m sulfur colloid scan.[12] In no case with adequate follow-up in this series has there been late segmental collapse of the femoral head.

Displaced Fractures

Closed reduction and internal fixation is the procedure of choice when the head is viable and there is little or no comminution of the posterior neck. Open reduction is performed if anatomical reduction is not possible by closed manipulation, or if there is severe posterior neck comminution. The muscle pedicle graft is utilized when the head is not viable and when there is severe comminution of the posterior neck.

Open reduction, internal fixation with multiple cancellous pins or screws (Asnis, AO, etc.), and a muscle pedicle graft is the treatment of choice for displaced fractures in the active vigorous adult with a long life expectancy, irrespective of the patient's age. Meticulous adherence to the principles of accurate reduction, firm fixation, impaction, use of iliac bone chip grafts to fill any gap created by comminution of the posterior neck, and use of the quadratus femoris muscle pedicle graft to enhance or restore circulation to the head fragment should give the best results of any surgical procedure.

A bipolar hemiarthroplasty is the treatment of choice in individuals with a short life expectancy, minimal activity, debility, Parkinson's disease, mental illness, hemiplegia, or spastic paralysis. Treatment of pathologic fractures depends on the extent and type of the disease process (see chapter 27).

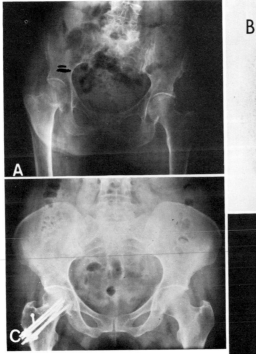
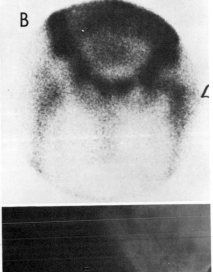
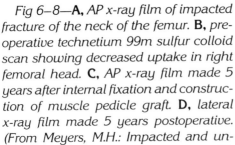

*Fig 6–8—**A,** AP x-ray film of impacted fracture of the neck of the femur. **B,** pre-operative technetium 99m sulfur colloid scan showing decreased uptake in right femoral head. **C,** AP x-ray film made 5 years after internal fixation and construction of muscle pedicle graft. **D,** lateral x-ray film made 5 years postoperative. (From Meyers, M.H.: Impacted and un-displaced femoral neck fractures, in The Hip Society (eds.): The Hip. St. Louis, C.V. Mosby Co., 1982. Reproduced by permission.)*

Nonambulatory or bedridden patients can be treated in traction for a short time until the pain abates. Nonunion is of no consequence in these patients. In some cases a Girdlestone procedure can be performed to relieve intractable pain.

REFERENCES

1. Pauwel E.: Der Schenkelhalsbruch: Ein mechanisches Problem. Grundlagen des mei-lungsvorganges Prognose und kausale Therapie. Stuttgart, Ferdinand Enke Verlag, 1935.
2. Garden R.S.: Low angle fixation in fractures of the femoral neck. *J. Bone Joint Surg.* 43B:647, 1961.
3. Crawford H.B.: Impacted femoral neck fractures. *Clin. Orthop.* 66:90-93, 1969.
4. Hillebee J.W., Staple T.W., Lanche E.W., et al.: The non-operative treatment of impacted femoral neck fractures. *South. Med. J.* 63:1103-1109, 1970.
5. Bentley G.: Impacted fractures of the head of the femur. *J. Bone Joint Surg.* 50B:551-561, 1968.
6. Burrata R.E., Fahey J.J., Drennan D.B.: Factors influencing stability and necrosis in im-pacted femoral neck fractures. *JAMA* 223:41-44, 1973.
7. Garden R.S.: Stability in subcapital fractures of the femur. *J. Bone Joint Surg.* 46B:630-647, 1964.

8. Hargedorn E.J., Pearson J.R.: Treatment of intracapsular fractures of the femoral neck with the Charnley compression screw. *J. Bone Joint Surg.* 45B:305-311, 1963.
9. Meyers M.H., Harvey J.P. Jr., Moore T.M.: The muscle pedicle bone graft in the treatment of displaced fractures of the femoral neck. *Orthop. Clin. North Am.* 5:770-792, 1974.
10. Scheck M.: Intracapsular fractures of the femoral neck: Comminution of the posterior neck cortex as a cause of unstable fixation. *J. Bone Joint Surg.* 41A:1187-1200, 1959.
11. Leadbetter G.W.: Treatment for fracture of the neck of the femur. *J. Bone Joint Surg.* 15:931, 1933.
12. Meyers M.H.: Impacted and undisplaced femoral neck fracture, in *Proceedings of the Tenth Open Scientific Meeting of the Hip Society,* C.V. Mosby Co., St. Louis, 1982.
13. Meyers M.H., Telfer N., Moore T.M.: Determination of the vascularity of the femoral head with technetium 99m-sulphur-colloid. *J. Bone Joint Surg.* 59A:658-664, 1977.

Chapter 7

Cervicotrochanteric, Intertrochanteric, and Peritrochanteric Fractures

Marvin H. Meyers, M.D.

Fractures in proximity to the intertrochanteric line occur most often in the elderly. The incidence of fracture in younger persons is significantly less because they have stronger bones. In young persons such fractures are most often associated with severe trauma.

The high mortality accompanying these fractures in the elderly is due to the shock of the trauma superimposed on (usually) preexisting medical complications. Cardiopulmonary failure, urinary disease, malnourishment, and immobilization caused by the fracture are debilitating and stressful factors that may lead to death.

Stabilization of the medically ill patient and rapid mobilization will decrease the frequency of additional life-threatening complications and thus improve the survival rate. The surgeon must select the simplest and safest method that will provide adequate fixation and stability of the fracture so as to permit early mobilization. Elderly patients respond to early mobilization with improved cardiopulmonary function, a decrease in life-threatening complications such as thromboembolism, and a decrease in the incidence of decubitus ulcers and limb contractures.

CLASSIFICATION

Boyd and Griffin classified fractures of the trochanteric region into four types for planning treatment and determining prognosis.[1] In type 1, the fracture runs between the greater and lesser trochanter. Boyd and Griffin stated that reduction was simple, the fracture was stable, and results were satisfactory (Fig 7–1). Type 2 fractures are comminuted fractures involving the intertrochanteric line and the cortex of the trochanter and proximal femur. Reduction is more difficult because of the comminution, which may be severe (Fig 7–2). Type 3 fractures are comminuted fractures that basically involve the subtrochanteric area and lesser trochanter. Achieving and maintaining reduction is difficult. Complications of fracture treatment are frequent (Fig 7–3). Type 4 fractures are comminuted and involve the trochanter and proximal shaft. Fracture lines run in several planes. Achieving and maintaining reduction is difficult. Fixation is complicated and sometimes requires osteotomy to gain stability (Fig 7–4).

The classification of Tronzo[2] is based on the type of reduction necessary to gain stability. There are five types of fractures, as follows. Type 1 fractures are in-

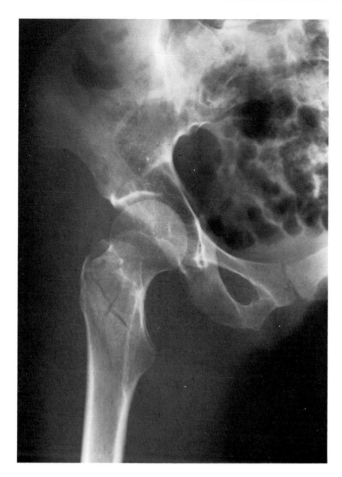

Fig 7–1—Stable in-tertrochanteric fracture, Boyd and Griffin type 1.

complete trochanteric fractures that can be reduced anatomically by traction, if necessary (see Fig 7–1). Type 2 fractures are simple trochanteric fractures with or without displacement, both trochanters are involved. Reduction is easily accomplished by traction (see Fig 7–2). Type 3 fractures are comminuted fractures with a large lesser trochanteric fracture. The posteromedial wall is disorganized and the inferior beak of the femoral neck is displaced into the femoral canal, producing a varus displacement. These are unstable fractures. There may be a displaced fracture of the greater trochanter (see Fig 7–4). Type 4 fractures are completely separated. The spike of the inferior neck is displaced and is not in the femoral shaft (Fig 7–5). In type 5 fractures, whereas the main fracture line usually runs obliquely from the medial femoral shaft proximally toward the greater trochanter, the obliquity of the fracture line is reversed. It runs from the medial femoral cortex distally to the base of the greater trochanter or subtrochanteric level.

Most trochanteric fractures are four-part injuries involving the greater and lesser trochanters. Stability of the fracture depends on the integrity of the posterior and medial regions of the intertrochanteric construct. Unstable fractures are associated with difficulties in reducing fractures in the intertrochanteric region and are responsible for most fracture complications at this level.

A successful reduction requires osseous stability of the medial and posterior cortices. A more practical classification than the Boyd and Griffin or Tronzo systems is simply to consider these fractures as stable or unstable.

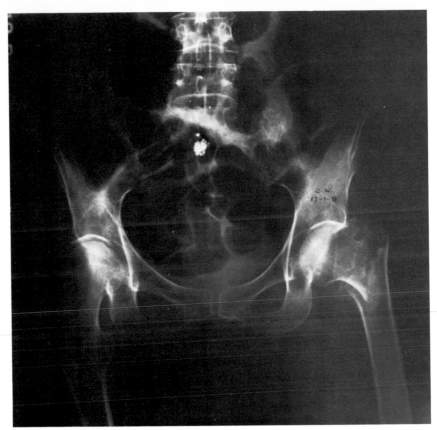

Fig 7–2—*Unstable intertrochanteric fracture, Boyd and Griffin type 2.*

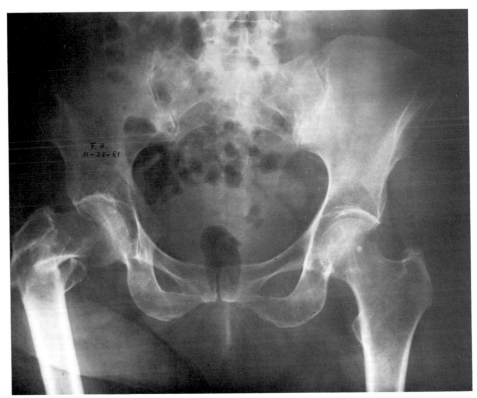

Fig 7–3—*Subtrochanteric fracture with fracture of the lesser trochanter, Boyd and Griffin type 3.*

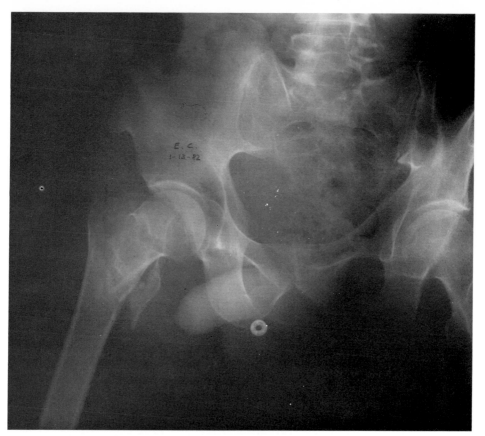

Fig 7–4—Unstable intertrochanteric, Boyd and Griffin type 4.

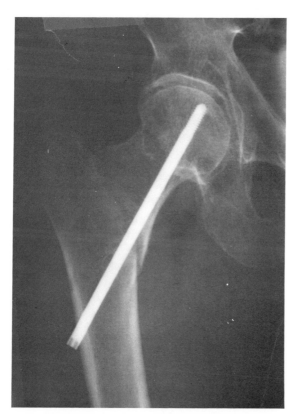

Fig 7–5—Tronzo type 4 fracture.

TREATMENT

Selection of treatment often depends on the fracture classification. The stability of the fracture is of utmost importance. A stable fracture may be defined as a fracture in which there is continuity of the bone of both the proximal and distal fragments. Stable fractures without displacement of the fragments may be treated nonoperatively. Anatomical reduction by manipulation and traction is possible when the fragments are displaced. Immobilization in a cast after reduction of the stable fracture has been recommended in the literature. Unstable fractures would be difficult to treat by this method.

Displacement of the lesser trochanter or comminution with displacement of the posterior and medial cortices is the hallmark of an unstable fracture.

The voluminous literature on fractures in proximity to the intertrochanteric line reflects the disagreement of surgeons about methods of reduction, surgical approaches, and choice of metallic fixation device.

The objectives of treatment are early mobilization, fracture fixation, and osseous union. In some cases, the advanced age of the patient, severity of the fracture, concurrent medical problems, and traumatic shock are overwhelming issues and surgery is inadvisable.

Treatment Options
Traction

Young patients can be treated successfully with traction, but surgery is preferable for economic and social reasons. Traction as a treatment option for elderly patients is ill-advised since they do not tolerate prolonged bed rest. Likewise, manipulation and immobilization in a cast is fraught with complications and rarely tolerated by elderly patients.

Skin traction is not tolerated by the elderly, and because of the prolonged time for osseous union of these fractures (12–16 weeks), it is a questionable choice for any patient. Skeletal traction through the proximal tibia is a choice if the traction method is selected. As much as 25–30 lb of traction may be required for reduction. I prefer the Neufeld traction method[3] (see chapter 11).

Cast

Hip fractures should not be treated with a spica cast. The elderly patient will not tolerate the cast or the prolonged inactivity that accompanies this method. Complications such as pressure sores and contractures due to the cast are frequent. The deleterious effects of prolonged immobilization lead to serious medical problems and death for many patients. In some cases younger patients can be treated with a cast because they tolerate cast immobilization better than the elderly.

In desperate situations the surgeon may want to resort to "well leg traction," advocated by Roger Anderson many years ago.[4] Well-padded short-leg casts are applied bilaterally and connected with wooden or metal bars attached by plaster bandages to each cast. The bars are attached after the uninvolved leg is pulled out to length and the hip is placed in abduction and neutral rotation. The result is abduction of the uninvolved hip and abduction of the good hip. Nursing care is simplified, the patient can be placed in a sitting position, and some degree of reduction can be maintained until union occurs.

Surgical Reduction and Internal Fixation

Many methods and many devices have been proposed for internal fixation. All are effective when used for the proper indications as long as one pays attention to the principles underlying each method. Some commonly used devices are the single-nail plate, the sliding nail or screw, the condylocephalic nail, and the Ender nail.

Internal fixation is the simplest and safest method to maintain stability of stable fractures. It permits early mobilization and ambulation of the patient. The patient will be more comfortable and complications less frequent. Nursing care is facilitated and hospital utilization and costs are reduced. There is a significantly lower mortality associated with surgical treatment of these fractures compared to non-surgical methods.

The disoriented, institutionalized, nonambulatory patient is treated best with the condylocephalic nail or with Ender pins. Insertion of the pins is less time-consuming, is accompanied by a significant decrease in blood loss, and allows an early return to the patient's home or institution.

All of the surgical methods mentioned are acceptable for treating the stable fracture. A successful reduction restores stability by medial cortical abutment, impaction of the major fracture fragments, and an anatomical or slight valgus position.

The unstable fracture, however, is best treated with the sliding nail or screw or on occasion by the "pushover" technique. Technical difficulty is increased by the frequency of osteoporosis when the solid single-nail plate is used. The common problems of loss of reduction, shortening, and difficulty with appropriate placement of Ender pins demand a high degree of technical skill for internal fixation of the unstable fracture.

Impaction of the fracture fragments is of paramount importance because 75% of the stress is absorbed by the impacted bony cortex and only 25% by the nail. If the nail were to bear most of the stress it would probably fail. Therefore, a sliding device must allow for impaction of the fragments in order to gain stability.

The angle of weightbearing across the hip approaches 160°. The closer the angle of the device is to 160° the more easily will the screw slide in the barrel. Due to the anatomical structure of the femur, accurate placement of a sliding nail with an angle more than 150° is practically unobtainable. In most instances, placement of a nail with an angle of 145° to 150° is possible. The higher the angle of the nail, the less chance there will be for jamming of the screw in the barrel. Thus, the factors preventing impaction and consequently stability are decreased with high angled nails.

A period of bed rest and traction is frequently necessary when the condylocephalic or Ender nails are used to treat unstable fractures, which is a disadvantage.

It is essential that the integrity of the medial buttress be maintained or restored, especially when early mobilization and weight-bearing is contemplated. Displacement fixation will provide a medial stabilizing buttress of cortical bone, thus permitting early mobilization and faster healing of the fracture.

The sliding nail and compression screw must be placed into the central portion of the head and neck or in the posteroinferior portion of the head, with the tip of nail within 0.5 cm of the subchondral surface of the head (Fig 7–6). Under no circumstance should the end of the device be placed anteriorly or superiorly in the head fragment. Penetration of the head will follow any shifting of the fragment or shortening due to postoperative impaction of the fracture fragments.

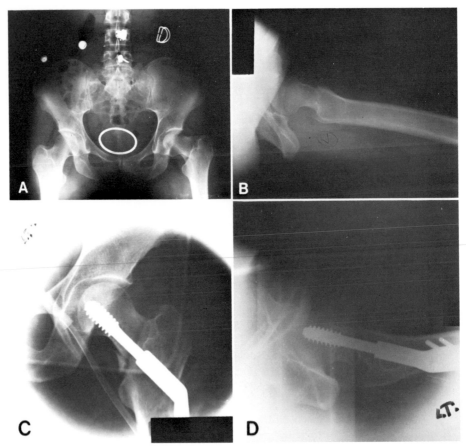

Fig 7–6—**A,** *anteroposterior roentgenogram of cervicotrochanteric (basal neck) fracture.* **B,** *lateral roentgenogram of cervicotrochanteric fracture.* **C,** *ideal placement of compression screw in inferior half of femoral head 0.5–1 cm from the articular surface.* **D,** *ideal placement of compression screw in posterior half of femoral head 0.5–1 cm from the articular surface.*

COMPLICATIONS

Complications are frequent following surgery of fractures in the region of the trochanters. These complications are related to the reduction and method of fixation and include (1) malunion and nonunion, (2) nail penetration of the femoral head, (3) nail failure (breakage, bending, or screw disengagement from the femoral shaft), and (4) loss of reduction.

A good reduction requires maximal bone-to-bone contact of the major fracture fragments to supplement the structural strength of the fixation device. Frankel has shown that 75% of the stress at the fracture site is borne by bone contact.[5] Maintenance of the reduction requires proper positioning of the metallic fixative in the femoral head and neck and impaction of the fragments to ensure cortical support. The device should rest in the center of the femoral head or the posteroinferior half, with the tip approximately 1 cm from the subchondral surface of the head. This will prevent nail penetration if the soft bone shifts, and further impaction will not be impeded as long as the sliding nail or compression screw does not fail.

Nonunion and malunion are probably due to loss of the reduction, incorrect nail placement, or failure of the device.

Frequently, complications from internal fixation devices are due to mechanical factors. Failure of the nail to slide in the barrel of the device because of excessive friction may result from imperfections in the quality of the device. Nail breakage, bending, and disengagement of the nail or screws are the result of cyclic loading. Poor bone quality, imperfections in the device, and improper placement and fixation are contributing factors. If bone-to-bone contact is insufficient, most of the stress is shifted to the metallic device, which leads to failure of the device or disengagement. Penetration of the femoral head or cutting out of the nail depend on the degree of osteoporosis, the position of the fixative, and the reduction.

REFERENCES

1. Boyd H.B., Griffin L.L.: Classification and treatment of trochanteric fractures. *Arch. Surg.* 58:853, 1949.
2. Tronzo R.G.: *Surgery of the Hip Joint.* Philadelphia, Lea & Febiger, 1973.
3. Mays J., Neufeld A.J.: Skeletal traction methods. *Clin. Orthop.* 102:144, 1974.
4. Anderson R.: New methods for treating fractures utilizing the well leg for countertraction. *Surg. Gynecol. Obstet.* 54:207, 1932.
5. Frankel V.H.: *The Femoral Neck Function: Fracture Mechanics and Internal Fixation.* Springfield, Ill., Charles C Thomas, Publisher, 1960.

Chapter 8

Subtrochanteric Fractures

Robert E. Zickel, M.D.

Fractures of the proximal shaft of the femur, often referred to as sub-trochanteric fractures, are frequently the result of high-velocity trauma such as that caused by motor vehicle accidents. In elderly patients, however, the cause of the trauma may be insignificant, often merely a fall at home. Although fractures in the elderly are more common at the femoral neck or intertrochanteric area, when the fulcrum of stress is transmitted below the lesser trochanter, it can cause a fracture in the upper shaft.

Subtrochanteric fractures may involve both areas, starting at the intertrochanteric line and extending down the shaft, usually in a spiral pattern, with or without comminution (Fig 8–1). The incidence of these fractures is quite low compared to that of other hip fractures varying from 8% to 20% in different reports, but they will probably account for less than one of every ten fractured hips in most hospitals. This explains why for many years the fracture was rarely appraised as a separate entity, but rather was considered a variation of the intertrochanteric fracture. It follows that internal fixation devices designed for intertrochanteric fractures were extended for use in the subtrochanteric area. Early recognition of the problems of management must be credited to Allis, who in 1891 described the difficulties of treating fractures of the upper femoral shaft by traction, showing the problems of varus deformity and nonunion. He recommended internal fixation to control the fracture and osteotomies to correct malunion.[1] It is particularly interesting that he published his findings before x-rays had been discovered. Lambotte in 1907 recommended open reduction and internal fixation in one of his many treatises on internal fixation techniques of fractures.[2] He combined hip nails with cerclage wires for fixation. Russell Hibbs, while still a resident, presented a paper to the New York Academy of Medicine, on subtrochanteric fractures. He recommended bringing the distal shaft in line with the proximal shaft and maintaining the alignment with traction. Most investigators prior to 1950 agreed with Hibbs and advised that subtrochanteric fractures be treated with traction or plastercast immobilization. The excellent circulation in the proximal part of the femur was believed to ensure a high rate of union. Many reports, however, emphasized the high complication and mortality rates, particularly in elderly patients, who could not tolerate prolonged traction or body casts.

With the development of the triflanged nail by Smith-Petersen and modifications of the nail by Johannson, the benefits of internal fixation of hip fractures quickly became evident. The triflanged nail alone could not be used for fractures that extended below the trochanters. The addition of the side plate by Thornton, Jewett, and Neufeld was a logical modification of the Smith-Petersen nail. While other open

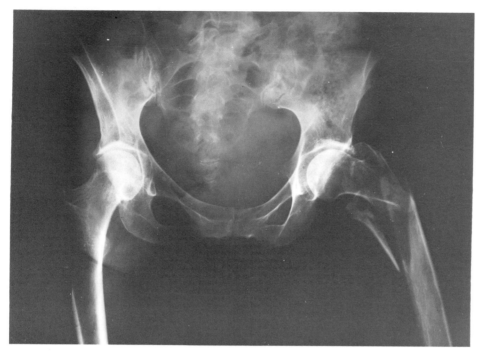

Fig 8–1—A subtrochanteric-intertrochanteric fracture.

methods have been reported, the nail plate became the most widely accepted device for trochanteric fractures, and indeed its use was extended to the subtrochanteric area by lengthening the side plate. Jewett, realizing the need for greater fixation, added an attached anterior plate to the standard Jewett nail.[3]

Kuntscher, in 1940, introduced a semitubular intramedullary nail for many fractures of the femur. The very first Kuntscher nailing was reportedly performed on a subtrochanteric fracture.[4] Shortly thereafter Kuntscher modified the tubular nail for hip fractures. This modified intramedullary nail received a second nail for the femoral neck which passed through a slot in the first. He referred to this appliance as a "doppelnagel" (double nail), which he initially used for trochanteric and subtrochanteric fractures, but admitted technical difficulties in aligning the appliance so that the second nail would engage the neck of the femur properly. He later modified this into a second doppelnagel, called a Y nail (Fig 8–2). It has a large, somewhat sled-shaped nail which is driven first into the neck of the femur from the lateral shaft, which then receives a long intramedullary rod inserted from above, passing through an opening in the femoral nail as it is driven down the femoral canal. Both of these appliances provide complete intramedullary support to the femur but have never gained wide endorsement because of intraoperative technical problems.

In 1949, Boyd and Griffin classified 300 trochanteric fractures into four types. Their patients were treated with Jewett nails, Neufeld nails, and Moore-Blount blade plates.[5] They noted a high complication rate in their type III fracture, a high transverse subtrochanteric fracture. Causes of failure of fixation in this group included medial migration of the shaft, protrusion of the nail into the hip joint, and appliance breakage. Watson, Campbell, and Wade in 1964 reviewed 100 subtrochanteric fractures and reported a high incidence of failure with different devices.[6] They inferred that intramedullary nails provided superior fixation to a variety of different nail plates but did not find sufficient cases treated with intramedullary nails to make a definite conclusion.

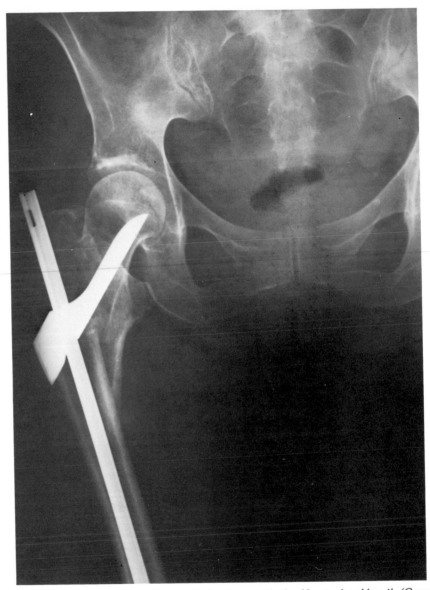

Fig 8–2—A healed subtrochanteric fracture with the Kuntscher Y nail. (Courtesy of H. Koenig, M.D., Pittsburgh.)

In 1966, Fielding and Magliato reported a high complication rate with the Jewett nail in 64 consecutive subtrochanteric fractures. Although the entire series had a failure of 25%, those fractures most distal to the lesser trochanter (Fielding and Magliato classification type III) had a failure rate of almost 50%. They advised surgeons to protect these patients with traction in bed until there was evidence of sufficient healing to provide stability.[7]

It was hoped that the development of stronger nail plate devices would provide a better solution. Although there is probably a wider margin of safety with these devices, they have not been that successful in treating subtrochanteric fractures (Fig 8–3). The screws that secure the plate to the femoral shaft may become the weakest link and fail (Fig 8–4). This was the reported experience with the Holt nail, which was probably the strongest nail plate appliance ever developed. Johnson, Lottes, and Arnot, after reviewing 146 fractures treated with the Holt nail, reported five significant complications in nine subtrochanteric fractures. They concluded that this appliance provided no advantage over other nail plates.[8]

The introduction of the sliding or telescoping nails by Pugh and Massie helped to correct the problem of joint penetration associated with medial migration of the shaft in hip fractures.[9] Although Pugh and Massie nails were not the first such devices designed, they quickly gained wide recognition because of their effectiveness in maintaining fixation while permitting impaction in fractures of the hip. They were to stimulate the development of a series of sliding nails or telescoping appliances,

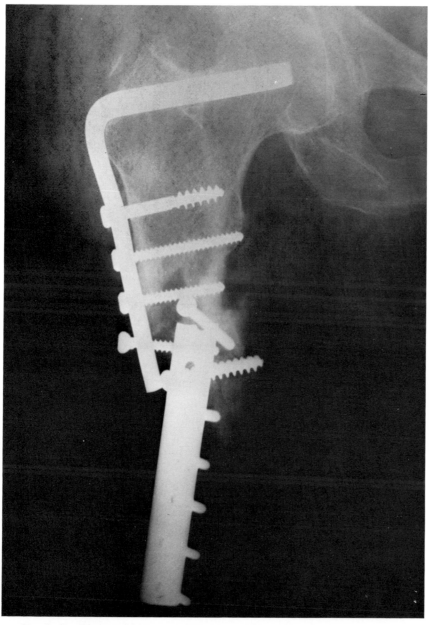

Fig 8–3—Broken blade plate from a comminuted medial buttress.

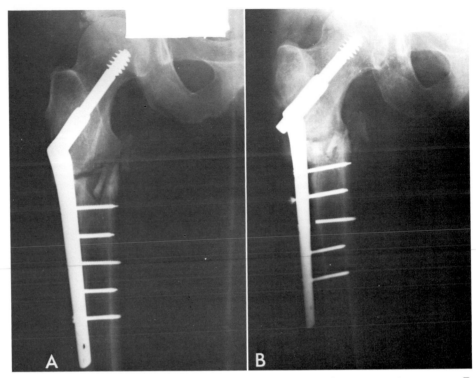

Fig 8–4—**A,** *unstable medial buttress in fracture with compression screw.* **B,** *with settling of the fracture, the screws failed although the plate did not break.*

the most popular of which today is the sliding compression screw. In subtrochanteric fractures these appliances are an improvement on fixed nail plates, by helping to prevent joint penetration when there is medial migration of the femoral shaft. The telescoping feature of the nail usually does not help in stabilizing fractures below the lesser trochanter, as fixation there is provided by the plate and not the nail.

Intramedullary fixation for subtrochanteric fractures was strongly advocated by Kuntscher, who developed modifications of the cloverleaf nail already mentioned. The Zickel subtrochanteric nail was developed in 1964 and was first used in 1966. This appliance was specifically designed to provide intramedullary support for a variety of fractures of the proximal shaft (Fig 8–5).[10] In concept, the appliance is similar to Kuntscher's original doppelnagel, but it differs in several design features, which will be described in chapter 20.

Standard femoral intramedullary rods such as the Kuntscher nail were designed for the midshaft, where the diaphyseal canal is narrow and uniform. Such rods did not provide sufficient fixation in the widened proximal metaphyseal canal with a short proximal fragment, as is often found in subtrochanteric fractures. Special intramedullary appliances were needed, such as the Kuntscher Y nail or the Zickel subtrochanteric nail. More recently the multiple flexible nails developed by Ender and Simon-Weider have provided another intramedullary approach.[11] The Ender nails are actually modifications of Kuntscher's condylocephalic nail developed in the early 1960s but are thinner and more flexible than their predecessor, not unlike Rush pins. Inserted into the medullary canal at the supracondylar area of the femur, they are driven proximally through the fracture site and up into the femoral head and neck after the fracture is reduced. Because they are thin and flexible, multiple pins are used to fill the medullary canal.

This procedure is usually performed with image intensification and without opening the fracture site, and has the advantage of eliminating surgical trauma and periosteal dissection at the area of fracture. Traction postoperatively for periods of 3–6 weeks has been recommended by Ender because of instability in subtrochanteric fractures associated with comminution.[12]

In 1978, Allen, Heiple, and Burstein reported preliminary experience with a fluted intramedullary rod.[13] This rod, which is round in cross-section, has longitudinal ridges or flutes which in bench testing were shown to have superior torsional strength when compared to other existing intramedullary rods. The fluted rods in addition are manufactured in sections which can be assembled during surgery to attain a desired overall length for a particular femur. This appliance was later manufactured with a special section (18 mm in diameter) which can be used for fractures of the proximal femoral shaft. This provides a large-diameter, cross-section rod to achieve better fixation in the widened trochanteric canal. The successful use of this appliance in 18 subtrochanteric fractures was reported by the same authors in 1979 (Fig 8–6).

Attempts at classifying subtrochanteric fractures have generally been too simple or too complex. Boyd and Griffin described all trochanteric fractures as of four types, and two of those types were subtrochanteric. Watson, Campbell, and Wade used a somewhat complex formula determined by measurements from reference points at the greater trochanter. Those fractures caused by severe trauma such as a gunshot wound or a fall from a very high elevation are so comminuted that no specific pattern can be identified. Fielding and Magliato described three types of subtrochanteric fractures: type I, at the lesser trochanter; type II, 1 inch below the lesser trochanter; and type III, 2 inches below the lesser trochanter (Fig 8–7). Zickel in 1976 described six types of subtrochanteric fractures, four that are oblique or spiral and two that are transverse (Fig 8–8). In the oblique fracture, the fracture begins proximally at or adjacent to the lesser trochanter with the obliquity extending laterally down the femoral shaft. These fractures may be accompanied by an inter-

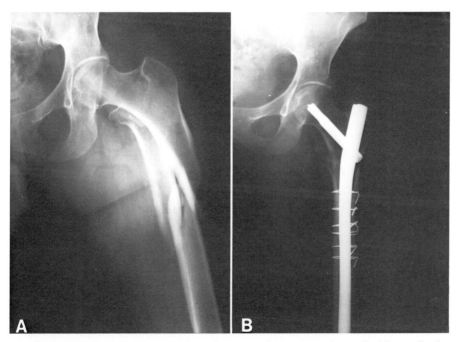

Fig 8–5—A, a long oblique subtrochanteric fracture with medial butterfly fragment. B, same fracture with Zickel nail and cerclage wires.

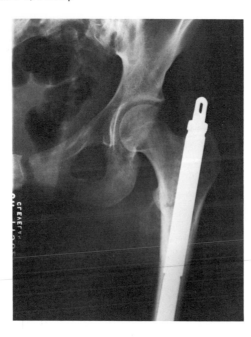

Fig 8–6—Sampson fluted nail. (Courtesy of K.G. Heiple, M.D., Cleveland.)

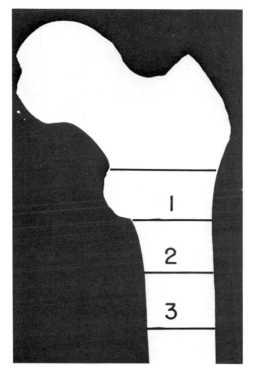

Fig 8–7—Fielding-Magliato classification of subtrochanteric fractures. (Courtesy of J.W. Fielding, New York.)

trochanteric fracture or a butterfly fragment off the shaft medially. The two transverse types are just below the lesser trochanter or just proximal to the femoral diaphysis.[10] In 1978, Seinsheimer discribed a classification system in which he divided these fractures into five major types and then subdivided each of the major groups into numerical and alphabetical subtypes (e.g., 2A, 2B, etc.), for a total of eight fracture types (Fig 8–9). He also attempted to correlate these fractures with clinical experience. He found type 3A, a somewhat short, oblique fracture with medial comminution and

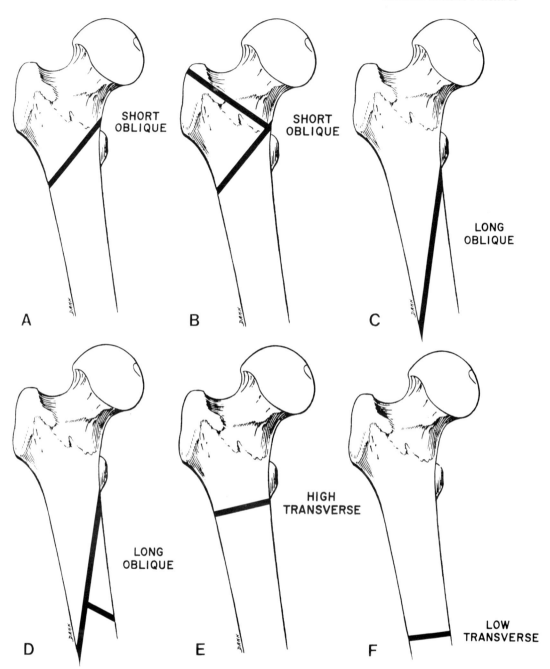

Fig 8–8—Zickel classification of subtrochanteric fractures. **A,** *short oblique;* **B,**
short oblique with intertrochanteric fracture; **C,** *long oblique;* **D,** *long oblique with*
butterfly fragment; **E,** *high transverse,* **F,** *low transverse.*

an intertrochanteric component, to have the highest incidence of failure with various
fixation devices.[14] While the Seinsheimer classification has been referred to by other
investigators, it is probably too complex to be practical for the clinician who must
first describe the fracture and then try to remember its category. Conversely, an
oversimplified system of classification such as that described by Fielding and Magliato
does not provide for spiral fractures which transcend two or more of the classification

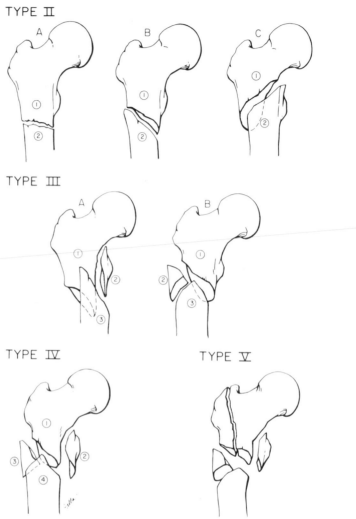

Fig 8–9—Seinsheimer classification of subtrochanteric fractures. (Courtesy of F. Seinsheimer, M.D., Silver Springs, Md.)

zones. There is probably no system of classification available that can describe all subtrochanteric fractures adequately. Comminution and loss of the medial buttress, as noted by Evans in 1949,[15] is probably the greatest cause of failure and must be considered the major threat to management.

BIOMECHANICAL CONSIDERATIONS

There are few areas in the skeletal system that more clearly demonstrate applied biomechanics than fixation of the proximal femoral shaft. As the longest and strongest long bone of the body, the femur must be structurally sound to endure the enormous stresses placed on it. Attempts to repair it must therefore be guided by concern for potential mechanical failure. If the femur was straight rather than angulated at approximately 135° at the junction of the neck and shaft, the problem would be much simpler. This, however, is not the case, and loads transmitted from the body to the femoral head reach the proximal shaft not in a straight line but through a cantilevered femoral neck. This leverage by the femoral neck causes bending of the shaft through compression stresses medially and tension stresses laterally. The leverage or bending moment is very high because of the long lever arm created. Koch, in 1917, using measurements of the cross-sectional area of the femur from a 200 lb male cadaver, analyzed theoretically the mechanical stresses on the femur during weight-bearing and calculated the stresses placed on weight-bearing with muscle pull. Assuming 100-lb load on the femoral head, he found that compression stresses were greater than 1,200 lb per square inch along the medial cortex, 1–3 inches below the lesser trochanter, while tensile stresses on the lateral cortex were about 20% less (Fig 8–10).[16]

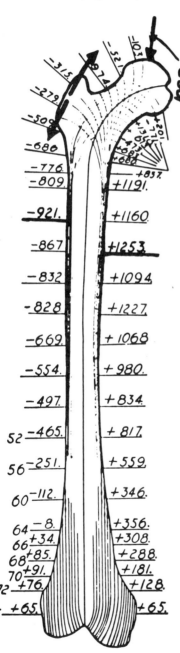

Fig 8–10—Koch diagram showing stresses on the proximal femoral shaft in static loading.

Froimson described the additional forces projected on the subtrochanteric area by powerful muscles that act on the proximal femur (Fig 8–11).[17] It is well known that during stance these muscles create forces on the head of the femur equal to two to three times body weight. This position increased the forces by Koch, which were computed in static loading. More recent investigations by Rybicki et al. using a mathematical computer model and by Cochran et al. using strain gauges in vitro not only substantiated Koch's findings but predicted that in vivo, forces placed on the femur are two to three times greater when the hip muscles are active. Some hip muscles such as the tensor fascia lata may act to neutralize part of the bending forces under certain conditions. In subtrochanteric fractures, the forces are unbalanced and the unopposed muscle action produces the characteristic abduction, rotation, and flexion deformity demonstrated by Froimson. These unopposed forces are extremely difficult to control by nonoperative methods of traction or casts. These same muscle forces are very active even in a patient confined to bed. Rydel instrumented a femoral prosthesis with a strain gauge and demonstrated that flexion or extension of the hip while the patient was in bed caused as much pressure on the femoral head as slow walking with or without crutches.[18] Frankel and Burstein instrumented a nail plate used in subtrochanteric osteotomies and reported similar forces generated by muscle pull alone. Frankel's "telltale nail" revealed the large stresses at the nail plate junction caused by high bending movement even in a patient in traction (Fig 8–12).[19]

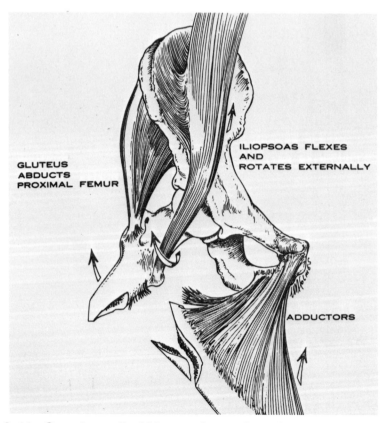

Fig 8–11—Opposing pull of hip muscles on the subtrochanteric region. The proximal fragment is flexed, abducted, and externally rotated, while the femoral shaft is shortened and adducted. (From Froimson.[17] Reproduced by permission.)

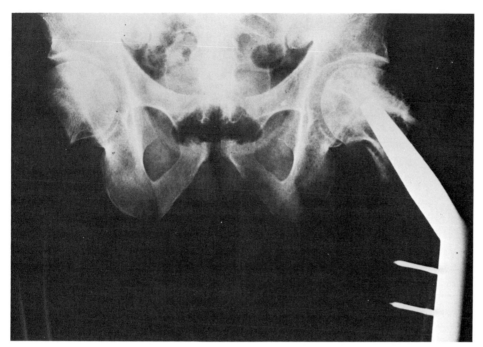

Fig 8–12—Frankel "telltale" nail. (Courtesy of V. Frankel, M.D., New York.)

How then can any fixation device deal with the enormous stresses described? Many fractures fixed with mechanically inadequate devices may heal because the biologic healing process was rapid enough to provide stability before the appliance failed. The implant will fail from fatigue if healing is slow or if there is a delay in union. It will also fail if the the device is subjected to one large stress that exceeds its yield strength before healing is complete. Although improved alloys with superior yield and fatigue strength offer greater protection, no device can consistently withstand the stresses in the proximal femoral shaft unless the bone itself shares part of the load. Load sharing between bone and appliance should be the goal of successful internal fixation of the femur. Stronger and more rigid appliances do not guarantee success and may well be detrimental. Osteopenia from stress shielding has been well recognized as a problem in recent years. Conversely, the more flexible or ductile implants may not adequately immobilize the fracture in the early stages of healing and so may also fail. The concept not of the device alone but the device-bone union is paramount in treatment (Fig 8–13).

TREATMENT
Nonoperative

Fractures of the proximal femoral shaft may be managed without internal fixation. Traction has long been an acceptable method of treatment and may well be indicated as the primary method of treatment in some cases. Skeletal traction with balance suspension requires insertion of a pin in the proximal tibia or the distal femur. If traction has been selected as the method of total treatment, the distal femur is probably the best site, as greater pull may be exerted directly on the fractured femur. Proximal tibial traction should be reserved for temporary treatment when the plan calls for eventual use of internal fixation. The hazard of introducing infection

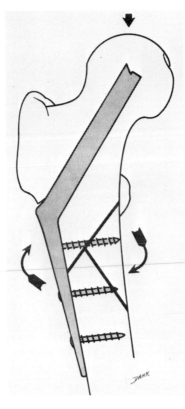

Fig 8–13—Comminuted subtrochanteric fracture puts stress on plate and not the nail.

through a pin tract must be considered; infection is more of a problem if it is initiated in the femur, further complicating the management of the fracture. Skin traction has little place in the management of subtrochanteric fractures, as the force of pull required cannot be safely attained by this method.

One must consider whether traction is indicated as a primary or as a secondary method of management. Some open fractures with large wounds and soft tissue contamination, the multiply injured patient or ill patient who cannot be taken to the operating room, and severely comminuted fractures that defy open reduction and internal fixation (Fig 8–14) should be treated nonoperatively.

Our experience with traction in subtrochanteric fractures has not been favorable. Varus and rotational deformity, malunion, and nonunion have occurred too frequently, even in the most carefully managed cases. Cardiopulmonary complications (usually due to emboli), deterioration of the sensorium, and stiffness of both hip joint and knee joint may cause permanent and severe disability. Perhaps one of the most important considerations when selecting a plan of treatment for comminuted fractures of the proximal femur is later options for salvage of a malunion or nonunion. Healed fragments in malalignment may preclude the use of intramedullary fixation later because of ablation or distortion of the medullary canal. Extramedullary nail plates may become difficult to use because of gross distortion of the cortical bone surface. Reconstructing the femur anatomically, even if it results in nonunion, makes future salvage procedures a more rational option, as the major anatomical configuration of the femur has been preserved.

Plaster immobilization is another nonsurgical approach. Total body spica casts may provide adequate immobilization once satisfactory alignment has been achieved. This method is rarely used today because of the consequences of permanent loss of joint mobility, muscle atrophy, and the necessity of confining patients to bed for prolonged periods. Modified hip spicas have been described in some reports to permit ambulation. Such a method should only be attempted in very youthful patients who can control these cumbersome supports.

The use of the cast-brace has been controversial in the treatment of subtrochanteric fractures. Most advocates of cast-brace treatment have been reluctant to recommend this method for fractures of the proximal femur. Bulky thigh muscles and short proximal femoral bone fragments make immobilization difficult. In 1981, DeLee et al. reported results in a series of 15 patients treated with a long quadralateral socket cast-brace and a pelvic band. These fractures were initially treated in traction for 3.5–7 weeks (average, 4.8 weeks) before application of the body cast.[20] In this series all fractures united, with an average return of knee motion of 130° and return of almost all hip motion. It should be noted that the average age of patients in this group was 27.4 years, and the authors emphasize the importance of meticulous attention to detail to avoid unacceptable shortening, angulation, or malrotation, which are common complications of the cast-brace method.

It is my opinion that most subtrochanteric fractures should be managed by reduction and internal fixation. The contraindications to surgery, already mentioned, are usually temporary. The possible complications of shortening, varus, malrotation, and nonunion with closed methods are reasons for planning surgical repair.

Internal Fixation

The concept of establishing a load-sharing relationship between the bone and the appliance should be the guide when selecting an operative method of fixation of fractures of the proximal femur. The nail plate and its later modifications with

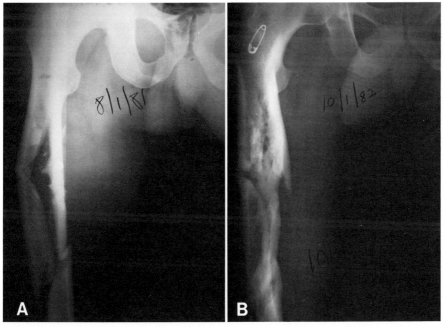

*Fig 8–14—**A,** comminuted proximal femoral shaft fracture treated in traction with hip spica. **B,** same fracture 1 year later was healed, but leg was externally rotated and shortened, with stiffness of both hip and knee.*

sliding nails or compression screws are widely used for subtrochanteric fractures of the femur. If the nail or compression screw component of these appliances provides intramedullary fixation of the fracture so that impaction from settling can occur, then fixation is probably sound. This type of fixation can be achieved in some high subtrochanteric fractures or intertrochanteric fractures with a short subtrochanteric component. This *intertrochanteric-subtrochanteric* fracture, in which the major portion of the fracture is intertrochanteric, should be reduced and nailed in valgus, with the nail entered somewhat distally on the shaft so the nail or screw part of the device provides intramedullary fixation. In those femora where most or all of the fracture is below the lesser trochanter, nail plates are no longer providing intramedullary fixation but perform as extramedullary plates. The nail or sliding screw anchoring the end of the plate to the head and neck of the femur does not permit settling or impaction of the fracture because of its location; instead, it simply fixes the end of the plate.

A load-sharing relationship may be achieved with a nail plate in an ideal situation such as a subtrochanteric osteotomy. If bone cuts are properly made and if the device is properly applied, then there is excellent medial bone contact with good stability. Such ideal fixation is rarely achieved in a fracture because of obliquity and comminution. The addition of extra bone plates on the anterior surface of the femur offers little more security. Reconstructing a lost medial buttress with bone grafts may provide faster healing but little mechanical support in the early phases of healing. If the surgeon has selected a nail plate for fixation of a true subtrochanteric fracture, then he or she would be wise to protect it by keeping the patient in postoperative traction for a number of weeks until there is roentgenographic or clinical evidence of stability from sufficient healing.

Intramedullary fixation should be used whenever possible in stabilizing fractures of the proximal femoral shaft. By establishing a load-sharing relationship between the bone and appliance by decreasing the mechanical lever arm because of its position in the medullary canal, the intramedullary nail has a distinct advantage over the nail plate.

A transverse, low subtrochanteric fracture at the junction of the proximal and middle thirds of the femur can often be treated with a standard intramedullary rod such as a Kuntscher cloverleaf nail, which was actually disigned for the midshaft. There is usually sufficient proximal bone stock for good fixation. More proximal subtrochanteric fractures are better treated by appliances designed specifically for that area, as the trochanteric medullary canal cannot afford sufficient stability to these nails.

The Ender intramedullary nail is a flexible, somewhat curved nail similar in size to the Rush pin. One end is modified to accept a special driver or extractor, and the sled shape of the tip permits tracking in the medullary canal. The nail can be modified intraoperatively by bending it, and it is inserted through a hole in the supracondylar area above the knee. Multiple nails can be inserted to provide better stability by nesting them in the narrow part of the medullary canal. The nails are usually driven through a hole in the medial supracondylar cortex in a retrograde manner to achieve fixation in the proximal femoral neck and head after crossing the fracture site. Ideally the nailing is performed without opening the fracture, so an image intensifier is necessary to ascertain maintenance of the fracture and position of the nail. Although the nailing is usually performed by insertion through the medial supracondylar cortex, with seating of the nails in the head and neck of the femur, additional nails may be driven through the lateral supracondylar cortex and fixed proximally in the greater trochanter of the femur. Both Ender and Bohler have suggested that postoperative traction be used for a number of weeks until there is sufficient stability to enable mobilization of the patient.

This technique provides total intramedullary support of the fracture by closed nailing. Disadvantages reported include backing out of the nail, external rotation deformity, and the necessity for postoperative traction. Difficulty in achieving satisfactory alignment of a comminuted fracture intraoperatively sometimes forces the choice of open reduction.

The Zickel intramedullary subtrochanteric nail was designed specifically to provide intramedullary fixation for a variety of fractures of the subtrochanteric and proximal femoral shaft areas. The appliance consists of a specially designed and contoured intramedullary rod which is inserted through the tip of the trochanter and into the medullary canal, after the canal has been reamed and the fracture reduced. The intramedullary rod has a round tunnel at its proximal end which can receive a triflange nail, which, when driven through the tunnel, engages the neck and head of the femur and provides anchorage for the intramedullary rod. This appliance, which was first used in 1966, is discussed at greater length in chapter 20.

REFERENCES

1. Allis O.H.: Fractures in the upper third of the femur exclusive of the neck. *Med. News* 59:585, 1981.
2. Lambotte A.: *L'intervention operatoire dans les fractures: Recentes et ancienées Envisagee.* Brussels, Lamertain, 1907.
3. Jewett E.L.: A new approach for subtrochanteric and upper femoral shaft fractures using a dual phlange nail plate: A preliminary report. *Am. J. Surg.* 81:186-188, 1951.
4. Kuntscher G.: A new method of pertrochanteric fractures. *Proc. R. Soc. Med.* 63:1120, 1970.
5. Boyd H.B., Griffin L.L.: Classification and treatment of trochanteric fractures. *Arch. Surg.* 58:853, 1949.
6. Watson H.K., Campbell R.D., Wade P.A.: Classification, treatment and complications of the adult subtrochanteric fracture. *J. Trauma* 4:457, 1964.
7. Fielding J.W., Magliato H.J.: Subtrochanteric fractures. *Surg. Gynecol. Obstet.* 122:555, 1966.
8. Johnson L.L., Lottes J.O., Arnot J.P.: The utilization of the Holt nail for proximal femoral fractures: A study of 146 patients. *J. Bone Joint. Surg.* 50A:67, 1968.
9. Massie W.K.: Extracapsular fractures of the hip treated by impaction using a sliding nail-plate fixation. *Clin. Orthop.* 22:180, 1962.
10. Zickel R.E.: An intramedullary fixation device for the proximal part of the femur: Nine years' experience. *J. Bone Joint Surg.* 58A:866, 1976.
11. Ender J., Simon-Weider R.: Die fixierung der trochanterem Beicle nil remden elastichen Condylemagelin. *Acta Chir. Austr.* 1:40, 1972.
12. Ender H.G.: Treatment of pertrochanteric and subtrochanteric fractures of the femur with Ender pins, in *The Hip (Proceedings of the Hip Society).* St. Louis, C.V. Mosby Co., 1978, p. 187.
13. Allen W.C., Heiple K.G., Burstein A.H.: A fluted femoral intramedullary rod: Biomechanical analysis and preliminary clinical results. *J. Bone Joint. Surg.* 60A:506, 1978.
14. Seinsheimer F. III: Subtrochanteric fractures of the femur. *J. Bone Joint. Surg.* 60A:300-306, 1978.
15. Evans E.M.: The treatment of trochanteric fractures of the femur. *J. Bone Joint Surg.* 31B:190-203, 1949.
16. Koch J.C.: The laws of bone architecture. *Am. J. Anat.* 21:177, 1917.
17. Froimson A.I.: Treatment of comminuted subtrochanteric fracture of the femur. *Surg. Gynecol. Obstet.* 131:465-472, 1970.
18. Rydell N.W.: Forces acting on the femoral head prosthesis: A study on strain gauge supplied prosthesis in living persons. *Acta Orthop. Scan. Suppl.* 88:37, 1966.
19. Frankel V.H., Burstein A.H.: *Orthopedic Biomechanics.* Philadelphia, Lea & Febiger, 1970.
20. DeLee J.G., Clanton T.O., Rockwood C.A.: Closed treatment of subtrochanteric fractures of the femur in a modified cast brace. *J. Bone Joint Surg.* 63A:773-779, 1981.

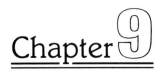

Chapter 9

Trochanteric Fractures

Marvin H. Meyers, M.D.

FRACTURES OF THE GREATER TROCHANTER

Isolated fractures of the greater trochanter or separation of the epiphysis of the greater trochanter are uncommon injuries. They are the result of direct injuries such as a fall on the lateral aspect of the hip (Fig 9–1), a kick, or avulsion by muscle pull. The symptoms are tenderness, swelling in the region of the greater trochanter, and pain on rotation or active abduction of the hip. Usually the patient can bear weight on the affected limb but limps because of pain.

The diagnosis is made by x-ray examination. Separation of the fragments is usually slight. Epiphyseal avulsion of the entire trochanter is usually proximal. In the adult, fracture of the greater trochanter is almost always comminuted, and displacement, when it occurs, is usually proximal and medial.

Treatment options are immobilization in a plaster of Paris jacket, weight-bearing as tolerated with external support (crutches or cane), and internal fixation. Early ambulation as tolerated on crutches or with a cane is the treatment of choice when the fracture is minimally or slightly displaced. Wide separation of the fragment (>1 cm) may require reduction and fixation of the fragment. Displacement can be reduced by wide abduction and internal rotation to counteract the action of the hip abductor muscles. Approximation of the trochanter and shaft of the femur often follows the latter maneuver. This position can be maintained in a double hip spica cast. On rare occasions, especially in young patients, when the fragments are widely separated and cannot be reduced by closed reduction, open reduction through a straight lateral incision directly over the trochanter is the advised treatment. Reduction is achieved and maintained by screws or a tension band wire. Weakness in hip abduction may be the result of nonunion or malunion of the trochanter in a proximal direction.

Weight-bearing as tolerated with external support for 6–8 weeks is the recommended regimen for the patient with an undisplaced fracture. If a hip spica cast is utilized to protect the fracture after reduction it can be removed in 4–6 weeks and protected weight-bearing resumed. After open reduction and internal fixation, a hip spica cast is advisable for 4–6 weeks for protection. However, protected weight-bearing can be considered for cooperative, reliable patients.

Nonunion in untreated cases is extremely rare. If the patient has weak hip abduction, open reduction and internal fixation is the treatment of choice, especially in the young patient. Impacted fractures of the greater trochanter are frequently missed since they may be difficult to identify radiographically, or the greater trochanter may be overexposed by poor technique. If necessary, tomography will demonstrate the cortical disruption clearly.

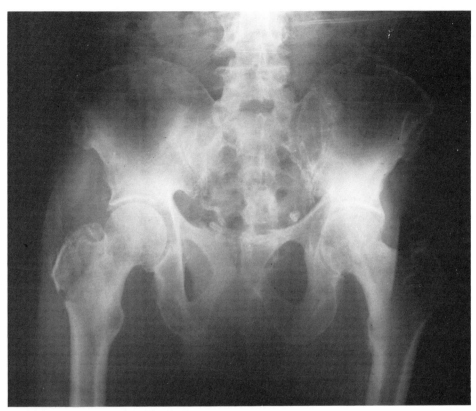

Fig 9–1—Communited undisplaced fracture of the greater trochanter in an adult following a fall on the right hip.

FRACTURE OF THE LESSER TROCHANTER

An isolated fracture of the lesser trochanter is a rare injury. These fractures are isolated avulsions of either the lesser trochanter in adults or the lesser trochanteric apophysis in adolescents (Fig 9–2). Most often the fracture occurs in association with intertrochanteric fractures in older adults.

Isolated fractures are the result of violent contraction of the iliopsoas muscle complex, which inserts into the lesser trochanter. Violent muscle contraction while the hip is hyperextended or abducted produces the fracture. The fragment is pulled proximally by the iliopsoas muscle.

The diagnosis is based on the history, symptoms, and radiologic findings. It is more frequent in adolescent boys than in adults. Young persons sustain the injury while running or kicking. Injury is accompanied by pain, tenderness, and swelling in the proximal, medial aspect of the thigh. There is weakness of hip flexion in the sitting position (Ludloff's sign) and pain can be elicited by passively hyperextending the hip on the affected side. X-ray films made with the leg in slight external rotation will reveal the fracture or epiphyseal separation.

Treatment depends on the degree of separation of the fragment. Separation of less than 2 cm can be treated by early weight-bearing as tolerated, with or without external support. Strenuous activity must be avoided until healing occurs.

Open reduction and fixation with a screw should be considered with avulsions of 2 cm or more. Cast fixation after closed reduction is a treatment option. Flexion

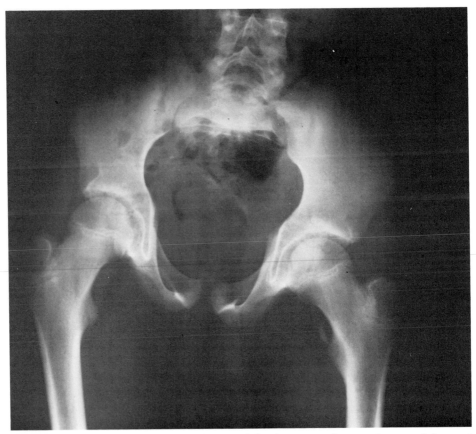

Fig 9–2—Avulsion of the apophysis of the lesser trochanter in an adolescent hurdler.

of the leg to 90° and external rotation of the leg may bring the base of the fragment close to the femur. The cast is removed in 4–6 weeks. Weight-bearing with the aid of a cane or crutches is resumed for an additional 4 weeks, after which the external support can be discontinued.

Fractures of the lesser trochanter that are part of an interochanteric fracture seem to do well without replacement.

Chapter 10

Fractures of the Hip in Children

Marvin H. Meyers, M.D.

Fractures of the hip in children are rare. The reported incidence is low, probably because the force required to fracture the bone in childhood is of great magnitude. The bone is tough and growing at this age, which makes the upper end of the femur very strong. These injuries occur in severe accidents or as a result of excessive force, such as that incurred in a fall from a height, in automobile accidents, or in physical assault (battered child).[1]

Although no one individual has accumulated a series large enough to be statistically significant with respect to results and guidelines for treatment,[2,3] many published papers on these rare fractures report similar trends in results with various treatments, so that reasonable treatment guidelines have been established.[3-7]

Delbet's classification of hip fractures in children, as reported by Colonna,[8] is accepted by most authors. Subtrochanteric fractures are here added to Delbet's classification, since they should be considered in a discussion of hip fractures. The list then reads as follows: transepiphyseal, transcervical, cervicotrochanteric, intertrochanteric, and subtrochanteric.

Rang listed several important differences between children and adult hip fractures,[9] as follows:

1. Displaced fractures are less frequent in children, probably because the periosteal tube is thicker and stronger.

2. The anatomical difference in the blood supply makes the femoral head more vulnerable to osteonecrosis.

3. The high incidence of shortening of the femoral neck after transcervical fractures is due to premature closure of the epiphysis, a result of osteonecrosis.

4. Coxa magna may occur and result in an increase in leg length due to the hyperemia of fracture repair.

5. Children tolerate cast immobilization better than adults; therefore, this method can be used in undisplaced fractures, with an excellent chance for osseous union.

6. The hardness of the bone as well as the small size of the femoral neck make treatment with standard Smith-Peterson nails impossible. Rang advises the use of threaded pins or screws.

7. Prosthetic replacement is not available as a solution for problems after femoral neck fractures in the child.

Other differences that hamper the treatment of hip fractures in children include:

1. There is a greater curvature of the femoral neck, which decreases the tolerance for placement of internal fixation devices.

2. Attempts at internal fixation of femoral neck fractures may damage the growth plate.

3. Vigorous manipulation may be an additional source of trauma to the blood supply.

TRANSEPIPHYSEAL FRACTURES

These injuries are usually Salter type I separations of the proximal femoral epiphysis. The incidence is greater in children less than 8 years.

It may be difficult to distinguish between a true traumatic separation and epiphysiolysis with increased symptoms following a minor injury or a slipped capital femoral epiphysis. Severe trauma is the basis for the diagnosis. Miller stated that separation of the proximal femoral epiphysis without a history of violent trauma should not be considered in a study of hip fractures in children.[5] The injury has been reported in battered children,[1] and physical abuse should be considered the cause in a child with transepiphyseal fracture of the hip without a history of severe trauma.

The injury is complicated by dislocation of the epiphysis from the joint in some patients. Canale and Bourland reported on five patients, all of whom had dislocation of the epiphysis.[3] I have treated six children with fractured hips, none of whom had dislocation from the joint.

The prognosis as reported in the literature is poor. Morrissey stated that avascular necrosis seems guaranteed.[6] Canale and Bourland reported a similar result no matter what treatment was given.[3] (It must be kept in mind that the epiphysis was completely dislocated in their series.) I have a more optimistic attitude toward transepiphyseal hip fractures in children, based on treatment of a small number of children, none of whom had joint dislocation. In general, transepiphyseal fractures associated with dislocations must be viewed with gravity.

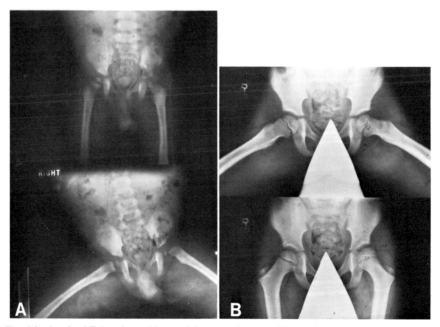

*Fig 10–1—***A,** *AP (top) and lateral (bottom) x-ray films showing displaced transepiphyseal fracture in a 2-year-old boy injured in an automobile accident. The child was treated in a spica cast for 8 weeks.* **B,** *lateral (top) and AP (bottom) x-ray films 5½ years later show a normal growth plate and epiphysis.*

Complications of Transepiphyseal Fractures

Lam noted that avascular necrosis occurs in almost all cases, closure of the epiphysis occurs in a high incidence, and coxa vara may occur.[4] There are reports in the literature which suggest that gentle closed reduction and immobilization in a cast is favored over manipulation with in situ pinning or open reduction and pinning as the treatment of choice. Avascular necrosis, closure of the epiphysis, and coxa vara were complications in most reported cases of internal fixation. In some reports gentle manipulation and cast immobilization produced good results and no complications.[1,5] My experience supports the latter treatment. Vigorous manipulation is not advised. As in most Salter type I epiphyseal injuries, remodeling occurs readily (Figs 10–1 and 10–2). Manipulation and surgery conceivably could damage the already precarious circulation of the epiphysis (Fig 10–3).

Figures 10–1 and 10–2 demonstrate that remodeling can occur if the fracture is not reduced and that undesirable complications such as avascular necrosis, premature closure of the growth plate, or coxa vara may not take place. Internal fixation and manipulation may result in avascular necrosis[3] as well as displacement of the epiphysis (see Fig 10–3). Manipulation may add to the trauma and damage to the epiphysis and produce avascular necrosis, premature closure of the epiphyseal growth plate, and neck shortening.

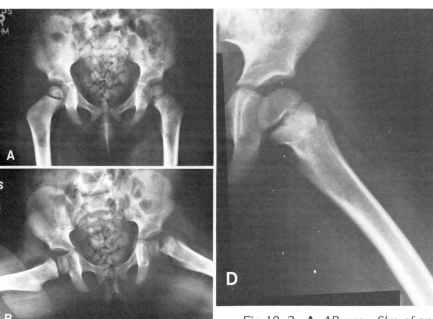

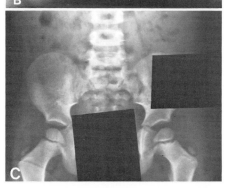

*Fig 10–2—**A,** AP x-ray film of an untreated transepiphyseal fracture of the left hip in a 2-year-old boy, 3½ weeks after injury. **B,** lateral x-ray film demonstrating Salter type I displacement of the proximal femoral epiphysis with evidence of early callous formation. **C,** AP x-ray film obtained 1½ years later. There is a slight shortening of the femoral neck. **D,** lateral x-ray film obtained 1½ years after injury shows normal appearance of growth plate and remodeled epiphysis.*

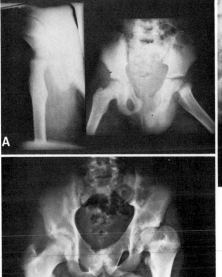
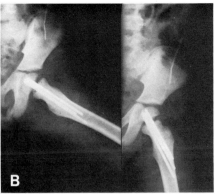

*Fig 10–3—**A**, AP (left) and lateral (right) x-ray films of a 3-year-old boy injured in a fall from a second-story window. There is a displaced transepiphyseal fracture. **B**, lateral (left) and AP (right) views after manipulation and internal fixation. Note widening of the growth plate. **C**, AP view 9 years later. Pins have been removed. Note marked shortening of neck and coxa vara.*

My preferred treatment for transepiphyseal fractures with displacement but without dislocation of the proximal fragment is immobilization in a spica cast for 2–3 months. Closed reduction of the fracture is not necessary (see Fig 10–1).

Manipulation or open reduction may be necessary when the head fragment is dislocated. The prognosis for these patients is grave.[3]

TRANSCERVICAL FRACTURES

Transcervical fractures are rare but occur more often than transepiphyseal fractures. Patients with undisplaced fractures have a good prognosis (Fig 10–4). Immobilization in a spica cast is the recommended treatment,[3-7] although displacement may occur in the cast.[7] Internal fixation is not warranted except in very unusual circumstances when compliance with follow-up care is in doubt.

Traction as a form of treatment is indicated only when there are other injuries that require hospitalization and treatment. Traction should be utilized until a spica cast can be applied. Traction requires meticulous attention to skin care, maintenance of the mechanical aspects of the traction system, and proper positioning of the fracture fragments. Traction for treatment of an undisplaced transcervical fracture with no other injuries is expensive since it necessitates a long hospitalization.

Displaced transcervical fractures are difficult to manage. There is a high incidence of nonunion, malunion, shortening of the femoral neck, and avascular necrosis with this fracture (Fig 10–5).

Manipulation followed by traction is not a suitable treatment for displaced transcervical fracture. Manipulation and immobilization in a spica cast is accompanied by a high incidence of complications such as coxa vara, nonunion, and avascular necrosis.

The treatment of choice is closed reduction and internal fixation with multiple pins. The triflanged nail is usually too large for the femoral neck in children and the hard bone makes insertion of the nail very difficult. Multiple pins, however, allow

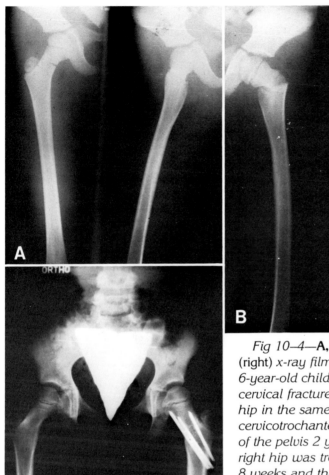

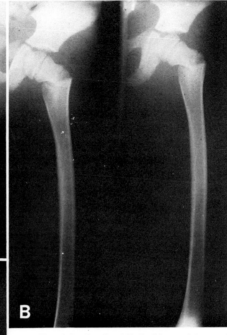

*Fig 10–4—**A,** AP (left) and lateral (right) x-ray films of the right hip in a 6-year-old child with undisplaced transcervical fracture. **B,** AP views of the left hip in the same patient show displaced cervicotrochanteric fracture. **C,** AP view of the pelvis 2 years after injury. The right hip was treated in a spica cast for 8 weeks and the left hip was treated by open reduction and internal fixation with multiple pins.*

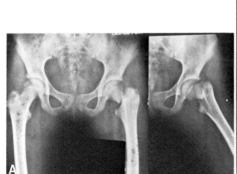

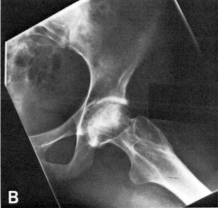

*Fig 10–5—**A,** AP (left) and lateral (right) views of the pelvis in a 13-year-old girl with a displaced transcervical fracture. **B,** lateral view 3 years after surgery and removal of pins. There is osseous union of the fracture with avascular necrosis and segmental collapse of the femoral head (Ratliff type I).*

modification in pin placement and are more versatile. I prefer threaded pins that do not cross the growth plate and lie in the neck portion of the proximal fragment. Threaded pins provide firmer fixation and do not tend to migrate.

Opening the capsule to obtain a good reduction has been advocated by some. Open reduction is not necessary unless closed reduction fails. The surgeon should not persist in manipulating the fracture if reduction is unsuccessful after one or two attempts, because of possible damage to the precarious circulation to the femoral head.

Attempts at aspirating the hip to remove a hemarthrosis within a few hours of injury in order to prevent aseptic necrosis are not warranted. Intra-articular bleeding is minimal after hip fractures.

There are several precautions to be taken with internal fixation. The threaded portion of the pin should cross the fracture line but not bridge the growth plate, and in younger children it should lie within the proximal fragment. Crossing the growth plate with pins is acceptable in older children (13 years or older), in whom growth of the proximal femoral epiphysis is nearing an end. The resulting minimal loss in length from premature closure of the growth plate is acceptable. In younger children, the degree of leg length shortening would be unacceptable. Impaction may not be possible if the threads bridge the fracture line, and therefore delayed union or non-union may be a consequence. The hardness of the bone has been mentioned before. Insertion of pins may be very difficult in some cases. In this event predrilling with a drill point that has a slightly narrower diameter than the threaded nail will permit easier insertion.

Ratliff advocates a primary subtrochanteric osteotomy in patients less than 10 years old because of the difficulty encountered in fixing these fractures internally.[7] Canale and Bourland[3] and I believe that a primary subtrochanteric osteotomy is not necessary but should be considered if internal fixation cannot be readily accomplished.

Complications of Femoral Neck Fractures
Avascular Necrosis

There is an unacceptably high rate of avascular necrosis of the femoral head following displaced transcervical fractures in children, no matter what method of treatment is used. Ratliff has divided avascular necrosis into three types (Fig 10–6):

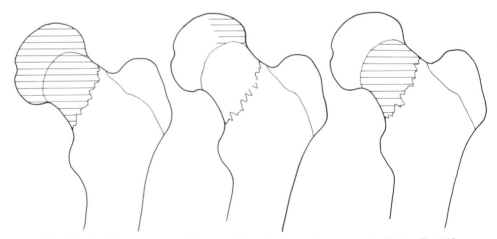

Fig 10–6—Three types of femoral head avascular necrosis (after Ratliff).

type I, diffuse involvement of the femoral head and neck with subsequent collapse; type II, involvement of only the superior portion of the head; and type III, involvement of only the femoral neck. He found that type I necrosis developed in 50% of cases and types II and III in the remainder of cases in about equal proportions. A review of the literature suggests that the incidence of avascular necrosis is not related to the type of therapy. It appears to be a consequence of severe trauma in an area that has a precarious and vulnerable blood supply. Theoretically, vigorous manipulation or careless insertion of metallic fixation devices could further embarrass the circulation, but there is no evidence to support this view.

Premature Closure of the Epiphyseal Growth Plate

Closure is not related to the type of treatment except in certain circumstances. Threaded pins that penetrate the epiphysis may produce premature closure.[3] There is a higher incidence of premature closure when avascular necrosis is present, probably because of the sudden decrease in oxygen tension due to vascular insufficiency. Greater shortening of the involved extremity can be expected in the younger patient because of the greater potential for growth of the proximal epiphysis. The older child nearing maturity may have an insignificant leg length discrepancy as a consequence of premature closure of the epiphysis.

Nonunion and Malunion

Nonunion is not as common as in adults with displaced transcervical fractures. On the other hand, coxa vara is frequently reported in the literature.[3-5, 7] Poor reduction, displacement after cast immobilization, and inadequate or poor fixation are probably the responsible factors. Early recognition of coxa vara may be a reason to consider subtrochanteric osteotomy, as advocated by Ratliff.[7]

CERVICOTROCHANTERIC FRACTURES

The cervicotrochanteric fracture, sometimes referred to as a basal neck fracture, is partially intracapsular and partially extracapsular. Undisplaced fractures can be treated successfully in a spica cast. Displacement in a cast is unusual. If it should occur, traction can be utilized to restore anatomical position, followed by internal fixation. If traction does not eliminate the coxa vara and there is a more than 10% deformity, a subtrochanteric osteotomy with internal fixation should be seriously considered.

Displaced fractures should be treated by open reduction and internal fixation (Fig 10–7; see also Figs 10–4, B and C). The high incidence of coxa vara reported in the literature following traction or manipulation and immobilization in a cast supports the recommendation for surgery.[4, 7] However, in most reports there is a higher incidence of avascular necrosis of the femoral head following manipulation and internal fixation. The added trauma of these procedures may be detrimental to the delicate circulation to the femoral head (see Fig 10–7).

INTERTROCHANTERIC FRACTURES

Intertrochanteric fractures are best treated by traction, cast immobilization, or both. Internal fixation is an alternative for displaced fractures when the anatomical position cannot be restored and maintained by traction. There is a danger of com-

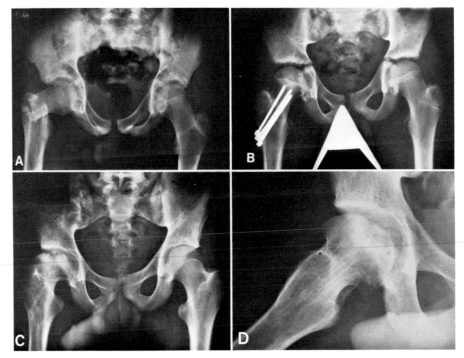

*Fig 10–7—**A,** cervicotrochanteric fracture of the right hip in a 13-year-old boy. **B,** the fracture healed in 3 months following open reduction and internal fixation. **C,** AP view shows premature closure of the epiphysis and avascular necrosis with segmental collapse of the femoral head 2 years following injury. **D,** lateral view.*

plications such as avascular necrosis and premature closure of the epiphysis with this method.[3] Fractures at the intertrochanteric level are the simplest and easiest of all children's hip fractures to treat.

Undisplaced fractures can be treated effectively in a spica cast with little danger of displacement. Traction is an acceptable method but requires an expensive hospital stay.

Displaced fractures can be treated by skin or skeletal traction for about 3 weeks and then the patient can be placed in a spica cast until solid union occurs (Fig 10–8). If anatomical reduction cannot be obtained or if the fracture slips back to a coxa vara position, open reduction and internal fixation with a nail plate should be resorted to early. Later a subtrochanteric osteotomy may be necessary if the deformity is severe.

SUBTROCHANTERIC FRACTURES

Some may question the inclusion of subtrochanteric fractures in a discussion of hip fractures. However, these fractures are in close proximity to the intertrochanteric or peritrochanteric area and therefore are legitimately in the region of the hip. These are rare fractures in children.

In children, subtrochanteric fractures, like other hip fractures, are the result of a violent injury. The proximal fragment is almost always flexed, abducted, and externally rotated. Thus, when traction is used as the treatment of choice the distal fragment must be brought into line with the proximal fragment. Flexion of the distal

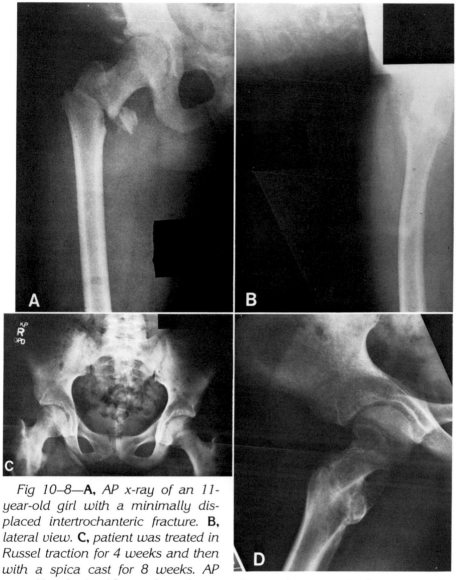

*Fig 10–8—**A,** AP x-ray of an 11-year-old girl with a minimally displaced intertrochanteric fracture. **B,** lateral view. **C,** patient was treated in Russel traction for 4 weeks and then with a spica cast for 8 weeks. AP x-ray film obtained 2 years later shows union with minimal shortening of femoral neck. **D,** lateral x-ray film obtained 2 years after injury.*

limb to conform with the amount of flexion present in the proximal fragment as well as abduction and external rotation to reduce the fracture anatomically require care and persistence.

Traction should be continued for 4–6 weeks before switching to a spica cast. The forces concentrated in the subtrochanteric area are of great magnitude, and a strong callus is required to prevent angulation in the cast (Fig 10–9).

As in other hip fractures in children, undisplaced fractures can be treated in a cast or by a combination of traction followed by immobilization in a cast.[1, 10, 11]

Displaced fractures can be treated successfully in traction (Figs 10–10 and 10–11). Open reduction and internal fixation has been advocated as the choice of treatment.[12]

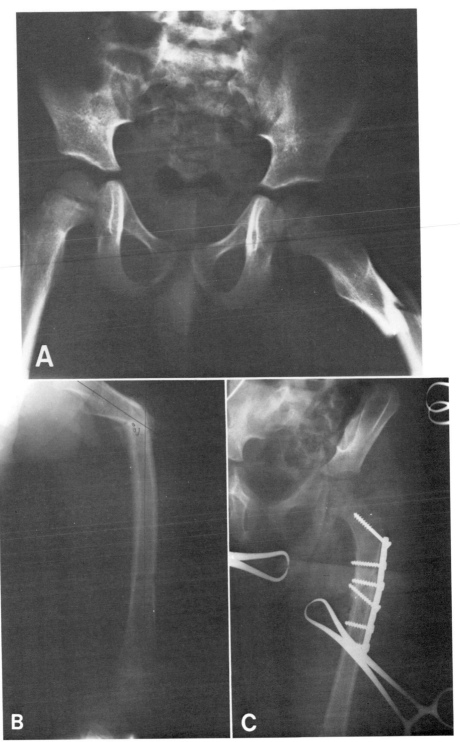

*Fig 10–9—**A,** AP view of the pelvis showing a subtrochanteric fracture of the femur in a 9-year-old boy. Patient was treated in traction and switched to a spica cast at 19 days. X-ray films taken at 6 weeks show 80° angulation at the fracture site. **C,** osteotomy and internal fixation to correct deformity.*

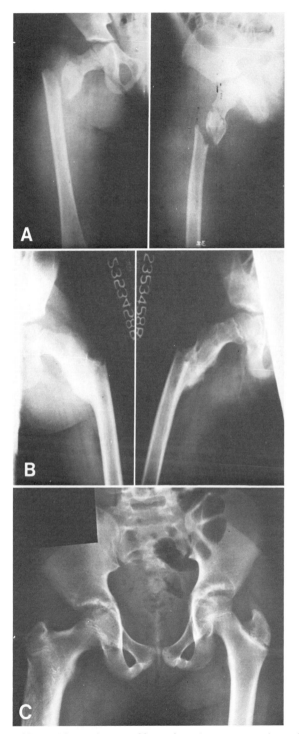

*Fig 10–10—**A,** AP and lateral x-ray films showing concomitant ipsilateral cervicotrochanteric and subtrochanteric fractures in a 6-year-old girl. Patient was treated in Russel traction. **B,** fractures united with malunion at the subtrochanteric level. **C,** 9 years after injury the fracture at the subtrochanteric level has remodeled. There is coxa vara at the cervicotrochanteric level.*

Bryant traction is a satisfactory method for treating displaced fractures in infants (see Fig 10–11). However, this traction method must be watched closely. Slippage of the traction may cause necrosis of the skin in the area of the achilles tendon. There is a possibility that Bryant traction applied too tightly may embarrass the circulation and cause gangrene, unless relieved. Buck or Russel traction is recommended for patients aged 2–10 years, while skeletal traction in the 90-90 position or with slight modification is preferred in older children.

Nonunion should not be a problem. There is little if any danger that avascular necrosis of the femoral head will follow treatment unless internal fixation is selected as the method of treatment, since the blood supply to the femoral head is at a significant distance from the fracture.

Malunion

Malunion in children's hip fractures is infrequent. The upper end of the femur in young children has the capacity to remodel if malunion occurs (Fig 10–10). However, the amount of correction that can be obtained with growth is not known.

Generally, more correction can be expected in the young patient than in the child who is closer to maturity. The closer the deformity is to the growth plate, the greater will be the correction. Angular deformities (e.g. coxa vara, anterior and posterior angulation) will correct to some extent depending upon the age of the patient.

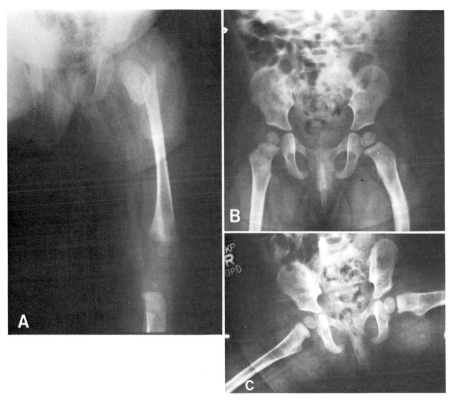

*Fig 10–11—**A,** AP x-ray film showing displaced subtrochanteric fracture of the femur in a 3-year-old girl. The patient was treated in Bryant traction. **B,** AP view of the pelvis. One year after injury fracture is united. **C,** frogleg lateral view 1 year after injury.*

On the other hand, rotational deformities will be corrected little if any in children. However, correction of malunion can be anticipated in infants.

REFERENCES

1. Milgram J.W., Lyne D.: Epiphysiolysis of the proximal femur in very young children. *Clin. Orthop.* 110:146-153, 1975.
2. Blount W.P.: *Fractures in Children.* Baltimore, Williams & Wilkins Co., 1954.
3. Canale S.T., Bourland W.L.: Fracture of the neck and intertrochanteric region of the femur in children. *J. Bone Joint Surg.* 59A:431-443, 1977.
4. Lam S.F.: Fractures of the neck of the femur in children. *J. Bone Joint Surg.* 53A:1165-1179, 1971.
5. Miller W.E.: Fractures of the hip in children from birth to adolescence. *Clin. Orthop.* 92:155-188, 1973.
6. Morrissey R.: Hip fractures in children. *Clin. Orthop.* 152:202-210, 1980.
7. Ratliff A.H.C.: Fractures of the neck of the femur in children. *J. Bone Joint Surg.* 44B:528-542, 1962.
8. Colonna P.C.: Fracture of the neck of the femur in children. *Am. J. Surg.* 6:795, 1929.
9. Rang M.: *Children's Fractures,* ed. 2. Philadelphia, J.B. Lippincott Co., 1983.
10. Dameron R.B. Jr., Thompson H.A.: Femoral shaft fractures in children: Treatment by closed reduction and double spica cast mobilization. *J. Bone Joint Surg.* 41A:1201, 1959.
11. Ireland D.C.R., Fisher R.L.: Subtrochanteric fractures of the femur in children. *Clin. Orthop.* 110:157-166, 1975.
12. Daum R., Jungbluth K.H., Metzger E., et al.: Subtrochantere und superakondylare Femur Fracturen im Kindersalter: Behandlung and Ergebrusse. *Chirurg* 40:217, 1969.

Chapter 11

Concomitant Ipsilateral Fractures of the Hip and Femur

Marvin H. Meyers, M.D.

Combined ipsilateral fractures of the hip and femur are infrequent. This fracture complex is seen several times a year in a busy emergency room. The injury turns up frequently in the multiply injured patient who has also sustained injury to other body systems from high-velocity motor vehicle accidents, falls from a height, or collisions between vehicles and pedestrians. Associated injuries are frequently major in scope. The primary problem often is resuscitation of the patient. Because physician efforts are devoted to life-saving measures, the diagnosis of the femoral neck fracture may be delayed or missed.

The patients are most often young adults. Concomitant ipsilateral fracture of the hip and femur is sometimes difficult to diagnose. The fractured femoral shaft may be obvious but the hip fracture is frequently missed.[1-3] An anteroposterior (AP) x-ray film of the pelvis is essential for diagnosis and should be obtained whenever there is a lower extremity femoral shaft fracture, especially in the mutiply injured patient. Other long bone fractures and ipsilateral knee injuries are frequently associated. Casey and Chapman reported a 43% (9/21) incidence of ipsilateral knee injuries,[2] which were thought to be responsible for disability after the fractures healed. The treatment of multiple fractures in the same extremity is complex.

DIAGNOSIS

An AP x-ray film of the pelvis is mandatory in all cases in which the femur is fractured. When the femoral shaft fracture is displaced the leg will lie in external rotation so that the femoral neck fracture may be difficult to see or may be obscured by the splint (Fig 11–1). Incomplete intracapsular fractures may be seen only on a cross-table lateral x-ray film of the hip. In order to visualize the femoral neck, in addition to a cross-table lateral x-ray film an AP x-ray film with the hip in internal rotation should be obtained, if possible. The knee must be thoroughly evaluated by physical and radiologic examination. There should be a high index of suspicion for knee injury if an effusion is present.

The hip fracture is frequently undisplaced. The obvious deformity in the shaft, pain, and external rotation of the lower extremity focus attention on the shaft fracture. Unless the examining physician is aware of the frequent association of hip fracture with a shaft fracture, he or she may not order an x-ray study of the pelvis

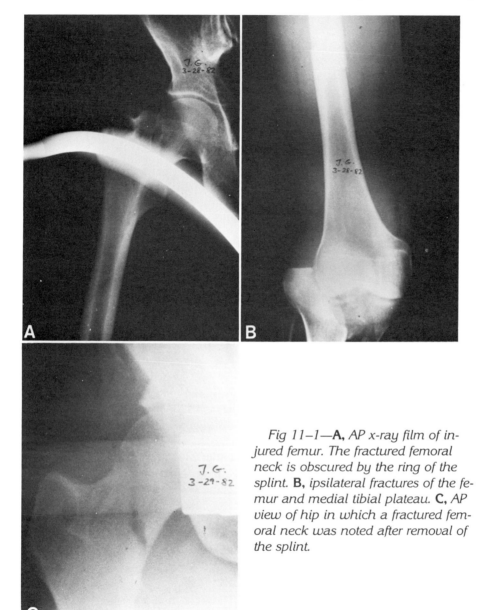

Fig 11–1—**A,** AP x-ray film of injured femur. The fractured femoral neck is obscured by the ring of the splint. **B,** ipsilateral fractures of the femur and medial tibial plateau. **C,** AP view of hip in which a fractured femoral neck was noted after removal of the splint.

when a shaft fracture is present. X-ray studies of the pelvis should be ordered routinely when the shaft of the femur is fractured.

FRACTURE COMBINATIONS

The following fracture combinations are possible: femoral neck and shaft, cervicotrochanteric (basal neck) and shaft, intertrochanteric and shaft, subtrochanteric and shaft, and femoral neck and intertrochanteric. The most frequent combination is fracture of the femoral neck and shaft. All the other combinations together occur about half as often. The combination of femoral neck and intertrochanteric fracture is rare.

PATHOMECHANICS OF INJURY

The injury follows a longitudinal compression force with the leg in abduction and the knee flexed.[4] Dislocation of the hip may occur if the leg is in adduction. The frequency of associated patella fractures supports the concept that longitudinal compression is the major cause. The direction of the fracture line in the neck is longitudinal (90°) in almost all cases (see Fig 11–1,C and 11–3,A).

TREATMENT

At the scene of the accident, the fractures should be splinted adequately to prevent further displacement of the fragments, minimize hemorrhage, and protect other soft tissues, including neurovascular structures. After the patient has been admitted to the hospital and stabilized, definitive treatment of the fractures can be carried out.

Many methods, including traction, casts, diverse metallic fixatives, and combinations of these, have been advocated to treat this fracture complex.[1-10] The reader may refer to the literature cited for details. Most methods of treatment of individual fractures of the hip or the femoral shaft are well known.

PERSONAL PREFERENCE FOR TREATMENT

I favor internal fixation of both the hip and femoral shaft fractures in the multiply injured patient to allow early mobilization. Overwhelming evidence indicates that there is a decrease in the incidences of respiratory distress syndrome and death when polytrauma victims are mobilized early.

Mobilization of the knee is facilitated when all fractures are internally fixed, thus reducing knee disability caused by stiffness following immobilization in a cast or traction. Early aggressive physical therapy to mobilize the knee and strengthen the muscle is possible following internal fixation of both fractures.

Occasionally the degree of comminution or the grave condition of the patient may preclude surgery. In such cases cast or traction methods may be the treatment of choice. Neufeld's roller traction method is a very satisfactory technique for traction of femoral shaft fractures (Fig 11–2).[9] It permits reduction of the fracture fragments to an appropriate length and allows maintenance of accurate alignment. Physiologic stresses are sustained at the fracture site, which enhances osseous healing. At the same time the patient has freedom in bed and nursing care is facilitated. This traction method is suitable for treating comminuted femoral shaft fractures in the adolescent or adult and in the patient for whom internal fixation may not be suitable because of serious medical problems.

Internal fixation of the hip fracture takes precedence over treatment of the shaft fracture. Nonoperative treatment of the hip fracture is unlikely to be successful when the fracture pattern is unstable. The condition of the patient may permit only one operation. Traction or a cast brace are acceptable methods for treatment of shaft fractures when further surgery may jeopardize the patient.

Intracapsular and Femoral Shaft Fractures

There are several principles for the treatment of this combination. The femoral shaft component must be fixed so that it is stable and permits early ambulation

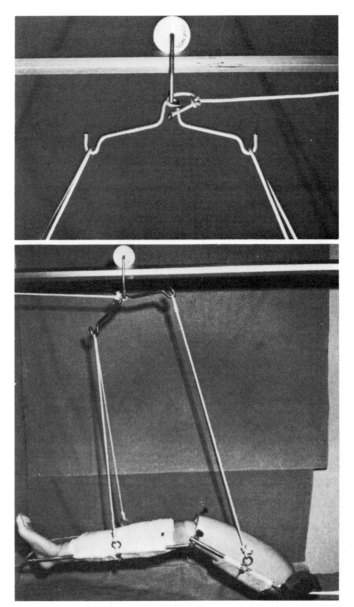

Fig 11–2—Neufeld's roller traction method. (From Mays J., Neufeld A.J.: Skeletal traction methods. Clin. Orthop. *102:144, 1974. Reproduced by permission.)*

(Figs 11–3, A, B, and D). The femoral neck component must be anatomically reduced, rigidly fixed with multiple pins, and impacted (Figs 11–3,C and D).

Transverse fracture patterns in the shaft are rare and can be fixed by closed intramedullary nailing if the femoral neck component is subcapital or transcervical. Closed nailing of the femoral shaft fracture is contraindicated when intertrochanteric or basal neck fractures are also present since further comminution is likely to occur during nail placement. Therefore, pinning of the hip fracture is technically more difficult and firm fixation may not be obtained. Displaced fractures of the shaft with a vertical fracture pattern probably are less likely to lose reduction with other types

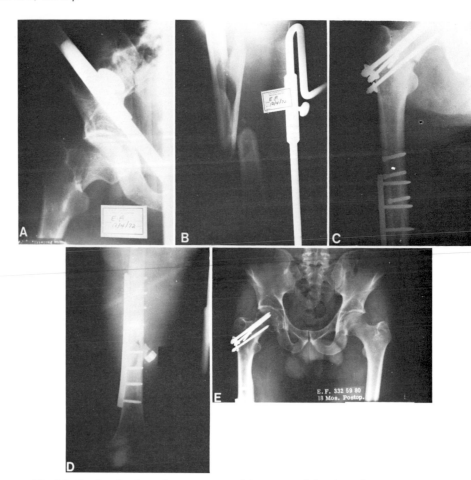

*Fig 11–3—**A,** displaced transcervical fracture of the hip. **B,** ipsilateral commi-nuted femoral shaft fracture. **C,** hip fracture reduced and fixed with multiple pins. Augmentation was with a muscle pedicle graft. **D,** metal plate fixation of the shaft fracture. **E,** united fractures.*

of fixation. A basal neck fracture is a contraindication for intramedullary nailing of the shaft fracture because of the danger that further comminution will occur during metal insertion and because basal neck fractures are less stable (Fig 11–4). Severely comminuted and oblique fracture patterns are best fixed with open reduction and a rigid metal plate (see Fig 11–3,B and D). The latter is also advisable when a basal neck fracture is present.

I request a technetium 99m sulfur colloid scan to ascertain the status of the femoral head circulation. The intracapsular component is fixed rigidly with multiple pins. If circulation in the femoral head is lacking, a muscle pedicle graft is added (see chapter 17). If the scan demonstrates evidence of adequate femoral head circulation, a muscle pedicle graft is not necessary. Usually a radioisotope scan cannot be obtained prior to surgery in the polytrauma patient. The scan can be taken in the postoperative period after the fracture has been internally fixed. The patient can be returned to surgery 1–2 weeks later, when he is stable, for the muscle pedicle graft, if indicated.

Femoral shaft and basal neck fractures are fixed with a sliding nail plate for the femoral neck fracture and a separate metal plate for the shaft. Multiple pins are a poor choice for unstable basal neck fractures since the fixation may not be adequate to prevent varus deformity and malunion.

Intertrochanteric and Femoral Shaft Fracture

I prefer a sliding nail plate for the hip fracture and a metal plate for the shaft fracture. An alternative method of fixation for the undisplaced, stable intertrochanteric fracture pattern and a shaft fracture which is transverse and not comminuted is fixation with multiple Ender nails (Fig 11–5). The surgical incision is small and blood

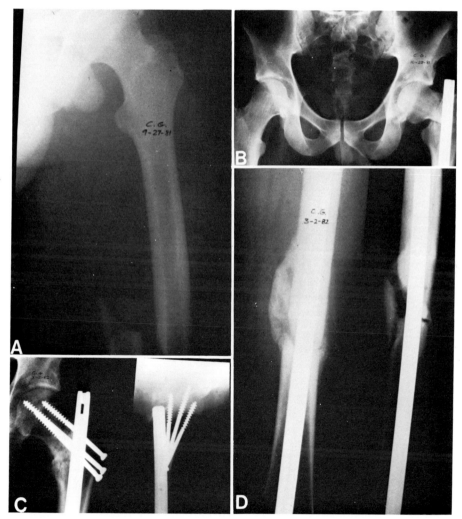

*Fig 11–4—**A,** concomitant ipsilateral fractures of the basal neck and femoral shaft. The closed fracture of the basal neck was not diagnosed prior to surgery. **B,** insertion of intramedullary nail caused displacement of the basal neck fracture. **C,** healed fracture of neck of the femur after reduction and multiple screw fixation. **D,** healed shaft fracture.*

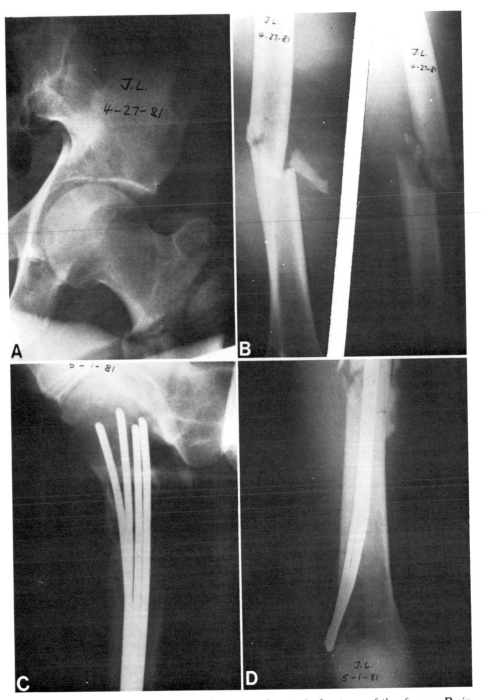

*Fig 11–5—**A,** stable undisplaced intertrochanteric fracture of the femur. **B,** ipsilateral midshaft fracture of the femur. **C,** hip fracture nailed with Ender pins. **D,** femoral shaft fracture nailed with Ender pins.*

loss is minimal, which is an advantage in the polytrauma patient requiring immediate fixation.

Subtrochanteric and Femoral Shaft Fracture

The preferred treatment is with an intramedullary nail (Fig 11–6). If comminution at either or both fracture sites is present, an interlocking nail is a satisfactory solution. The latter type of fixation is new and requires a surgeon who is familiar with the exacting surgical technique. Otherwise an acceptable solution is an intramedullary nail with cerclage wires and a bone graft or multiple plates.

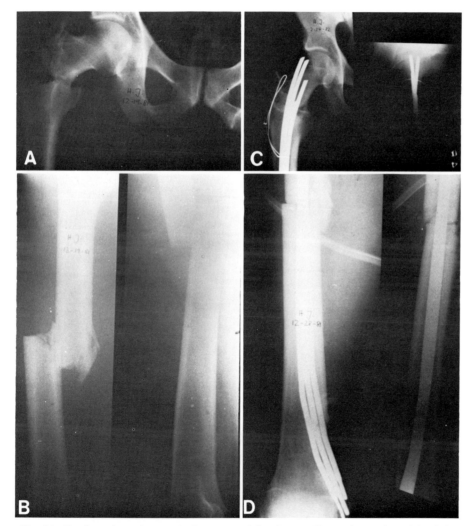

*Fig 11–6—***A,** *subtrochanteric fracture of the femur.* **B,** *ipsilateral midshaft fracture of the femur.* **C,** *healed subtrochanteric fracture after Ender nailing and tension band wiring for greater trochanteric fracture fragment.* **D,** *Ender nailing of the shaft fracture.*

Femoral Neck and Intertrochanteric Fractures

This combination of ipsilateral fracture is rare (Fig 11–7). I prefer a sliding nail plate augmented with additional pin fixation as required. The muscle pedicle graft is utilized when circulation to the head fragment is impaired.

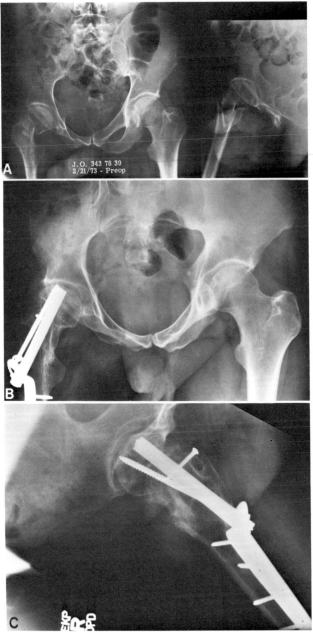

*Fig 11–7—**A,** AP and lateral x-ray views of concomitant ipsilateral fractures of the femoral neck and intertrochanteric level. **B,** AP x-ray film showing healed fractures 3 years following internal fixation with a Smith-Peterson nail and Thornton plate augmented with a Hagie pin and muscle pedicle graft. **C,** lateral x-ray film showing healed fractures.*

A concomitant ipsilateral fracture of the hip and femur requires careful patient assessment and a detailed plan for treatment, as well as meticulous surgical technique, followed by intensive rehabilitation to prevent severe disability of the injured limb.

REFERENCES

1. Bernstein S.M.: Fractures of the femoral shaft and associated ipsilateral fractures of the hip. *Orthop. Clin. North Am.* 5:799-818, 1974.
2. Casey M.J., Chapman M.W.: Ipsilateral concomitant fractures of the hip and femoral shaft. *J. Bone Joint Surg.* 61A:503-509, 1979.
3. Schatzker J., Barrington T.W.: Fractures of the femoral neck associated with fractures of the femoral shaft. *Can. J. Surg.* 11:297-305, 1968.
4. Richey S.J., Schönholtz G.J., Thompson M.S.: The dashboard femoral fracture: Pathomechanics, treatment and prevention. *J. Bone Joint Surg.* 40A:1347-1358, 1958.
5. Ashby M.E., Anderson J.C.: Treatment of fractures of the hip and ipsilateral femur with the Zickel device: A report of three cases. *Clin. Orthop.* 127:156-160, 1977.
6. Delaney W.M., Strett D.M.: Fracture of femoral shaft with fracture of neck of same femur: Treatment with medullary nail for shaft and Knowles pins for neck. *J. Int. Coll. Surg.* 19:303-312, 1953.
7. Kimbrough E.E.: Concomitant unilateral hip and femoral-shaft fractures—a too frequently unrecognized syndrome: Report of five cases. *J. Bone Joint Surg.* 43A:443-449, 1961.
8. MacKenzie D.B.: Simultaneous ipsilateral fracture of the femoral neck and shaft: Report of 8 cases. *South Afr. Med. J.* 45:459-467, 1971.
9. Mays J., Neufeld A.J.: Skeletal traction methods. *Clin. Orthop.* 102:144, 1974.
10. Wright P.E., Becker G.E.: Results of treatment of simultaneous hip and femoral shaft fractures. *Orthop. Trans.* 3:43-44, 1979.

Chapter 12

Stress Fractures of the Hip

Marvin H. Meyers, M.D.

A **stress fracture** results from a physiologic process that produces bone fatigue. Biologic processes change the modulus of elasticity of trabeculae, which increases the fatigue properties. The fracture, partial or complete, follows repetitive stress and is the result of a subclinical accumulation of stress that exceeds the structural strength of the bone. These stresses are not normally experienced by the patient. Initially there is localized bone resorption at the fracture site with subsequent reparative new bone formation.

Stress fractures of the hip are seen most commonly in athletes (runners and joggers) and military recruits. Individuals who enter the armed forces usually embark on extensive exercises to which they are unaccustomed. This increase in exercise commonly produces stress fractures.

Many believe that fatigue is the underlying cause of fracture in the osteoporotic femoral neck of elderly patients. An accumulation of trabecular fatigue fractures has been demonstrated in the same region of the femoral neck in which subcapital fractures occur.[1] A stress fracture may occur at this site without a preceding violent injury.

Fatigue fractures are sometimes found in patients on renal dialysis or prolonged systemic steroid therapy. Other diseases that cause generalized osteoporosis put the patient at risk for fatigue fracture of the femoral neck.

Stress fractures are more common at the subcapital and transcervical areas than at the basilar neck or at the intertrochanteric or subtrochanteric levels.

DIAGNOSIS

Early recognition of a stress fracture is important so that treatment can be started in order to prevent displacement of the fragments. Displacement of the femoral neck stress fracture can be disastrous, especially in young patients, because of the high incidence of nonunion and avascular necrosis in this age group. Rarely is there history of an injury.

Signs and Symptoms

Patients complain of the gradual onset of groin pain or pain on the medial side of the knee. Pain may be increased by active or passive motion. The patient walks with an antalgic limp. Aching and morning stiffness are accompanying symptoms. There is no obvious deformity. Shortening or external rotation of the limb do not occur unless there is displacement. There may be muscle spasm involving the muscles about the hip. Frequently tenderness over the anterior aspect of the hip can be elicited. Concomitant fatigue fractures of other bones are not uncommon.

Radiologic Findings

The spectrum of radiologic changes visible on x-ray films varies from none to the classic picture of a stress fracture. On standard skeletal radiographs there must be an approximately 50% change in bone density before trabecular lesions can be diagnosed. Therefore, minor stress fractures may never show radiographic changes.

The earliest radiographic sign of fracture is a small crack in the cortex (see Fig 12–2, C). Unless the limb is held in internal rotation when the x-ray film is made, minimal changes in the femoral neck may be obscured by the greater trochanter.

Devas classifies femoral neck stress fractures into transverse and compression types.[2] The transverse type tends to displace, while the compressive type is less likely to collapse. The compression type is more common in young patients. The earliest sign is a barely perceptible fluffy appearance in the inferior neck (Fig 12–1), probably due to the formation of interosseous callus around trabeculae. This

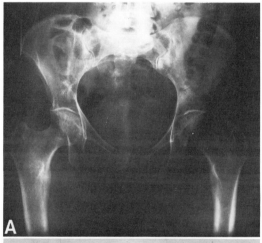

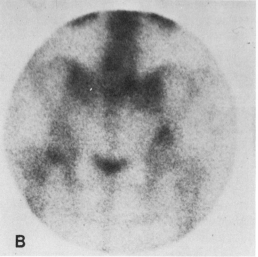

*Fig 12–1—**A,** AP x-ray film of the pelvis in a case of stress fracture. Note the fluffy appearance in the inferior aspect of the right femoral neck and subcapital region. **B,** technetium 99m MDP scintigram showing increased activity in area of fluffiness.*

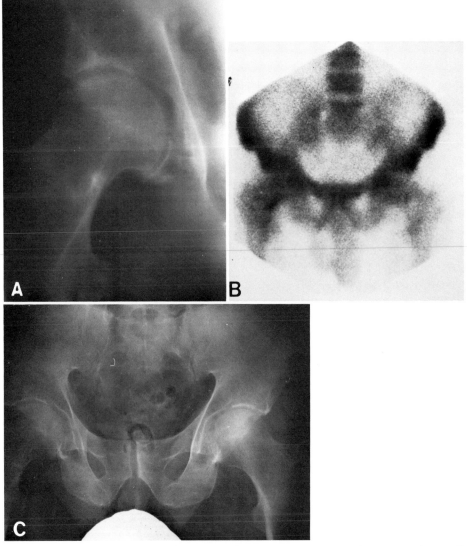

*Fig 12–2—**A**, AP x-ray film (tomogram) showing increased density, with small-est area of decreased density (cyst) in inferior aspect of femoral neck. **B**, tech-netium 99m MDP scintigram showing increased activity. **C**, AP x-ray film obtained 4 weeks later showing compression stress fracture of the right hip.*

appearance may remain unchanged or progress to a crack in the inferior cortex of the femoral neck, which later becomes sclerosed (Fig 12–2). This type of fracture has little tendency to displace if stress is removed.

The transverse type of femoral neck stress fracture occurs more often in the elderly. The first radiologic sign is a small crack in the upper surface of the femoral neck (Fig 12–3). The crack gradually widens and the fracture becomes obvious. Displacement frequently follows unless the fracture is rigidly immobilized. Therefore, internal fixation is required to prevent displacement.

Distinction From Other Entities

The differential diagnosis includes osteoid osteoma, osteogenic sarcoma, osteomyelitis, and Paget's disease. The clinical history is different for osteoid osteoma. Stress does not increase the pain, and night pain is frequent. Tomograms may be helpful in distinguishing osteoid osteoma from a stress fracture. Osteogenic sarcoma may be difficult to differentiate from stress fracture early in the course of the disease. Osteomyelitis can usually be differentiated by an increased blood sedimentation rate and an elevated white blood cell count.

Scintigraphy

Technetium 99 MDP scintigraphy is an early and highly sensitive test for the detection of stress fracture of the femoral neck, even in the absence of radiologic findings. The bone scan shows abnormalities about 3 weeks before changes can be seen on radiographs.[3] It is more sensitive than computerized tomography in the early stage.

Greaney et al., in a study of stress fractures in Marine recruits, concluded that "a focally abnormal scintigram, in the proper clinical setting, establishes the diagnosis of stress fracture, with radiography to be performed at the time of initial workup to rule out a non-stress injury."[4]

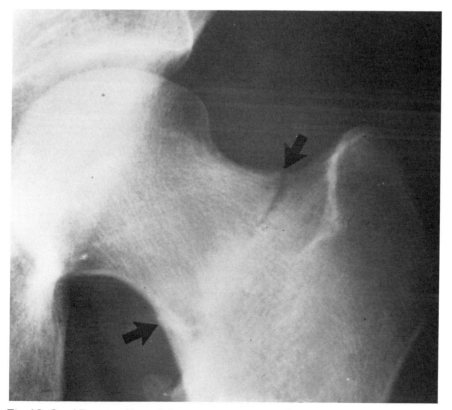

Fig 12–3—AP x-ray film of the transverse type of stress fracture of the femoral neck.

TREATMENT

Recognition of the transverse type of fatigue fracture in the femoral neck is imperative so that adequate internal fixation can be performed to prevent displacement. It should be considered a surgical emergency.

Nonoperative treatment for the compression type of stress fracture of the femoral neck is acceptable so long as the patient is cooperative in following the treatment regimen. Non-weight-bearing for 6–8 weeks on the affected side until all pain has subsided is the recommended treatment, to be followed by gradual resumption of weight-bearing and normal activities if function can be accomplished without pain. Internal fixation should be considered in compression-type stress fractures of the femoral neck in the uncooperative patient, since fracture displacement is a danger and poor results are the consequence of disimpaction.

Nondisplaced stress fractures in the intertrochanteric or subtrochanteric area can be treated by non-weight-bearing ambulation for 6–8 weeks, to be followed by the gradual resumption of normal activities if the patient remains free of pain. The patient must be cautioned to watch for signs of refracture, such as groin pain, loss of range of motion, or knee pain, in the rehabilitation period.

Displaced fractures at the intertrochanteric or subtrochanteric level require treatment. Traction is an acceptable method to reduce the fracture until healing takes place. However, it is not an attractive alternative because of the long hospitalization required. Open reduction and internal fixation will permit early discharge from the hospital and mobilization on crutches. Weight-bearing should be withheld until there is radiologic evidence of adequate healing, which occurs in 8–10 weeks in most cases.

REFERENCES

1. Freeman M.A.R., Todd R.C., Pirie C.J.: The role of fatigue in the pathogenesis of senile femoral neck fractures. *J. Bone Joint Surg.* 56B:698-702, 1974.
2. Devas M.P.: Stress fracture of the femoral neck. *J. Bone Joint Surg.* 47B:728-738, 1965.
3. Wilcox J.R. Jr., Monoit A.L., Green J.P.: Bone scanning in the evaluation of exercise-related stress injuries. *Radiology* 123:699-703, 1977.
4. Greaney R.B., Gerber F.H., Laughlin R.L., et al.: Distribution and natural history of stress fractures in U.S. Marine recruits. *Radiology* 146:339-346, 1983.

Chapter 13

Fractures of the Acetabulum

Robert W. Bucholz, M.D.

The word "acetabulum" is derived from the Latin *acetum,* meaning vinegar, and *abulum,* meaning cup. Pliny and Celsus were the first to use this term for the hip socket, which to them resembled a small vinegar cup.[1] Trauma to this cup-shaped structure has remained a formidable challenge to physicians over the ages.

Orthopedic principles dictate that fractures involving weight-bearing joints be anatomically reduced for optimal functional recovery. Surgeons have been willing to violate this rule for acetabular fractures, in contrast to their management of comparable intra-articular fractures of the knee and ankle joints. Unfamiliar complex pelvic anatomy makes surgical exposure difficult. Fracture comminution may be overwhelming. Associated abdominal and thoracic injuries frequently influence the surgeon's perception of the risks and benefits of operative reduction of pelvic fractures. Indeed, compromise of basic surgical tenets often seems justified. Nevertheless, precise surgical restoration of displaced acetabular fractures, whenever feasible, remains the treatment of choice.

RADIOLOGIC EVALUATION

The acetabulum is located at the confluence of the ilium, pubis, and ischium. Two well-defined columns of bone, the anterior or iliopubic column and the posterior or ilioischial column, converge at a 60° angle to form the arch of the acetabular dome (Fig 13–1).[2] The thick posterior column provides support for the posterior acetabular facet and much of the normal weight-bearing surface of the joint. Although it buttresses the anterior articular surface of the joint, the narrower anterior column is of less structural importance. The acetabular dome is seated in the thick compact bone of the ilium.

Proper treatment of displaced acetabular fractures depends on an accurate preoperative evaluation of the pathologic anatomy of the injury. The pattern of injury and the extent of comminution can generally be determined by careful inspection of an anteroposterior (AP) pelvic radiograph.

A good-quality, well-centered AP radiograph reveals several osseous landmarks. The cortical margins of the anterior and posterior rims of the acetabulum can be identified overlying the femoral head (Fig 13–2). The posterior border is traced from the lateral cortex of the ischial tuberosity superiorly and laterally toward the iliac crest. The anterior lip is less distinct and more horizontal in configuration. It may be obscured on poor-quality radiographs. The subchondral bone of the ace-

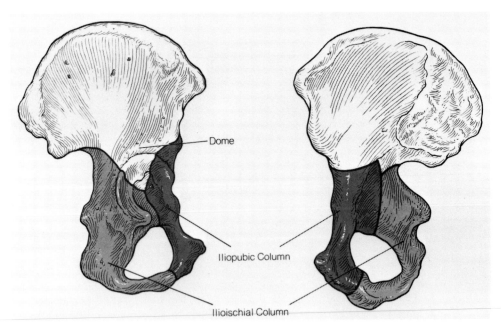

Fig 13–1—Medial and lateral views of the anterior and posterior acetabular columns.

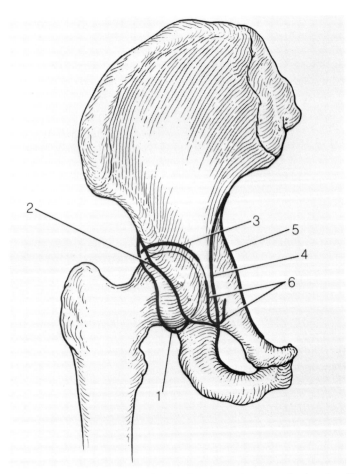

Fig 13–2—Radiographic landmarks for the posterior acetabular rim (1), anterior acetabular rim (2), dome (3), posterior acetabular column (4), anterior acetabular column (5), and teardrop (6).

tabular roof is easily visualized on the AP radiograph but the structural integrity of the entire dome can only be established by examination of the supporting columns.

The ilioischial line defines the medial border of the posterior acetabular column. It represents a tangential view of the quadrilateral surface of the ischium. Any break in this cortical line implies a fracture of the posterior column. The anterior column can be traced by following the anterior three quarters of the cortical line forming the pelvic brim. The lateral limb of the radiographic teardrop of the acetabulum delineates the acetabular fossa of the hip joint, the medial limb delineates the quadrilateral surface of the ischium.

Oblique or Judet views should standardly supplement the AP radiograph (Fig 13–3). On the obturator-oblique radiograph, the x-ray beam is directed 45° toward the midline. Structures more easily identifiable in this radiograph include the pelvic brim (anterior column), the posterior acetabular rim, and the obturator foramen. This view is best for judging the size of posterior acetabular rim fractures, the degree of displacement of the anterior column, and the presence or absence of vertical fractures into the obturator foramen. This latter finding is crucial for distinguishing simple transverse acetabular fractures from complex T-shaped fractures.

The iliac-oblique radiograph is obtained by aiming the x-ray beam 45° away from the midline. The iliac crest is thereby brought into full view. Structures clearly visualized include the posterior column, the ischial spine, and, to a lesser extent, the anterior acetabular rim. This view is most helpful in assessing the degree of posterior column and iliac crest displacement.

Pelvic inlet and tilt radiographs, routinely requested in pelvic ring disruptions, may also assist in the evaluation of some acetabular injuries. Severely displaced

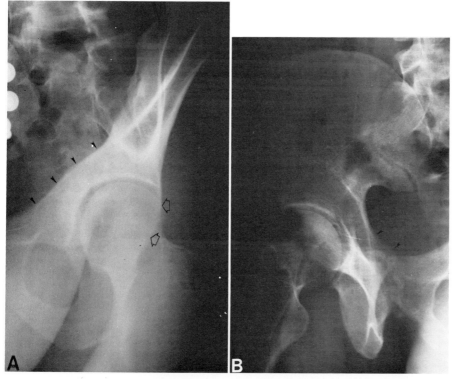

*Fig 13–3—**A,** obturator-oblique radiograph showing the anterior column* (solid arrowheads) *and posterior rim* (open arrows). **B,** *iliac-oblique radiograph demonstrating the posterior column* (arrowheads).

acetabular fractures frequently are associated with concomitant ipsilateral or contra-lateral injuries to the sacroiliac joint. The planes of displacement of this joint may not be evident on plain AP radiographs.

Polytomography of acetabular fractures has been largely supplanted by com-puterized tomographic (CT) scanning. Traditionally polytomography was employed to detect interposed osteochondral fractures in the joint and acetabular dome com-minution.

The improved resolution of CT has made it the preferred technique not only for identifying trapped joint fragments, but also for precisely demonstrating the patho-logic anatomy of complex acetabular fractures. Using 5-mm contiguous axial cuts, the entire acetabular dome and socket can be studied with eight to ten sections. Additional levels may be studied as indicated. Extensive comminution and multiplanar displacement of fracture fragments, often unrecognized on plain radiographs, are easily delineated on CT (Fig 13–4). Sagittal and frontal reconstructions of the axial views may be helpful, depending on the resolution and computer capabilities of the scanner.

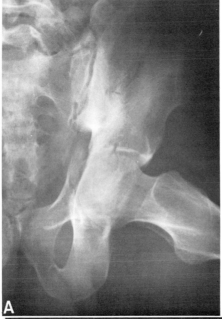

*Fig 13–4—**A,** AP radiograph of an acetabular fracture suggesting only minimal joint disruption. **B,** CT scan of the same patient discloses marked dome comminution with central dis-placement of multiple fragments.*

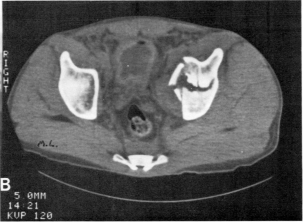

CLASSIFICATION

Numerous classification schemes have been devised to categorize fracture patterns. Letournel and Judet distinguished elementary from complex injuries.[3] The former include (1) fractures of the posterior acetabular rim, (2) fractures of the posterior column, (3) fractures of the anterior acetabular rim, (4) fractures of the anterior column, and (5) transverse fractures. Complex fractures are defined as a minimum of two of the elementary fractures in the same acetabulum. The most common associated fractures are (1) T-shaped fractures, (2) fractures of the posterior column and posterior rim, (3) transverse and posterior fractures, (4) fractures of the anterior column or anterior wall associated with a hemitransverse fracture posteriorly, and (5) fractures of both columns. Each complex pattern may have individual variations in fracture location, comminution, and additional fracture lines.

Such classifications are cumbersome and unwieldy. Tile simplified the grouping of acetabular fractures by stressing the "personality" of the fracture.[4] First, one differentiates simple from complex injuries. Simple fractures include the five types listed in the Judet-Letournel classification. Second, if the injury appears complex, the radiographs are closely inspected for four findings: a T-shaped component, acetabular dome involvement, extension into the iliac crest, and associated sacroiliac joint disruption. A T-shaped extension of a transverse, central fracture into the obturator foramen signifies that the anterior and posterior columns are separated from one another. Such dissociation of the two columns significantly alters the preferred surgical approach, often requiring independent fixation of each column. Major disruption of the acetabular dome carries a very poor prognosis. Burst injuries may result in multiple displaced, malrotated fragments necessitating reduction. Failure to restore this weight-bearing surface of the joint guarantees a poor functional result. Concomitant iliac wing fractures must be reduced and stabilized prior to any attempt at acetabular reconstruction. Finally, ipsilateral sacroiliac disruptions may cause similar difficulties in operative reduction of acetabular fractures.

Emphasizing pathologic anatomy and potential surgical pitfalls, the Tile system is a workable approach to acetabular injuries. Whatever classification is used, however, the single most important goal is to define preoperatively the full extent of damage to the joint.

EMERGENCY MANAGEMENT

Acetabular fractures are the result of high-energy impacts. Abdominal and thoracic visceral injuries frequently accompany these pelvic injuries. Blood loss from the acetabular fracture alone may amount to 4–6 units, more than enough to cause profound hemorrhagic shock. As with other major musculoskeletal injuries, general resuscitative measures and diagnostic evaluation of potentially life-threatening visceral injuries must take precedence.

Pelvic radiographs should be obtained with minimal patient movement and manipulation. A single AP radiograph suffices in disclosing if closed reduction of a dislocated hip must be performed. Nondisplaced or hairline acetabular fractures in an otherwise congruous joint may be easily managed with bed rest and protected weight-bearing. Displaced fractures in which the femoral head has remained well centered under the acetabular dome merely require gentle longitudinal traction through a distal femoral or proximal tibial Steinmann pin until a decision regarding the optimal definitive treatment is made. Further radiographs and CT scans can be ordered on an elective basis.

Subluxation or dislocation of the femoral head demands emergency closed reduction.[5] Performance of the reduction under fluoroscopic control aids in assessing the stability of associated acetabular fractures as well as the congruity of the joint. Frequently the medial acetabular wall in central fracture dislocations will not reduce, as the femoral head is centered under the acetabular dome fragment. In addition, independent movement of the anterior and posterior columns may be noted during fluoroscopic examination. Once the most stable position of the hip is determined, the extremity is placed in longitudinal skeletal traction. Lateral traction through trochanteric pins should be avoided since pin traction drainage at this site greatly increases the risk of a direct surgical approach to the fracture. Maintenance of the reduction by longitudinal traction simplifies any anticipated surgery.

As long as the femoral head is centered under the dome, surgical reconstruction can be postponed for several weeks. The ideal timing for surgery is generally 3–7 days following injury. This delay allows stabilization of the patient, the procurement of supplemental radiographs and a CT scan, and the ordering of any custom implants. Major acetabular fractures should not be surgically tackled under less than optimal conditions unless absolutely necessary. Delay of surgery beyond 2 weeks increases the difficulty of achieving anatomical reduction of the acetabulum.

NONOPERATIVE TREATMENT

Satisfactory results from nonoperative treatment can be anticipated for three types of acetabular fractures. As previously mentioned, nondisplaced hairline fractures through the medial wall of the acetabulum are amenable to short periods of bed rest followed by protected weight-bearing. If the fracture line extends into the acetabular dome, weight-bearing should be delayed for 2–3 months to avoid late displacement of the fracture.

Stable, congruently reduced hip dislocations with small acetabular rim fractures similarly may be managed nonoperatively. Following immediate closed reduction of a posterior dislocation, the hip should be flexed to 90°. If the hip does not sublux or redislocate and a congruent reduction is documented radiographically, the presence of a posterior acetabular rim fragment per se does not justify surgical fixation. Redislocation implies that the fragment is sufficiently large to compromise joint stability. Anterior dislocations rarely are unstable. Figure 13–5 outlines a treatment algorithm for hip dislocations.

A third fracture pattern that may be treated conservatively is the central fracture-subluxation in which an anatomical or near-anatomical closed reduction of all acetabular fragments has been achieved. Care must be taken to ascertain that the joint is congruent and remains so during the healing phase. Adjunctive lateral traction through trochanteric pins is warranted in these situations. This nonsurgical approach is especially appealing in elderly patients, osteoporotic patients, and patients with low functional demands.

RATIONALE FOR SURGERY

The results in incompletely reduced acetabular fractures involving the weight-bearing portions of the joint are mixed.[6,7] Elderly patients with low activity levels may function amazingly well. Younger patients unfortunately do not fair well with hip joint incongruity, and often demonstrate rapidly progressive degenerative joint disease.

Surgical reduction of unstable acetabular fractures yields several potential benefits. First, restoration of joint congruity minimizes the likelihood of joint degen-

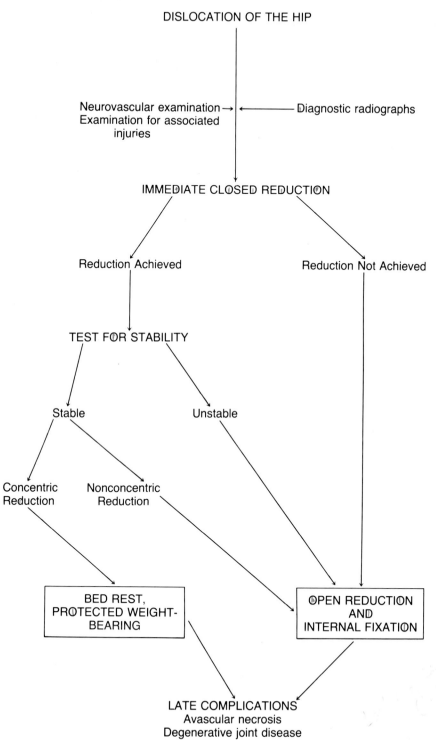

Fig 13–5—Treatment algorithm for hip dislocations.

eration. Even if cartilaginous damage destines the joint to osteoarthritis, reconstruction of the osseous anatomy may postpone the appearance of symptoms for years. Second, rigid fracture fixation allows early mobilization of the patient out of bed. Prolonged traction treatment is not well tolerated by polytraumatized patients. Third, early joint motion following joint stabilization stimulates fibrocartilaginous ingrowth into osteocartilaginous defects, thus enhancing the gliding motion of the joint. Early motion also reduces joint stiffness. Finally, even if symptomatic degeneration of the joint occurs, restoration of the acetabulum simplifies future reconstructive procedures such as total hip replacement or hip arthrodesis.

Surgery is therefore the treatment of choice in (1) unstable or inadequately reduced anterior and posterior hip dislocations and (2) fractures with incongruous joint surfaces secondary to dome comminution, persistent anterior or posterior column displacement, or entire medial wall displacement. In each case, the risks of surgical intervention must be weighed against the probable benefits of anatomical restoration of the joint.

SURGICAL APPROACHES

The ideal surgical approach to a given fracture is dictated by its pathologic anatomy.

Isolated Posterior Rim Fractures With Hip Dislocation

All posterior fracture dislocations necessitating operative treatment should be exposed through a standard posterior approach. Following transection of the short external rotators at the trochanter, the hip capsule and any attached acetabular rim fragments are carefully preserved. Detachment of the fracture fragments from the capsule will devascularize them as well as compromise the stability of the joint. The hip must be gently redislocated and the joint debrided thoroughly. Anatomical reduction of the posterior acetabular rim can be judged either by aligning the cortical fragments along the posterior column or by direct inspection of the joint surface through a small capsulotomy.

Interfragmental screws should be directed medially, away from the articular surface (Fig 13–6). Supplemental buttress plate fixation along the posterior column may be required in cases with extensive comminution of the rim. Intraoperative radiographs, postfixation ranging of the joint, and direct examination through a capsulotomy are all helpful in ensuring that none of the screws traverse the joint.

Isolated Anterior Rim Fractures

Anterior fracture dislocations of the hip rarely require operative reduction. Surgery is indicated most often for debridement of interposed bony or soft tissues from the joint or for reattachment of large anterosuperior femoral head fragments. Unlike posterior rim fractures, joint instability is not a problem. A standard Smith-Peterson or Watson-Jones approach will provide ample exposure of the joint and the anterior acetabular rim.

Simple Posterior Column Fractures

Through a southern approach, the posterior column should be exposed as described for posterior rim fractures. Dissection is extended down to the ischial tuberosity where the stout sacrotuberous ligaments and the origins of the hamstring muscles are subperiosteally elevated. Superiorly, the ilium is exposed sufficiently for

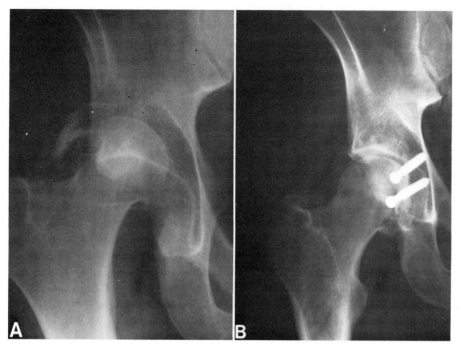

*Fig 13–6—**A,** AP radiograph of a posterior hip dislocation with a large, slightly comminuted acetabular rim fragment. **B,** postoperative radiograph demonstrating restoration of a normal joint space with proper direction of the screw heads away from the joint surface.*

the application of a plate. The knee must be flexed during this dissection to avoid stretch injury to the sciatic nerve. A blunt retractor inserted beneath the external rotator muscles in the sciatic notch around the posterior column offers additional protection to the nerve (Fig 13–7).

Most posterior column fractures occur between the sciatic notch and the ischial spine. There may be associated comminution of the posterior acetabular rim. The fracture site must be cleansed of all interposed tissue. Reduction can be achieved by manual elevation of the column using a bone hook or by utilizing a pelvic reduction clamp. This latter device must be positioned in such a fashion so as not to block the application of the plate. The adequacy of the reduction may be judged digitally by feeling the quadrilateral surface in the true pelvis or visually through a small capsulotomy.

The preferred implants for posterior column fixation are the 3.5-mm dynamic compression plate, the ASIF pelvic reconstruction plate, and the Letournel plate (Fig 13–8). A sufficiently long plate to span the fracture and provide adequate purchase on both the ilium and the ischial tuberosity should be selected. Plate contouring, always a challenge in the posterior column, can be simplified by the use of malleable templates. Precise contouring is imperative since slight malrotation or inaccurate bending of the plate will result in redisplacement of the fracture. All screws must be directed away from the joint surface.

Simple Anterior Column Fracture

Since the anterior column buttresses a less significant portion of the weight-bearing surface of the hip joint than the posterior column, greater degrees of fracture displacement may be accepted and treated nonoperatively. Grossly unstable anterior column fractures with central protrusion of the femoral head, however, demand surgical fixation.

Surgical exposure is difficult. A modified Smith-Peterson approach with elevation of the muscles from the inner wall of the ilium and the pubis allows only limited access to the pubic ramus. The ilioinguinal approach necessitates mobilization of the femoral vessels and the inguinal canal structures. While offering extensive exposure to the entire anterior column, it involves unfamiliar dissection to most orthopedists.[3] I have found surgical assistance from a general surgeon helpful when the ilioinguinal approach is indicated.

Lag screw fixation occasionally suffices, but plates similar to those used on the posterior column are usually needed. There is a high risk of maldirected screws penetrating the joint space, especially screws inserted at the level of the anterior rim.

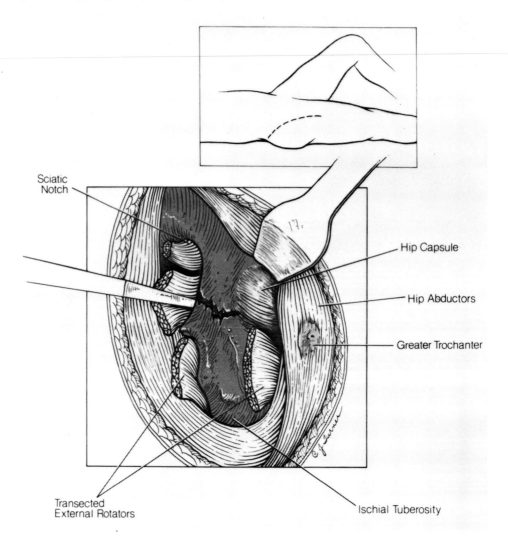

Fig 13–7—Wide exposure of a posterior column fracture can be achieved by a simple southern approach. A blunt retractor beneath the external rotators provides protection for the sciatic nerve. If additional superior exposure is required, the greater trochanter may be osteotomized.

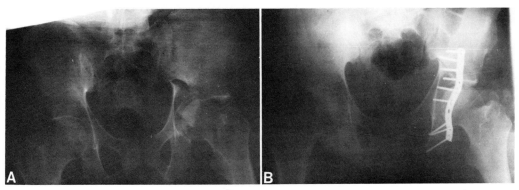

*Fig 13–8—**A,** AP pelvic radiograph of a combined anterior-posterior column fracture. **B,** satisfactory reduction was achieved by fixation of the posterior column alone using an ASIF 3.5-mm dynamic compression plate.*

It is therefore preferable to have the plate buttress the column with screws anchoring it in the ilium and the pubic ramus but leaving the central screw holes of the plate empty (Fig 13–9).

Simple Transverse Fractures

Simple transverse fractures, in which the anterior and posterior columns move as a unit, may be approached anteriorly or posteriorly. I prefer the more direct posterior approach. Methods of exposure, reduction, and plate stabilization are identical to those described for an isolated posterior column fracture. If any doubt exists about the adequacy of anterior column reduction, trochanteric osteotomy will yield greater anterior exposure. Supplemental lag screw fixation of the anterior column is then possible.

Complex Fractures

The surgical approach to any complex fracture must be individualized, based on which disrupted portions of the acetabulum require reduction and fixation. A CT scan is critical for preoperative planning. Special attention should be focused on dome fractures, vertical iliac crest fractures, T-shaped extension of a transverse fracture into the obturator foramen, and sacroiliac disruptions. A number of extensile approaches aimed at exposing these associated injuries have been described.

Osteotomy of the greater trochanter increases significantly the exposure afforded by either a standard southern or Gibson approach to the posterior column (Fig 13–10). With subperiosteal dissection of the gluteus medius and gluteus minimus, much of the acetabular dome is visualized. A Gibson incision also allows access to the iliac crest for fixation of crest fractures. Burst fractures of the dome and comminuted anterior column fractures cannot be adequately seen in this approach.

Senegas et al. devised a transtrochanteric approach that improves exposure of the entire dome.[8] Following splitting of the gluteus maximus fibers, the tensor fasciae latae are transected anteriorly to the level of the femoral sheath. By elevation of the abductors off the ilium, wide exposure of the posterior column and dome is achieved. A recent modification of this approach through a triradiate incision has been described.[9] Unfortunately, only limited access to the full length of the anterior column is feasible.

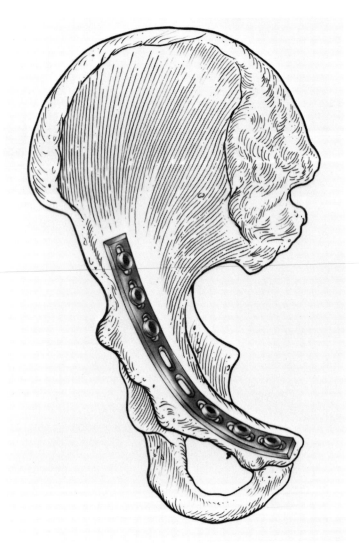

Fig 13–9—Anterior plates inserted through an ilioinguinal approach buttress anterior column fractures. The middle holes in the plates should be left empty, thereby avoiding screw penetration of the adjacent joint.

An extensile anterolateral approach has been proposed by Letournel and Judet.[3] The incision extends from the posterior superior iliac spine along the crest to the anterior superior iliac spine, and continues inferiorly down the anterolateral aspect of the thigh. All muscles are stripped from the lateral aspect of the crest, and then the abductors and external rotators are transected at the greater trochanter. The entire muscle mass is rotated posteriorly on its neurovascular bundle. Superb exposure of the crest and acetabular dome is provided, but the significant risk of ischemia and necrosis of the hip musculature has diminished enthusiasm for this approach.

Finally, separate posterior and anterior incisions and approaches can be made for complex fractures. Through a standard southern approach with or without trochanteric osteotomy combined with an ilioinguinal approach, access to all parts of the acetabulum is achieved. The prolonged operating time needed for both approaches is a major disadvantage. The procedures can be staged at a 3- to 7-day

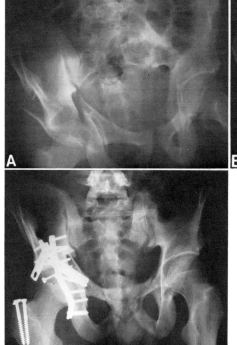
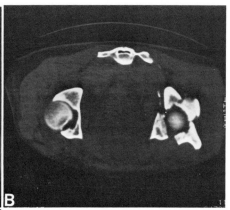

*Fig 13–10—**A,** AP radiograph of a complex fracture of the right acetabulum. **B,** CT scan discloses a burst injury to the dome with moderate displacement of all major fragments. **C,** surgical repair was performed through a posterior approach with osteotomy of the greater trochanter.*

interval in certain patients. This combined posterior and anterior approach is the only one that offers ideal exposure for osteosynthesis of T-shaped fractures with a comminuted anterior column.

COMPLICATIONS

Even in the hands of recognized experts in acetabular fractures, the incidence of complications from operative treatment is high. Letournel and Judet recorded a 28% complication rate in a series of 302 operations.[3] Early complications include deaths from associated injuries, infections, sciatic nerve palsies, thromboembolism, and secondary displacements of the fracture. Avascular necrosis of the femoral head, posttraumatic osteoarthritis, and heterotopic ossification in the hip musculature are the most common late complications. Given the severity of these injuries and the major complex surgery needed for their stabilization, the high frequency of these complications is easily understood. It is hoped that future developments in surgical techniques and implants will diminish their incidence.

REFERENCES

1. Dye S., van Dam B., Westin W.: Eponyms and etymons in orthopaedics. *Contemp. Orthop.* 6:100, 1983.
2. Judet R., Judet J., Letournel E.: Fractures of the acetabulum: Classification and surgical approaches for open reduction. *J. Bone Joint Surg.* 46A:1615-1675, 1964.
3. Letournel E., Judet R.: *Fractures of the Acetabulum.* New York, Springer-Verlag, 1981.
4. Tile M.: Fractures of the acetabulum. *Orthop. Clin. North Am.* 11:481-506, 1980.
5. Epstein H.: *Traumatic Dislocation of the Hip.* Baltimore, Williams & Wilkins, 1980.

6. Carnesale P., Stewart M., Barnes S.: Acetabular disruption and central fracture-dislocation of the hip. *J. Bone Joint Surg.* 57A:1054-1059, 1975.
7. Tipton W., D'Ambrosia R., Ryle G.: Non-operative management of central fracture-dislocations of the hip. *J. Bone Joint Surg.* 57A:888-893, 1975.
8. Senegas J., Liorzov G., Yeats M.: Complex acetabular fractures: A transtrochanteric lateral surgical approach. *Clin. Orthop.* 151:107-114, 1980.
9. Mears D., Rubash H.: Extensile exposure of the pelvis. *Contemp. Orthop.* 6:21-32, 1983.

Chapter 14

Surgical Impacted Fixation Over Plate and Resilient Multiple Pins for Immediate Weight-Bearing

William M. Deyerle, M.D.

The goal of treatment of hip fractures is bony union. However, the obstacles to achieving such union are so implanted in the minds of treating physicians that any method of treatment proposed to improve the results is regarded with skepticism. Frequently surgeons are tempted to choose routine treatment rather than a specific technique tailored to the patient. It is the surgeon's obligation to become proficient in new techniques that are based on the physiology of healing bone.

In January 1958, in an exhibit at the American Academy of Orthopedic Surgeons, I presented a new technique incorporating principles elaborated over the years. The technique entails impacted anatomical or translated reduction and absolute fixation. It allows immediate weight-bearing, stimulates early bony union, and minimizes the possibility of avascular necrosis. Fixation is accomplished with resilient multiple pins threaded deep into the cortex of the head. They are inserted accurately and held at a 140° angle by a plate guide combination, providing absolute fixation of the shaft end.[1,2] Cruciate head pins are used for ease of insertion. A smooth shaft permits the pin to be slid into the shaft portion when the fracture is impacted at the time of surgery. Vigorous impaction under direct vision collapses all comminuted fragments and provides contact compression while maintaining position in both planes.

FEMORAL NECK FRACTURES
Biophysics of Femoral Neck Fracture Healing

The hip is a weight-bearing unit composed of bone, surrounding soft tissues, muscle, fascia, and physiologic intrafascial pressure. This unit is capable of dissipating the stresses of weight-bearing. Efficient dissipation demands plasticity and bending, but sufficient resilience of the entire unit to avoid failure. It is an oversimplification to regard a fracture as two pieces of bone that must be held together rigidly. The same stresses that are borne by the intact weight-bearing unit must also be dissipated by the unit with its internally fixed fracture. Any fixation device must be sufficiently resilient that it remains stable on weight-bearing when combined with the natural intrinsic support of the impacted bone.[2-4, 6-7, 20-21, 23] As a result of percussion impaction at surgery, the unit will dissipate the stress without failure or permanent deformity (Figs 14–1 through 14–9). The bone and fixation share the stress.

Stress sharing is a unit concept. The impacted irregular bone surface must supply 75% of the fixation, to supplement the metal fracture fixation, which supports only 25% of the stress.[6, 7] The side plate with multiple pins allows the surgeon to perform percussion impaction at operation without dislodging the threads from the head of the femur. I insist on percussion impaction, which is essential to any technique of hip fracture fixation. Frankel demonstrated the need for impaction by using a "telltale" nail, an H-beam nail with a built-in strain gauge (see Fig 14–6).[6, 7] The nail-with-strain-gauge combination showed that mutual interdigitation of the bone fragments took 75% of the stress that was transmitted during weight-bearing. Only 25% was transmitted through the nail. It is essential that percussion impaction be completed at the time of fixation, measured visibly, and recorded on the chart (see Fig 14–5 and Fig 14–25).[8] Allowing collapse to occur over the first 6–8 weeks is not

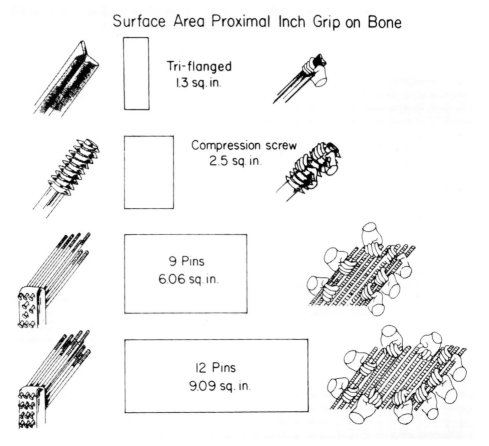

Surface Area Proximal Inch Grip on Bone

Tri-flanged
1.3 sq. in.

Compression screw
2.5 sq. in.

9 Pins
6.06 sq. in.

12 Pins
9.09 sq. in.

Fig 14–1—Comparison of the surface area of bone in the femoral head that grips the proximal inch of the common fixation devices. (From Deyerle.[2] Reproduced by permission.)

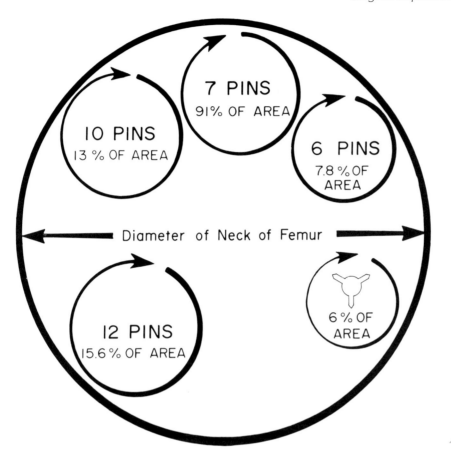

Fig 14–2—Spatial analysis of the cross-section of the neck. The compression screw and the triflanged nail both occupy 6% of the neck (see Fig 14–7). Each pin is %₆₄ inch in diameter. (From Deyerle.[2] Reproduced by permission.)

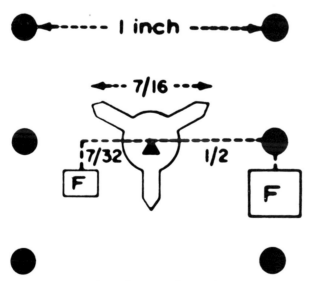

Fig 14–3—Leverage gives 3 to 5 times the resistance to rotary motion with peripherally placed pins compared to the triflanged nail and compression screw. (From Deyerle.[2] Reproduced by permission.)

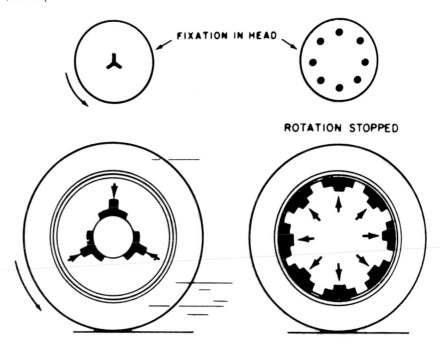

FIXATION IN HEAD

ROTATION STOPPED

BRAKE APPLIED TO AXLE   BRAKE APPLIED TO DRUM

Fig 14–4—Comparison of peripheral and central fixation in the head of the femur. The central fixation concentrates a large force over a small area of surface contact. The peripheral pins distribute less force over a larger area of surface contact. The surface area is 9 times greater (see Fig 14–1). (From Deyerle.[2] Reproduced by permission.)

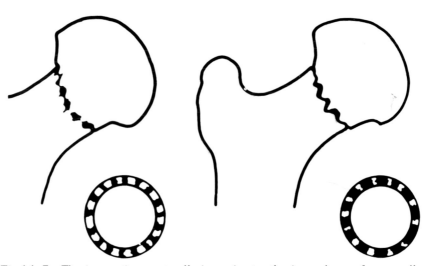

Fig 14–5—The impaction mutually invaginates the irregular surfaces, collapses the comminuted fragments, and increases the fracture area of contact. The area of contact before impaction is shown in black in the circle of the cortex, left. The increased area of contact after impaction is shown on the right. (From Deyerle.[2] Reproduced by permission.)

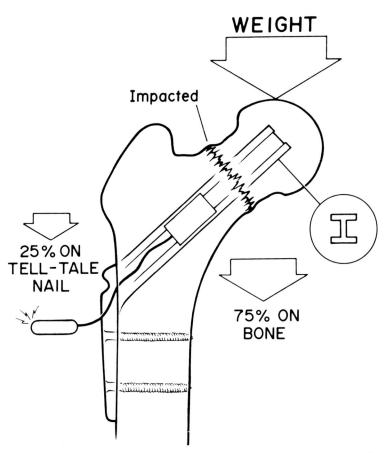

Fig 14–6—"Telltale nail" of Frankel with the built-in strain gauge shows that in well-impacted fractures, on weight-bearing only 25% of the stress was dissipated by the nail and 75% was dissipated by the bone. The fixation device and impacted bone act as an efficient unit. Impaction is essential to prevent failure or cutting out of the internal fixation under increasing stresses. (From Deyerle.[2] Reproduced by permission.)

acceptable. Collapse or shortening implies motion of the fragments. Our knowledge of primary bone healing predicts that motion leads to a secondary type of healing that passes through a fibrocartilaginous phase. This is a slower process and can lead to delayed union or nonunion, as reported by Anderson and others.[9-13]

The bone and metal unit, in a pliable relationship, and well impacted, permits weight-bearing treatment (see Figs 14–1 through 14–5, and 14–8). Frankel and Burstein state, "If multiple threaded pins are to be used to resist bending loads, they act in a manner analogous to a laminated structure. There must be present between the pins osseous material which will allow the formation of bending shear stress. The pin threads produce sufficient resistance to allow the transmission of the shear stress from the pins to the bone. With these two factors present the composite structure will have a strength many times the sum of individual pins."[7] This is corroborated by the mechanical analysis shown in Figures 14–1 through 14–5 and 14–8. Nine pins have nine times the strength of a compression screw. Twelve pins have 18 times the strength of a compression screw. Nine pins are four and one half times the strength of four Asnis screws and twelve pins are nine times as strong.

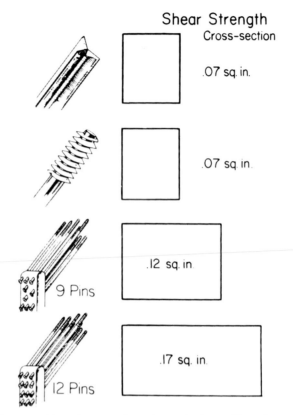

Shear Strength
Cross-section

.07 sq. in.

.07 sq. in.

9 Pins   .12 sq. in.

12 Pins   .17 sq. in.

Fig 14–7—Cross-sectional area of various devices. This figure only partially reflects the shear strength because the multiple pins have plastic resilient strength.[5,6,7] (From Deyerle.[2] Reproduced by permission.)

Walking stimulates the blood supply and healing. Contracting muscles and changing intrafascial pressures enhance the blood supply and aid in the physical support of the unit.[14] This accelerates primary fracture healing. Rydell's[15] and Frankel's[6,7] work show the advantages of weight-bearing. Non-weight-bearing is difficult, clumsy, and puts great stress on the hip. With weight-bearing, the surrounding musculature and fascia pump blood into the healing area and support the bone, with a dampening effect on the stresses that must be transmitted and dissipated across the fracture site.

Since interosseous healing is the primary mechanism of bone-to-bone healing (no cartilage), it alters the specific requirements of healing of the neck of the femur. Elderly patients are rehabilitated more efficiently if allowed to ambulate.[16] Walking is an essential part of postoperative care, decreasing the hospital stay, morbidity, thrombophlebitis, mental confusion, and depression. Crutches or a walker may be used for balance but not for weight-bearing.

Attention to detail in regard to timing of fracture treatment, reduction, internal fixation, and impaction is fundamental in treating fractures of the hip.

The neck of the femur requires an anatomical or slightly translated position to achieve maximum interdigitation of bone as well as to avoid the undue shear stress of the varus position.[1,3,4,17-21]

Many authors have reported good results with impacted reduction over plate and multiple pins.[19-23,40] Good results were related to accuracy of reduction and fixation.

Treatment should be prompt, with a minimal period of recumbency and with the hip fixed well enough to allow the patient to start immediate weight-bearing on the affected limb. Even those who are nonambulatory or avoid weight-bearing with a three-point gait put a stress on the hip equivalent to full weight-bearing.[6, 7, 15] To be considered effective, any treatment must provide sufficient fixation of the hip to allow immediate weight-bearing for a rapid physiologic and psychological return to normal activity.[16]

In the displaced fracture there are varying degrees of comminution and posterior displacement of the head, with posterior comminution of the neck.[24, 25] The joint capsule and synovia are usually intact, and there is blood within the capsule under pressure, which tends to collapse the synovial vessels (Fig 14–10) (other data dispute the presence of hemarthrosis following femoral neck fracture—see chapter 4). The longer these vessels remain collapsed, the more likely that thrombosis will occur and compromise the revascularization process of the head.[2, 26-28] If the fracture is several weeks old, the entire fracture surface is organized and fibrosis has begun, further delaying the healing process and revascularization of the head. This delay

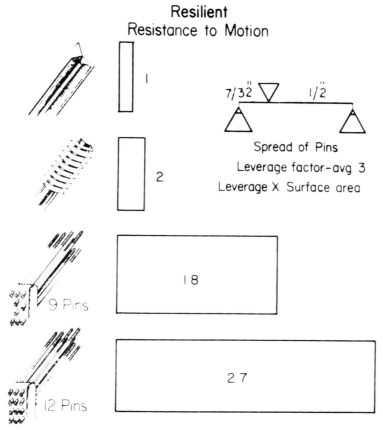

Fig 14–8—When the surface area (see Fig 14–1) is multiplied by the leverage factor of 3 (see Fig 14–3), resistance to motion is expressed in multiples of 1. The triflanged nail has a factor of 1. The compression screw has a leverage factor of 2. Nine pins have a leverage factor of 18, and 12 pins have a leverage factor of 27. The resilient plastic factor of the multiple pins plus the supporting bone as reported by Frankel and Burstein and Baril,[4, 5, 6] makes multiple pins even more efficient at dissipating the stresses across the fractured area. (From Deyerle.[2] Reproduced by permission.)

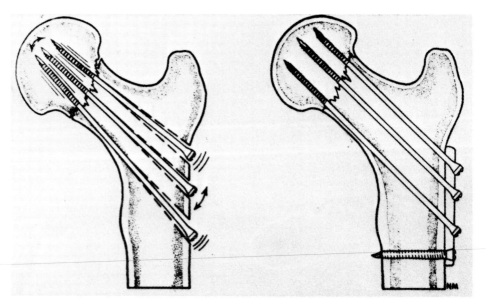

Fig 14–9—Comparison of multiple pins (left) and multiple pins with lateral shaft fixation. Pins alone tend to converge in the head.

may cause avascular necrosis on radiographs and possibly clinically, as reported by Garden et al.,[17] Brown and Abrami,[29] and others.[3, 4, 13, 26, 30]

Fractures of the neck of the femur are a 24-hour emergency. The longest reported interval between neck fracture and fixation is 7 days, the shortest is 3 hours. On average, these fractures have been repaired within 36 hours of injury. If for some reason postponement is required, the patient is placed in Buck traction and the hematoma is aspirated. In impacted fractures aspiration of the hip joint and identification of fat by staining will confirm fractures that may not be apparent initially. The diagnosis may be confirmed with a technetium 99m MDP bone scan. The impacted fracture is then treated by plate and multiple pins, without changing the position of the fracture. The impacted fracture is impacted further at surgery.[31] The pins usually back out ⅛ inch (see Fig 14–24). Hip joint aspiration is required in impacted fractures if there is to be any delay in treatment. At surgery, the capsule should be incised ¼ inch where it attaches to the anterior neck, for continuing evacuation of any hematoma. Aspiration of fractures of the neck of the femur was suggested by Albert Ferguson, Sr., in a personal communication.[27] Soto Hall et al.[28] and Calandruccio and Anderson[26] have done studies that substantiate the principle (see Fig 14–10).

Shortening of the Neck of the Femur

Since the capsule of the hip joint is intact, one can effect an excellent anatomical reduction with traction and internal rotation. Fixing the fracture anatomically without percussion impaction has led to one of the most tenacious and erroneous ideas concerning the normal healing of fractures of the neck of the femur. Many textbooks refer to the "normal shortening of the neck of the femur that occurs during the healing process." However, shortening is not a normal healing process and is almost completely preventable.[1-4, 20, 21, 30, 32-36] The attenuated, stretched-out capsule that permits reduction is also associated with attenuated and unsupported comminuted fragments that have no stability.[14, 24] The fracture surfaces of the major fragments are partially touching (see Fig 14–5). Since osseous healing in the neck of the femur is by endosteal bone formation, the size of this area of contact is of prime importance. Impaction is therefore necessary.

If there is no percussion impaction after fracture fixation, the comminuted fragments will collapse over the next 6–10 weeks.[9, 13, 37, 38] Failure to impact and mutually invaginate the fracture at the time of operation allows for motion. Motion may be rotary, shearing, or piston-like—all equally detrimental to primary fracture healing. Instead of primary bone healing, motion and collapse of the comminuted fracture produce cartilaginous healing.[9, 10, 12, 39] The cartilaginous phase may continue for several months, resulting in delayed healing or nonunion.

This cycle of events was so frequent with previous methods of fixation that it led to the mistaken conclusion that shortening of the femoral neck was normal in healing of fractures of the neck of the femur. Shortening stimulated the use of sliding nails to accommodate the "normal healing process." Such phrases as "dynamic impaction" were used, when in reality it was "dynamic collapse." Anderson has shown experimentally that primary bone healing without motion proceeds promptly, with no shortening.[9]

Fielding, in a paper on the telescoping Pugh nail that specifically delineated telescoping, stated, "The amount of telescoping could be accurately evaluated on roentgenograms in 80 patients with fractures of the neck of the femur."[37] The amount ranged from 7.9 to 19 mm, averaging 11.1 mm. Invariably most of the shortening occurred during the first 4 weeks. Gradual telescoping for longer than 4 weeks was associated with nonunion and avascular necrosis. In some patients absorption occurred at the fracture lines, but the nails failed to telescope and protruded into the hip joint. The healing time in this well-documented series was 6 months. Collapse in the first 4 weeks, and in some instances later, may account for the delayed healing time. One should expect union in 79% of displaced fractures at 9 weeks, and certainly all fractures should heal by 4 months.[19–20, 23, 40] If the fracture is surgically converted

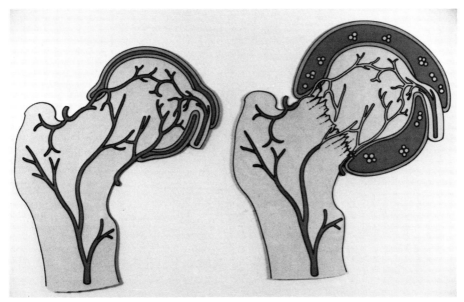

Fig 14–10—Intracapsular fractures have blood under pressure.[26, 27, 28] This collapses all the synovial vessels that may not have been injured during the initial injury. (From Deyerle.[2] Reproduced by permission.)

to an impacted fracture the healing time should be the same as in undisplaced impacted fractures, which is generally reported to be approximately 8 weeks.[31]

The necessity for prompt bony union of fractures of the neck of the femur with primary bone healing that does not go through a cartilaginous or fibrous stage can be appreciated when one considers that in many instances, the future blood supply to the head is largely derived from the healed fracture surfaces. The longer these surfaces are without blood vessels crossing them, the greater the chance that fibrosis will occur and avascularity of the head persist.[13, 26, 41-43]

One can conclude that union is not present when there is any change in the position between the head and neck or when shortening is seen on consecutive roentgenograms. Without vigorous percussion impaction at operation, the frequent course of events is collapse of the fractured fragments for 2–4 months.[2] This should be the golden period of healing in fractures, and in a series of patients I treated, the average time to bony union was 9 weeks.[2] Primary bone healing does not have a cartilaginous phase. The shortest time for histologic evidence of primary bone healing was in a man who died of aspiration pneumonia 25 days after surgery.[2, 39]

Bone Quality

In a few fractures, bone quality may be so poor that the plate and multiple pins and impaction of bone will not provide sufficient fixation to prevent motion and may put such strain on the fixation apparatus as to cause breakage. The poorer the bone quality, the greater the stress on the underlying fixation apparatus. Intrinsic support from the impacted bone is less. Rheumatoid patients have poorer bone quality. The poorer the bone quality, the more essential it is to increase the number of pins, even up to 13, always a minimum of 9.

EFFICIENCY OF INTERNAL FIXATION DEVICES
Single-Member Compression Screw Versus Plate and Multiple Pins

Although 75% of stress is applied to the impacted bone, it is nonetheless important to have the most efficient internal fixation device possible.[6, 7]

A compression screw with a side plate is more rigid and therefore puts more stress on the host bone. A multimembered plate and threaded pins is a more flexible and more resilient assemblage, as has been shown clinically and experimentally, and therefore is less destructive to the surrounding host bone.[5]

The rigid single member is in contact with one set of trabeculae. Once there is motion between the single member and the trabeculae, there is further crumpling of the trabeculae and further motion. Any crumpling of the surrounding trabeculae denotes complete failure, as has been shown by Baril et al.[5] Any motion around this rigid fixation which overstresses the gripping trabeculae is likely to induce total failure.

In the plate with multiple pins assemblage, the pins are distributed throughout the head, and each pin is in contact with a separate group of trabeculae. There are at least 9 and often as many as 13 different sets of gripping trabeculae. Failure of one group does not predispose to failure of another or to total failure. These trabeculae are widely separated and promote greater resistance to motion on the basis of the leverage involved. The average spread of the pins is over 1 inch at the periphery, whereas the compression screw puts stress on a more centrally placed half inch (see Figs 14–1 through 14–5 and 14–7 through 14–9). Any fixation device in the head is more firm if it is also fixed to the shaft. For that reason, when multiple pins are used they should be positioned through the plate so as to achieve maximum fixation at the shaft. This avoids the centrally placed pins, as shown in Figure 14–9, and provides more stability and allows for impaction. Sagging of the head and loosening of the pins in the head result from loosening of the pins in the shaft. Two factors are at work here. The shaft laterally is quite thin, and if break-off pins such as Knowles or Neufeld pins are used, the breaking-off process itself will partially loosen the pins laterally. Often the bending force is transmitted to the bone, and either the pins are loosened or a stress riser is created by the break-off maneuver. Whenever one uses a break-off pin it is essential to maintain the rigidity of the proximal portion of the pin with a pair of pliars so that no force is exerted on the surrounding bone. In many cases the pins are loosened in the shaft at the completion of the procedure. Schwab and Karr[25] reported four cases of subtrochanteric fractures at the level of the stress riser that resulted from insertion of either Knowles pins or Neufeld pins without a side plate to act as a tension band.

Delayed Treatment of Fractures

Because of potential problems with blood supply and organization of the fracture surfaces bathed in synovial fluid and blood, I have arbitrarily bone grafted any fracture more than 7 days old. Revascularization is decreased enough to warrant cancellous bone grafting followed by multiple plate and pin fixation. It is acceptable if some of the pins go through the cancellous bone graft. The cancellous graft should be 1/2 inch in diameter and 1½ long, to cross the fracture site. (The graft may be transfixed with one or more pins.) I also use the Meyers-Judet pedicle graft with plate and pins. This assemblage is more certain to produce union because of improved blood supply.

Attention to Detail With Plate and Multiple Pin Fixation

The need for attention to detail is pointed out by experiences reported by other orthopedists. Metz et al. reported meticulous care in following the proper technique.[40] With a 2-year follow-up of 63 patients, they reported that 81.4% had excellent functional and roentgenographic results, 11.6% had avascular necrosis, and there was a 4.7% incidence of nonunion. The average recorded pin backout was ½ inch.

In a later series of 38 patients treated at the same institution, 40.9% had excellent results. There was an 18.1% incidence of avascular necrosis and a 31.8% incidence of nonunion. The authors stated that "no basis for the difference in the results in the two groups could be determined."[44] There was no report of percussion impaction or of the number of pins inserted. They did state that "lack of parallel orientation prevented easy backing out of the pins when there was resorption or collapse at the fracture site." This is evidence that hammer percussion impaction was not carried out at operation. They accepted 6–8 weeks of delayed union and motion. If one does not pay attention to details, the results are predictable (Table 14–1).

Chapman et al. reported two series of cases that were examples of failure to apply detailed technique.[45] Pin counts varied from 6 to 12, with an average of 9 in one group and 7 in the other. They stated that "the author's requirements for reduction could not be met by most orthopaedic surgeons" and that "there was no relation between the adequacy of reduction and end results." Impaction was not recorded in their operative notes. Their report included only patients in whom 2-year follow-up was available unless the devices failed prior to 2 years. Their statistical

TABLE 14–1.—Expected Results in Displaced Neck Fractures Treated With Deyerle Device

Study, Year	No. of Cases	Nonunion (%)	Avascular Necrosis With Union (%)
Deyerle, 1965[30]	111	1.8	10
Metz et al., 1970[40]	63	4.7	11.6
McCutchen et al., 1982[23]	34	6	13
Thorling et al., 1980, 1981[19-21]			
12 mo.	235	7	7
2 yr.	117	8	17
Chapman et al., 1975[45]			
Attendings	26	11.5	4.1
Residents	51	15.6	27
Baker and Barrick, 1978[44]	38	31	18
Total	675		

data for the last 2 years noted that 16 patients treated by residents and four treated by attending physicians had excellent or satisfactory results. All these patients were excluded from the final reporting (end results), whereas patients with poor results from the same period of time were included. Notice the poorer results in the residents' series (see Table 14–1).

TECHNIQUE IN DISPLACED INTERCAPSULAR FRACTURES

All patients are operated on, usually within 24 hours. On admission the leg is placed in 5 lb of Buck traction. If there is any delay, the hip should be aspirated once or twice with a large 18- to 15-gauge needle to decompress the intracapsular hematoma (see Fig 14–10).

Positioning

The patient is placed on a fracture table with the opposite limb well out of the way so that good lateral roentgenograms can be obtained. The foot must be taped in such a way that the bindings do not loosen during the procedure. Strong traction is applied with the leg parallel with the body and the foot in midposition or slightly externally rotated.

Radiologic Monitoring

The efficacy of image intensification or of multiple radiographs is directly related to the efficacy of the entire procedure. Use of an image intensifier and a series of stored still images that can be reproduced later is the ideal method. Use of a fluoroscope increases by a factor of 20–40 the amount of exposure that can be delivered, whereas the electronic image intensification system has an automatic cutoff. One must have reproducible anteroposterior (AP) and lateral views. On the straight lateral view the neck should be parallel with the floor (see Figs 14–13 and 14–16). The surgeon must check these two positions with the image intensifier before proceeding.

If the foot has been turned the correct degree, the lesser trochanter will be just visible on the AP view. If the neck is not parallel with the floor, the foot should be rotated until the radiograph shows the neck parallel with the floor. This allows placement of the guide pin parallel to the floor (Fig 14–16).

Reduction

What are the pros and cons of varus, anatomical, overreduction (translated reduction), or valgus reduction? (see Figs 14–11 and 14–13). With an anatomical reduction in the lateral view and overreduction in the AP view a small price must be paid. There is not as much contact of the fracture surfaces. After the fracture has healed, the lever arm of the abductor to the weight-bearing portion of the head of the femur is shortened. This places greater stress on the head and neck and requires more muscle action of the abductors.[46]

This type of reduction with 9 or more pins and good hammer percussion impaction will provide sufficient contact and fixation to allow immediate weight-bearing and a rapid union (see Figs 14–5, 14–6, 14–24, and 14–25).

If a valgus reduction should allow a line extended from the parallel trabeculae in the head of the femur to fall medial to the calcar, this will increase the chance of avascular necrosis.[17, 47, 48] Although the stability of the fracture is good in the valgus position, it is preferable to have an anatomical or slightly translated reduction (see Figs 14–11,C and 14–16).

In the AP view the Garden angle should not be in excess of 180°.[17, 18] One should not accept any varus reduction in displaced fractures. This is the most unstable position from a standpoint of both the 75% of the stress that is received by the bone as well as 25% that is received by the internal fixation apparatus. A slightly superior translated reduction is preferred (see Fig 14–11,C.)

Stable Impacted Fractures of the Neck

In impacted stable fractures, however, one may accept a valgus position and even an anatomically aligned, slightly translated reduction inferiorly (see Fig 14–11, C).

The first set of radiographs should be AP and lateral views. If after reduction the head of the femur is tilted too far in valgus, the leg may be in too much abduction.

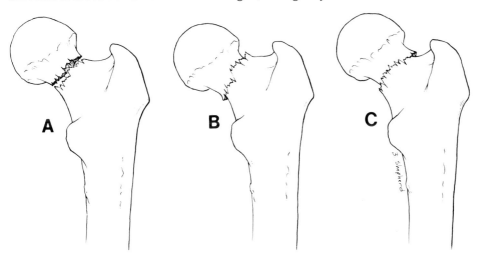

Fig 14–11—A, anatomical alignment before impaction; B, impacted varus reduction (acceptable in stable impacted fractures, not acceptable in displaced fractures); C, superior translated reduction.

It should be brought into adduction to the midline parallel with the body. To place the head in a normal alignment with the neck, pull laterally on the upper end of the femur. The objective is a slightly overreduced or anatomical position of the head in the AP view. One should rarely disimpact a stable fracture.

Reduction in the Lateral Plane

It is essential that the pelvis on the opposite side from the fracture be held firmly downward against the fracture table, especially when the oposite leg is elevated and abducted for x-ray exposure. If pressure is not firmly applied by an assistant at the moment of the reduction the pelvis will rotate and one will lose the straight posterior thrust that provides an anatomical reduction in the lateral plane.

The assistant directs posterior pressure over the greater trochanter with two hands, resisted by the firmly held pelvis on the opposite side (Fig 14–12). An anatomical or slightly overreduced position is seen in the lateral views (Fig 14–13). If one thinks of the head as a scoop of ice cream in a cone, it is essential to place the ice cream directly on top of the cone rather than leaving it hanging out of the posterior portion. A crunch can usually be heard or felt if this maneuver is performed with vigor, directly posterior, and if the pelvis is held down on the opposite side. This maneuver is described by Montgomery, and the orthopedic grapevine in Memphis reports that it is called the "Stewart jiggle."[49]

Reduction in the AP Plane

The next maneuver is to achieve an overreduced position of the head but without valgus rotation or tilting of the head. This is accomplished by placing traction on the leg parallel to the body and direct pressure laterally over the greater trochanter while pushing toward the centerpost of the fracture table and stabilizing the knee. If the leg is in traction and parallel with the body, the result will be an excellent reduction,

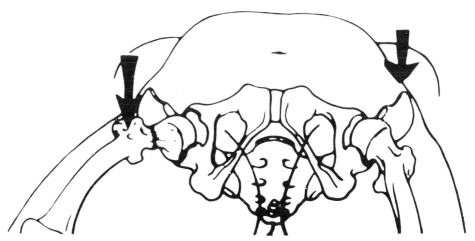

Fig 14–12—Applying direct pressure over the greater trochanter with two hands produces an anatomical or slightly overreduced position in the lateral plane (see Fig 14–16). It is essential that the assistant apply equally firm posterior pressure over the opposite iliac crest to prevent the patient from rocking on the fracture table. (Described by W. Montgomery[49] in a personal communication.) (From Deyerle.[2] Reproduced by permission.)

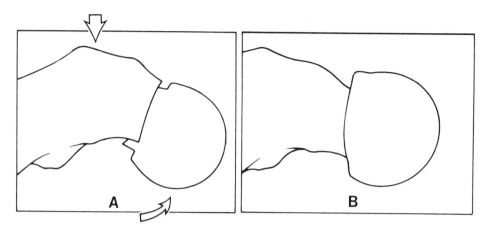

Fig 14–13—Outline of radiographs on the fracture table, lateral view **A,** *before reduction,* **arrow** *shows force applied in Figure 14–12.* **B,** *final anatomical or slightly overreduced (translated) reduction*

with the head of the femur slightly above the calcar (see Figs 14–11,C, 14–12 and 14–13). Do not attempt a valgus or tilted position in a displaced intracapsular fracture. After the traction is tensed and the fracture is overreduced, the foot is internally rotated until it is at an angle of approximately 45° with the floor. The assistant rotates the knee in as the foot is rotated to take some of the strain off the ligaments of the knee. Manipulation may be repeated as needed.

Surgical Approach

A 7-inch incision is made from the tip of the trochanter down the lateral shaft of the femur. Cutting, current, and coagulation are done generously to achieve hemostasis. The flare of the greater trochanter is carefully identified and a point 1 ¼ inches distal to the flare is selected as the site for insertion of a guide pin. An additional landmark helpful in selecting the proper distance down the femur is located by dissecting posteriorly on the femur to identify the well-delineated strap-like insertion of the lower third of the gluteus maximus into the femur. This proximal edge is at approximately the right distance distally to locate the hole for the guide pin. A Langenback dissector can be placed to mark this upper edge and to act as a retractor. A ¼-inch hole is drilled at this level of the femur midway between the anterior and posterior cortices. Placement of this hole is important. Two 9/64-inch guide pins, 5 inches long (identical in length) should be available. The surgeon places the guide pin through a 140° angle guide plate or jig (Figs 14–14 and 14–15) and inserts it parallel with the neck just across the fracture site (Fig 14–16). When the pin is inserted, it is essential that the plate or jig be flush with the shaft of the femur.

In older patients there may be an overgrowth of the lateral flare of the greater trochanter. If the overgrowth can be seen on a radiograph, the distance distal to the flare for guide pin insertion may be shortened accordingly. Thus the pin can be placed in the center of the neck in both views, or at least near enough the center for 1 of the 7 center holes (proximal to distal) to be used. If one of the 7 center holes cannot be used, the guide pin should be reinserted (Fig 14–17). The hole in the plate should be selected to allow the maximum number of pins to be inserted into the head (Figs 14–18 and 14–19). At times, in smaller patients, pins cannot be inserted into the anterior 3 or the posterior 3 holes. In most instances, at least 1 of

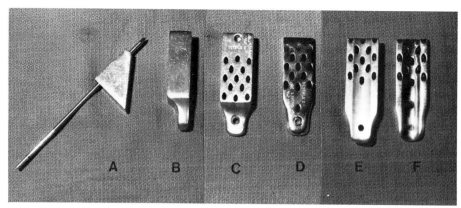

Fig 14–14—A, guide pin in 140° angle guide plate; B and C, drill guide jig with identical pattern and angle of all Deyerle plates; D, short plate for neck fractures (1 hole for transverse shaft pin, 1 hole for impacting punch, 13 holes for fixation pins); E, pattern of drilling jig; F, pattern of short plates.

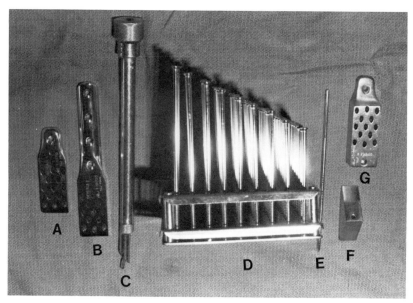

Fig 14–15—A, Deyerle 2 plate for neck fractures (13 holes for fixation pins, 1 hole for impacting punch, 1 hole for transverse shaft screw); B, Deyerle 2 plate for trochanteric fracture (4 holes for shaft; remaining pattern same as A); C, impacting punch; D, tray with pins in ¹/₄-inch increments; E, ⁹/₆₄-inch guide pin, 5 inches long; F, 140° angle jig; G, drill guide and jig. All plates, jig, and guides are at a 140° angle.

these 3 anterior or 3 posterior pins can be inserted along with the remaining pins in the plate.

Calculation of Pin Lengths

The proper length of pins is calculated by determining the length of the guide pin inserted in the neck. An estimate of the proper pin length is made preoperatively by obtaining an AP roentgenogram of the opposite hip, for a displaced fracture, or of the fractured hip, for an impacted fracture. Place all the pins in the plate and lay it over the x-ray film. Two variables must be taken into consideration: one, there is approximately 20% enlargement of the roentgenography shadow of the femur, and two, there will be ¼- to ½-inch impaction obtained by hammer impaction of the displaced fracture at the time of surgery. Bearing in mind these two factors, the surgeon superimposes the plate and pins on the roentgenogram of the normal femur. The proper-sized pins lie approximately 1 inch from the top of the head of the femur at the center of the head of the femur. In a stable impacted fracture, there will be less impaction if one superimposes the plate and pins deeper than 1 inch. The pins are approximately ¾ inch short of the articular surface of the head of the femur.

The preoperative pin length estimation is checked at the time of surgery. Using an identical guide pin, the surgeon determines the length of pin in the neck. After viewing this in two views on the image intensifier, the surgeon calculates what length of pin is needed to place the tip ¾ inch short of the articular surface of the

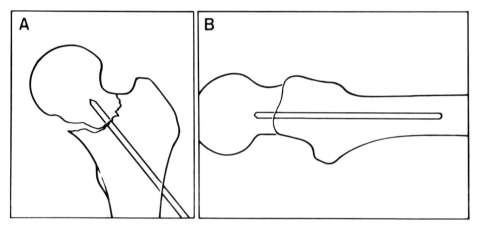

Fig 14–16—The ⁹⁄₆₄-inch guide pin in place. A, AP view. Foot is rotated 45° and lesser trochanter is just visible. B, lateral view. Neck and guide are parallel with the floor—a good position. AP view shows translated reduction; lateral view shows anatomical reduction.

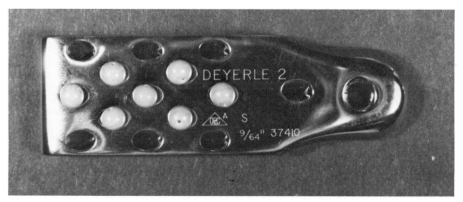

Fig 14–17—The guide pin must be in a position that allows one of the 7 center holes to be placed over it and a minimum of 9 pins to be inserted into the head.

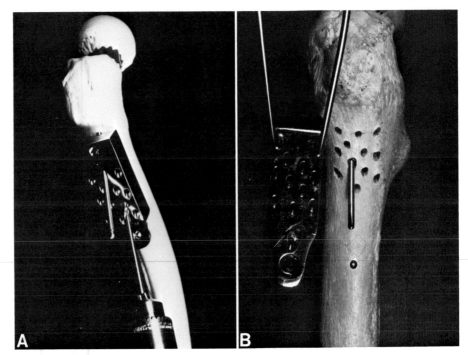

*Fig 14–18—**A**, thick guide plate screwed into place to put the maximum pins into the head. Here, the guide pins are in the superior middle hole. Figure 14–16 suggests that one of the center holes would be preferable. All holes to be used are drilled through this plate with the %64-inch drill bit. Do not drill beyond the fracture site. Always use a minimum of 9 pins. **B**, appearance of lateral shaft after drilling through jig with guide pin in one of the middle center holes. Plate will be screwed in place over the guide pin. Note that anterior and posterior holes enter the shaft at an angle but the pins remain parallel.*

head of the femur (see Figs 14–14 and 14–16). The length of the guide pin in place in Figure 14–16 is 5 inches. The length of guide pin in the bone is 2¾ inches and is approximately at the fracture site. The pin that will ultimately replace this guide pin should extend ¾ inch farther into the head, and the plate will take up ½ inch. The length of the pin that will replace the guide pin in the center hole will be 2¾ inches plus ¾ inch plus ½ inch, or 4 inches (see Fig 14–20).

Once the pin length is selected, the remaining pins have a constant relationship. In our example, since the guide pin is centrally placed, the centermost hole will be placed over it, and the relationship will be as follows: All 5 of the middle holes will also be 4 inches. The top 3 holes will be ½ inch shorter, or 3½ inches. The bottom 5 holes will be ½ inch longer, or 4½ inches deep (Fig 14–21). After the guide pin is removed, and based on the AP and lateral images on the intensifier screen, sometimes any or all of the 5 center holes may accept pins increased by ¼ inch. The surgeon should err on the short side to avoid overdrilling. One can always insert a longer pin (Fig 14–22). The strongest support on each pin is that support immediately at the top of the pin, and an overdrilled pathway will always be less efficient. The guide pin is not removed until all other pins are inserted. A minimum of 9 pins should be inserted.

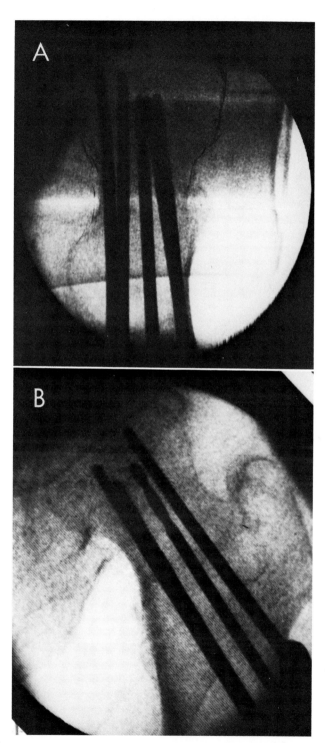

*Fig 14–19—**A,** lateral view with 4 corner pins. Guide drill is in center. **B,** AP view with 4 corner pins. Guide drill is in center.*

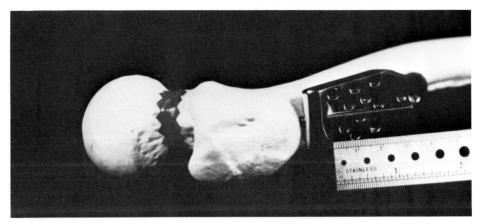

Fig 14–20—The exact length of the pin in the neck or head is calculated by subtracting the length outside of the plate, which is 1½ inches in this figure.

Use of the Guide Plate Jig

The guide plate jig is a thicker replica of the side plate. It is attached to the femur by inserting the cross screw and anchoring it firmly to the femur to act as a guide for the drill. It is screwed over the guide pin in the ideal position for the final insertion of the plate. The hole over the guide pin is one of the 7 center holes (see Figs 14–17 and 14–18), which permits placement of the maximum number of pins into the head (always a minimum of 9). With this drill guide screwed firmly in place with one transverse screw, the cortex is predrilled with the 9/64-inch drill bit. During this drilling a large amount of irrigating fluid should be used to keep the drill point cool. If there appears to be some resistance to the drilling the surgeon should remove the drill and cool it off, or use another drill and drill in another area. This avoids necrosis of surrounding bone and breakage of drills. The guide pin and transverse screw will hold the jig firmly in place during the drilling process. All of the holes to the fracture site are predrilled with a 9/64-inch drill bit. The surgeon should not drill beyond the fracture site, and should use irrigation fluid freely to keep the drill point cool. When all of the holes are drilled, the guide plate is removed. The guide plate is more accurate, being thicker, and it directs the drill in a more parallel fashion. In drilling through the guide plate and into the cortex it is essential to have fast spin and not too much pressure in the anterior and posterior holes because the drill is striking the lateral shaft of the femur at a slight angle, and too much pressure will force the drill to angle away from the femur rather than penetrate it. If the drill does not penetrate the superior or inferior holes easily, the surgeon should drill through the plate and spin the drill in the hole to mark the site of the eventual entrance into the femur. The drill is removed from the plate and the cortex drilled from superiorly or inferiorly in order to break the cortex at a better angle. The drill is then reinserted through the jig and will penetrate the cortex and advance to the fracture site. The guide plate is removed and a regular plate is screwed to the shaft, using the same screw tract in the femur and placing the same hole over the guide pin (see Fig 14–18). The pins are temporarily inserted in an extra plate to facilitate insertion of the pins in the correct holes (Fig 14–23).

An alternative technique that requires an extra set of radiographs is preferred by some. The four corner pins are inserted and their positions checked (see Fig 14–19).

The pins may be tapped to the fracture line with a hammer. If the pins advance with difficulty, drilling should be repeated.

After at least 9 pins are seated, the surgeon releases the traction, places the impactor in the impacting hole or any other vacant hole, and strikes four or five firm hammer blows. This will impact the fracture, collapse the comminuted fragments, and mutually invaginate the irregular surfaces of the fracture while the head is lowered down to the shaft, being held in proper relationship by the 9 pins (Fig 14–24; see also Fig 14–5). The percussion impaction can be evaluated by watching the screw

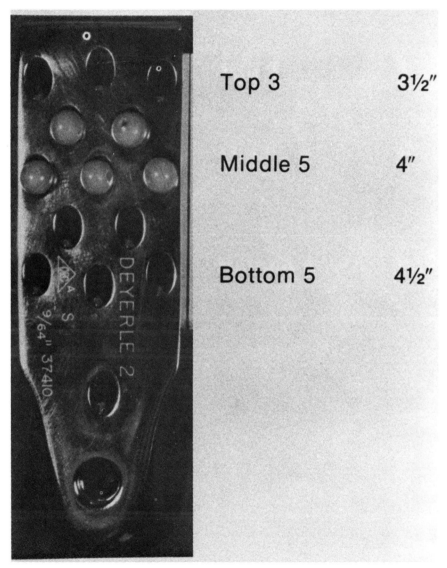

Top 3	3½"
Middle 5	4"
Bottom 5	4½"

Fig 14–21—Pin of proper length is selected by measuring the guide pin in the x-ray view (see Fig 14–17). Plan to insert the pins with ¾ inch of the top of the head before impaction. Once the length of any one pin is calculated, the remainder have a constant relationship. The top 3 are always ½ inch shorter than the middle 5, and the bottom 5 are ½ inch longer than the middle 4. The lengths shown are only examples and are not routinely used. Pin lengths must be calculated individually for each case. (From Deyerle.[2] Reproduced by permission.)

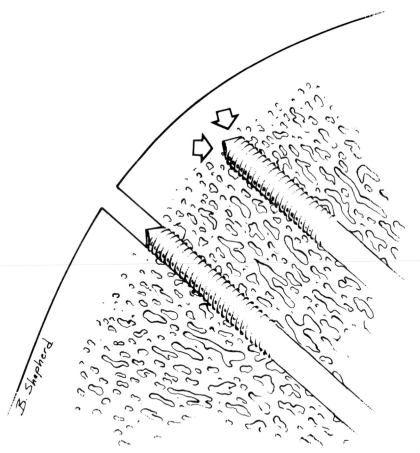

Fig 14–22—Overdrilling through the head removes the best bony support. It is better to insert the pins short and gradually insert them deeper either by radiographic or image-intensifier control. If necessary, insert a longer pin. There can never by any lag-screw effect. The conical top of 9 $^{9}/_{64}$-inch pins has an area of 0.156 square inches; of 12 pins, 0.211 square inches. A $^{1}/_{2}$-inch Holt bolt has an area of 0.197 square inches on the flat top.

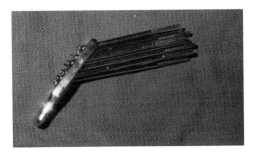

Fig 14–23—Plate set up with proper lengths of pins. Pins will be transferred to plate fixed to patient's femur.

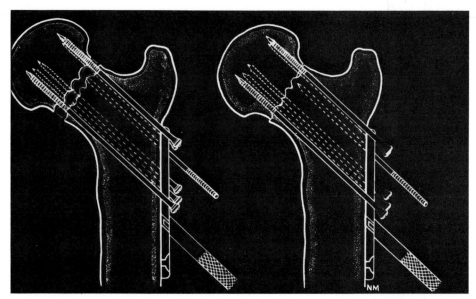

Fig 14–24—The plate fixed in place over the guide pin. The heads of the fixation screws back out of the plate ¼ to ½ inch. (From Deyerle.[2] Reproduced by permission.)

heads back out approximately ¼ inch or ½ inch. They are then tightened by hand. The pin backout must be recorded. The third and final set of views is then made (Figs 14–25 and 14–26). On the final radiographic views obtained after impaction, the pins should be ¼ to ½ inch from the joint surface. It is better to put pins a little short and exchange them for longer pins than to put a pin through the head and then have to replace it with a shorter one (see Figs 14–20 and 14–22). A pin should never be tightened with the power drill. The last two or three turns must be done by hand. No effort should be made to draw the head down on the femur. There is no lag screw effect.

STABLE IMPACTED FRACTURES

Stable impacted fractures are those fractures still in contact and still impacted at the time of first x-ray. The degree of stability may vary. A history of having walked on the fracture suggests stability. All impacted fractures should be treated by plate and multiple pins, with the same principles applied as for displaced fractures. There are a few minor variations in technique.

Reduction

Usually, the position of an impacted fracture should be accepted, providing it remains impacted. The surgeon should accept any valgus position and any posterior tilting less than 30°. If the posterior tilting is more than 30° it must be reduced. With the patient on the fracture table and the foot internally rotated, a reduction maneuver in the lateral plane, as described earlier, is performed (see Figs 14–12 and 14–13). The posterior pressure applied over the greater trochanter as the pelvis is held fixed will improve the reduction. This is the only impacted fracture in which one should attempt to change the position. All other impacted fractures should also be fixed in

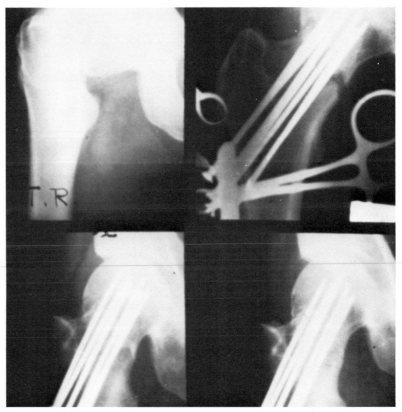

Fig 14–25—Displaced fracture. **A,** *reduction before impaction;* **B,** *after percussion impaction at surgery;* **C,** *healed solid at 8 weeks. (From Deyerle.[2] Reproduced by permission.)*

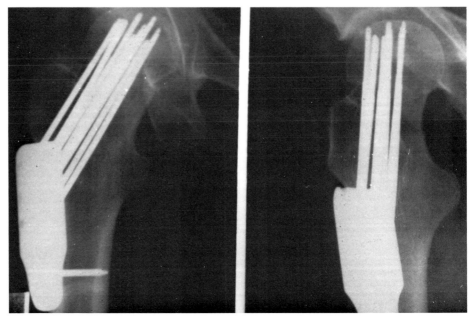

Fig 14–26—Translated reduction with ideal positioning of plate and pins.

place with plate and multiple pins followed by additional impaction (see Fig 14–11, B). Treating an impacted fracture nonoperatively risks disimpaction and a poor result. Disimpaction can occur very easily with nothing more than movement in bed, getting on a bed pan, or a slight twist of the foot. With 9 pins and additional impaction at surgery, union can be assured, with an 8% possibility of avascular necrosis. Avascular necrosis may require additional surgery.[50, 51]

At surgery after the 9 pins are in place following the previously described technique the fracture is further impacted with the impactor and the pins back out approximately 1/8 inch. They are then gently tightened down by hand.

Variations

It is ideal to have the guide pins parallel with the neck, firmly in the neck, and centrally in the head. It is acceptable if the guide pin runs slightly posterior in the neck, as this places the maximum fixation in the middle and posterior thirds of the head and neck. The usual comminution in the neck is posterior. After impaction the pins tend to buttress the posterior part of the neck and prevent posterior tilting of the head, the usual direction of deformity or displacement (see Fig 14–26). Generally, one should never drill beyond the fracture site with the 9/64-inch drill bit. It is preferable to have the threads of the pins cut their way into the area proximal to the fracture. If the drilling is very difficult, and after drilling to the fracture site with the 9/64-inch bit, the surgeon may wish to insert a 7/64-inch drill bit, the size of the root diameter of the pins. This bit can be used to drill across the fracture site approximately 3/4 inch. The surgeon then places the pins. This maneuver may be necessary in very young adults or in patients with very hard bones, such as those with Paget's disease or previous degenerative arthritis.

In Pauwell's type 3 fractures, if the fracture force occurs with the hip flexed, the inferior spike of the calcar may impale the capsule. This is usually ascertained on x-ray when the AP view appears abnormal. In these cases it is essential to open the capsule and free the impaled calcar and allow it to drop down in line with the femur. This is an absolute indication for opening the capsule.

POSTOPERATIVE CARE

No narcotics or barbiturates should be administered postoperatively. Pain is controlled with Bufferin or Darvon. Sleep is facilitated with 50 mg of Benadryl. On the first postoperative day, while the patient is still in bed, the limb should be held and pressure applied firmly proximally on the heel. This gives the patient confidence that the hip is firm and well fixed. Suction drainage, if used, is removed on the second or third day. A patient who is reluctant to ambulate should be placed in a Hubbard tank to gain confidence and for mobilization. The surgeon or physical therapist should assure patients they can put full weight on the fractured limb and may walk with either crutches or a walker for balance, and should point out in detail the advantages of early walking to build up the muscles around the hip and avoid the complications of pulmonary embolus, thrombophlebitis, and mental depression. We prefer below-knee antiembolism stockings. Salicylates help prevent venous thrombosis and embolism. The patient starts weight-bearing on the second or third day and should be bearing full weight with a four-point gait or step to gait with the crutches or walker by the seventh day. The surgeon should not be disturbed by patient reports of local discomfort laterally in the incision area. Anticoagulants are not used.

COMPLICATIONS

The only pain that causes concern is groin pain or pain referred to the knee. Unless this type of pain develops, the hip should not be radiographed for 6 weeks. Postoperative AP radiographs should be made with the foot rolled in, to place the neck exactly parallel with the underlying film. Either a cross-table lateral or frogleg lateral view is satisfactory. If pain develops in the groin or knee and radiographs show evidence of any motion or further collapse of the fracture, one should conclude that percussion impaction was insufficient at the time of surgery. Breakage of a pin in the first 6–8 weeks occurs because prior to breakage the total unit of fixation, muscles, bone, and internal fixation was insufficient to withstand the stress. Once a pin is broken, total fixation is decreased. This pin must be replaced, and one or two additional pins should be placed in other holes left vacant at surgery. If necessary, a pin should be placed into the head that does not go through the plate. This can be done by angling the pin over the anterior edge of the plate.

Fortunately, when a pin breaks, it is under stress and it is pushed sufficiently away from the original pin tract to allow replacement of the broken pin. Another pin can be inserted that will bypass the retained broken piece.

At surgery, the decision as to which pin is broken requires careful study of the radiographs. One or two pins may have to be eased out slightly before the broken pin is identified on the image intensifier. Since I began using %64-inch pins 12 years ago, I have seen no breakage problems.

Additional percussion impaction and gentle tightening of all pins will improve the intrinsic bone stability and the pin fixation.

The surgeon should decrease the patient's activity and allow only a touch-down gait with 30 lb of weight on the fractured hip.

If the original operation goes well, there will be no change in appearance between the immediate postoperative radiograph and the end result radiograph (see Fig 14–25). Very little callus is seen because the fracture is so impacted that the fracture line is not visible. The fracture behaves as all other impacted fractures that do not become dislodged. It heals by primary endosteal bone healing (Table 14–2; see also Figs 14–25 and 14–26).[44, 52]

There were no pulmonary emboli in the series of patients I treated. Thorling reported 2 instances in 319 patients.[19, 20]

Of the two cases of nonunion (see Table 14–2), one was porotic and the pins cut out. Satisfactory results were obtained with a Girdlestone resection. One patient fell at 6 weeks and the fracture went on to a nonunion, requiring a prosthetic replacement.

A third case of nonunion that has been reported, not from my series, was a Charcot joint that disintegrated.

TABLE 14–2.—Complications in 238 Femoral Neck Fractures: Personal Series	
Complication	**No.**
Thrombophlebitis	2
Infections	2
Pulmonary embolus	0
Hospital deaths	5

TABLE 14-3.—Follow-up of Neck Fractures (2–13 Years)

Type of Fracture	No.	Nonunion	Avascular Necrosis
Displaced intercapsular	111	2 (1.8%)	10 (9%)
Impacted:			
Displaced before surgery	4	0	1 (27%)
Stable	59	0	1 (7%)
Basilar neck	31	0	0
Combined neck and intertrochanteric	8	0	0

TABLE 14–4.—238 Consecutive Fractures

Type of Fracture	Total no.	No. With Follow-up	No. w/o Follow-up
Intercapsular:			
Displaced	129	18	111
Impacted	72	9	63
Basilar neck	26	2	24
Combined neck and intertrochanteric	9	1	8

Summary

Fractures of the neck of the femur require prompt treatment and anatomical or translated reduction on the fracture table, with traction applied parallel with the body. A valgus position is not satisfactory in displaced fractures. Use of a plate and a minimum of 9 pins, plus hammer impaction at surgery, coapts the irregular surfaces. It is essential to immediately secure the 75% support of the surrounding bone by impaction at surgery and by recording the degree of impaction on the chart. Shortening or collapse over the first 6–8 weeks means 6–8 weeks of secondary healing with a cartilage phase instead of healing per primum. Avascular necrosis, if it occurs, will not manifest until after 6 months. In this period the fracture site is vulnerable. One must promote primary endosteal bone healing with no cartilage and no motion at the fracture site. Resilient fixation dissipates the forces tending to displace the fracture yet holds it with sufficient rigidity to promote early, prompt union, typically within 9 weeks. Proper application of plate and pins allows full weight-bearing on the third to fourth postoperative days (Tables 14–3 and 14–4).

INTERTROCHANTERIC FRACTURES
Biomechanics

In elderly patients, many intertrochanteric fractures are of a fatigue type, and the architecture of the bone is sufficiently inadequate that fracture may occur with relatively minor trauma. These fractures occur in the same patient population as fractures of the femoral neck. In younger individuals with stronger bones, the fractures may result from a direct blow or twist on major trauma. The degree of comminution may vary from an undisplaced fracture, in which the periosteum is intact, to a severely comminuted peritrochanteric fracture.

The two major divisions of intertrochanteric fractures are stable and unstable. Stable fractures are those with two major fragments that are relatively easy to approximate in an anatomical position. In unstable fractures there is severe comminution, which makes bony continuity between the two major fragments difficult to achieve (Fig 14–27). The stability of the fracture is finally assessed at surgery. The greater the displacement, the less support is available from periosteum and the surrounding soft tissue. Impaction is essential (see Fig 14–16).

Owing to the length of the levers involved from the weight-bearing portion of the head through the fractured area, the mechanical stress on the internal fixation apparatus is greater than in fractures of the neck.[7, 12, 46]

The distance from the weight-bearing surface of the femoral head to the fracture surface in a neck fracture is 1½ or 2 inches, and as much as 3 or 4 inches in fractures of the trochanteric region. The stresses required for displacement are less because of the longer lever arm of the proximal fragment. Inherent stability of bone is more difficult to achieve in comminuted intertrochanteric fractures than in comminuted neck fractures.

In trochanteric fractures, it is possible to gather up the comminuted fragments and impale and impact them underneath the broad plate. Attachment of the plate in the trochanteric region and down the shaft of the femur provides a broad base for impacting the many fragments while maintaining proper alignment. The multiple pin distribution with its resilience and flexibility allows for the reduction and distributes the stress in the most efficient possible way in the multiplicity of fixation points within the head and neck as well as impaling the comminuted fragments in the region of the trochanter (Figs 14–28 and 14–29).

Intertrochanteric fractures heal better, often in spite of treatment, since there is a large amount of periosteal as well as endosteal healing. However, this should not dissuade the surgeon from the goal of anatomical alignment with early healing by well-disbursed resilient fixation. An example of massive periosteal bone healing is shown in Figure 14–30. Since the fracture is not intracapsular, there is no urgency for fixation of the fracture, as was the case with neck fractures. And since the intertrochanteric fracture is extracapsular, a hemarthrosis does not develop. Avascular necrosis rarely occurs after an intertrochanteric fracture.

Operative Technique
Reduction

The patient is placed on a fracture table, preferably with the normal leg elevated out of the way to facilitate obtaining lateral radiographic views. The fracture is reduced by placing the leg almost parallel with the body. The foot is internally rotated approximately 45°. It may be necessary to rotate the foot less in order to avoid opening the posterior surface of the fracture in the intertrochanteric area. Unlike the case with neck fractures, it is not always possible to reduce the intertrochanteric fracture and maintain the neck parallel with the floor, as seen on the lateral view. A 10-inch incision adequately exposes the shaft of the femur in the fracture area. Often, after opening the wound, it is necessary to use a supporting retractor under the neck of the femur to hold it upward and prevent it from sagging posteriorly. The surgeon should aim for an anatomical or slightly overreduced position, as seen on the first set of radiograph views (see Fig 14–28).

In intertrochanteric fractures there is no concern about a valgus reduction. If better radiographic exposure or image intensification can be achieved by placing the leg on the fracture table in some abduction, this is an alternate technique and

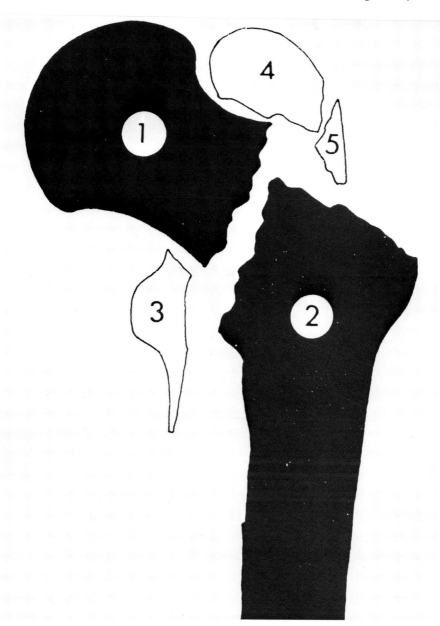

Fig 14–27—In intertrochanteric fractures the proximal fragment (1) *and distal fragment* (2) *are the important fragments to be fixed by internal fixation and impaction. (From Deyerle.[36] Reproduced by permission.)*

will usually create some valgus. The latter does not interfere with healing. It rarely causes any increase in length because the fracture will be impacted vigorously. The surgeon evaluates the reduction with traction applied and the foot in midposition or slightly externally rotated. The surgeon places a finger on the fracture site anteriorly and posteriorly. Any posterior displacement occurs as the foot is rolled into internal rotation. At times the fracture may be held in reduction by means of a bone clamp placed anteriorly and posteriorly completely around the femur and completely grasping the neck fragment. This requires some sharp dissection anteriorly and may require

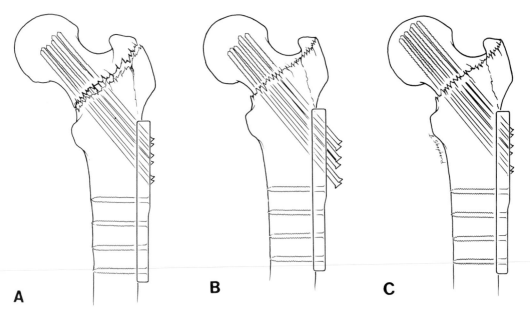

A   **B**   **C**

*Fig 14–28—**A,** the plate is held with 4 screws, and 9 or more pins are inserted into the base of the head. Impaction provides support for both bone and internal fixation. See Figure 14–24. **B,** vigorous impaction at surgery invaginates the irregular surfaces of the fracture. The pins guide the proximal fragment down onto the distal fragment. They can be seen to back out ½ to 1 inch. **C,** the inherent stability of the impacted fragments is maintained and the pins are carefully turned down flush with the plate as they enter the head.*

some resection posteriorly, even releasing a portion of the strap of the gluteus maximus insertion into the femur. The muscle should be reattached following fixation. If it is determined on palpation of the fracture that the posterior surface of the fracture is open, the foot is rotated externally. An alternative method is to use a forked elevator. The assistant holds up the neck of the femur, thereby closing the posterior surface of the fracture. This supporting retractor may be a bone skid held up against the neck by an assistant, or it may be a two-pronged fork in which the prongs are used to hold the neck upward.

The insertion of the guide pin is critical in intertrochanteric and neck fractures. A point is selected 1¼ inches below the flare of the greater trochanter on the lateral surface of the femur exactly halfway in the AP dimension. The guide pin is then inserted either through one of the fractured areas or by drilling or nibbling a ¼ inch hole, as necessary. A 9/64-inch guide pin or a drill 5 inches long is inserted into the neck of the femur using the 140° angle jig or the 140° guide plate. The second set of views determines the position of the guide pin in reference to the neck in anterior and posterior views. The surgeon decides which hole of the plate (or jig) is to be placed over the guide pin so that the maximal number of pins can be positioned in the neck of the femur (see Figs 14–17 and 14–18). From the guide pin, the proper length of the pin is determined. Once one pin length is determined, the remaining pins have a constant relationship. This determination is made in the same manner as described for fractures of the neck of the femur. However, in many comminuted intertrochanteric fractures the amount of impaction that is created at surgery will be greater than for neck fractures. For this reason, in severely comminuted fractures, calculations leave the pins 1¼ inches short of the subchondral head of the femur.

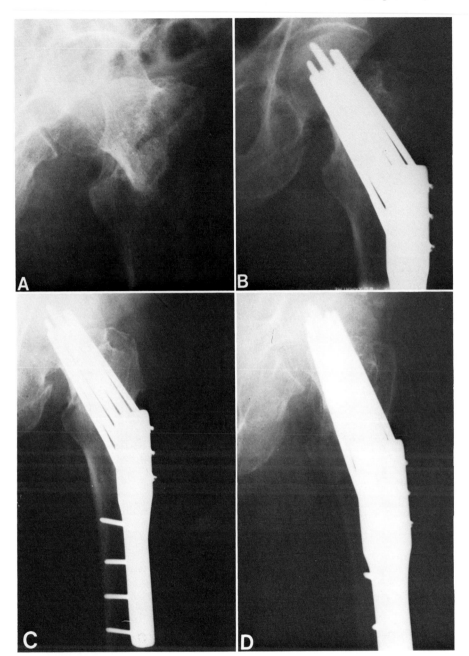

*Fig 14–29—**A,** stable type of intertrochanteric fracture. **B,** fracture has been well reduced, impacted, and fixed. **C,** AP view 8 weeks after surgery. The patient was walking unaided and the fracture had united. **D,** lateral view, 8 weeks after surgery.*

Example: It is calculated that 2½ inches of the guide pin is in the femur. One wishes to place the pin ½ inch deeper, and the plate is ½ inch thick. The pin length will be 3½ inches. All of the middle holes will be 3½ inches, the upper holes will be 3 inches deep, and the lower holes will be 4 inches deep. Many prefer to place the 4-hole side plate over the guide pin to drill one of the 4 holes to be sure that the long side plate

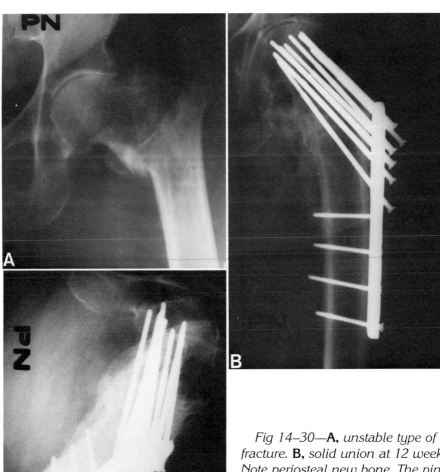

Fig 14–30—**A,** *unstable type of fracture.* **B,** *solid union at 12 weeks. Note periosteal new bone. The pins have backed out somewhat since surgery.* **C,** *lateral view showing solid union.*

will line up with the shaft once the short jig has been removed. One may drill through the plate that is to be inserted. Either the plate or the jig is bolted into place and the ⁹⁄₆₄-inch drill bit is used to drill through the lateral cortex. In many comminuted fractures holes must be drilled, in the fracture itself involves the area of the plate. All holes are drilled, the jig is removed, and the 4-hole side plate is attached with the 4 bone screws holding it over the proper guide pin so that the maximum number of pins can be inserted into the head and neck of the femur. A minimum of 9 pins is used, but often as many as 13 are used. The impaction hole may even provide space for a 14th pin. It is essential to leave the impaction hole open until after impaction. The ⁹⁄₆₄-inch pins may be drilled in, or tapped in, until they meet resistance, and then turned in by hand with a screwdriver. If a motorized screwdriver is used, the inserting screw must not be spun sufficiently to rip out the threads within the bone of the neck or head (see Figs 14–30 and 14–31).

Impaction

With the side plate attached by 4 screws and all pins inserted into the head and neck, traction of the foot is released slightly and the impacting punch is placed in the impacting hole. Vigorous, heavy, impacting blows are used to collapse all comminuted fragments and to ensure stable continuity between the proximal fragment and the shaft of the femur (see Figs 14–27 and 14–28). In severely comminuted fractures the pins may back out as far as 1 inch. They are then tightened down by hand, flush with the plate. If the backout appears to be in excess of the amount of space left in the head of the femur, slightly shorter pins must be used so that they do not enter the joint. In the intertrochanteric fracture it is not essential that the pins be any closer than ¾ inch to the joint space after impaction (Fig 14–31). It is acceptable if one or two pins leave the neck of the femur, provided they do not impinge on the edge of the acetabulum. This may occur in a very small neck. Ideally, all the pins should remain within the neck.

It is not necessary to do an osteotomy even in the most severely comminuted fractures. The vigorous impaction collapses the proximal fragment along the pins, which act as a guide. The intervening comminuted fractures are collapsed and impacted. The plate gathers up the comminuted fragments and maintains a large base

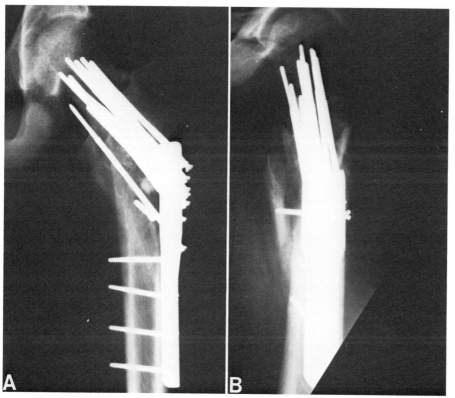

*Fig 14–31—**A,** severely comminuted peritrochanteric fracture. Patient was walking and bearing full weight with the aid of a cane. There was early union 8 weeks postoperatively. Note lowerst pin had been inserted in impacted holes. **B,** lateral view. Note an additional screw has been inserted in a transverse position anterior to posterior.*

of bony contact for union. Some of the more comminuted fractures will look as though a MacMurray osteotomy had been performed, but this is the result of the vigorous impaction. Ideally, all impaction can be achieved at surgery and visually assessed by watching the pins back out. The final set of radiograph films is made and the wound is closed in the routine manner over suction drainage tubes. In some of the more comminuted fractures and in osteoporotic patients, there may be further collapse, and the pins will back out of the plate a short distance. There may be some medial displacement as a result of the impaction.

Postoperative Care

Postoperative care is the same as for patients with neck fractures. There is some variation in monitoring their progress.

Patients frequently complain of lateral pain over the hip and occasionally complain of groin pain, which is related to motion of the lesser trochanter pulled by the iliopsoas. These are of no consequence in intertrochanteric fractures. Groin pain in neck fractures is considered to be a sign of motion at the fracture site. Radiographic views are taken in 2 months and often show bone healing.

If the fracture is severely comminuted, the lesser trochanter and the iliopsoas are attached thereto in the presence of a large amount of hemorrhage. These patients frequently have groin pain. I have satisfied myself as to the cause of this pain by injecting patients with Xylocaine in the region of the lesser trochanter and having them walk. This alleviates the pain, which will eventually subside without any specific treatment. The above-described injection was primarily done to satisfy my curiosity about the etiology of the groin pain in comminuted intertrochanteric fractures. The patient also can be reassured. Weight-bearing is increased to the patient's tolerance. Often the patient can progress to full weight-bearing in 2–3 weeks. The clinical progress determines when the patient dispenses with crutches or a cane. Patients with undisplaced intertrochanteric fractures usually discard their canes or crutches in 6–8 weeks, and those with badly comminuted fractures in approximately 3 months.

Breakage of Pins

Because of the longer leverage in intertrochanteric fractures, nine patients among those I have treated have experienced pin breakage. These patients required an alteration in postoperative weight-bearing. In all cases of pin breakage, 9 pins had been used to fix the fracture, which substantiates the view that 11 to 14 pins would decrease the chance of pin breakage. Breakage of a pin in an unhealed fracture signifies that the stress around the fracture was sufficient to break the pin. There is one less pin to neutralize the force across the fracture than at the time of pin breakage. Therefore, one must either replace the broken pin under local anesthesia and insert additional pins if possible, or decrease the weight-bearing. Once the fracture has healed, pin breakage indicates that the plasticity of the bone is greater than the plasticity of the metal, and the metal fractures because of fatigue.

Complications in Author's Personal Series

There were three cases of infection, probably due to the large amount of soft tissue damage and the possibility of wound contamination through a torn surgical glove while working with sharp fragments. All cases of infection were eradicated, but two patients required removal of the plate and pins before the drainage stopped.

TABLE 14–5.—Results in Intertrochanteric Fractures

Feature	No.
Consecutive cases	204
Lost to follow-up	19
Reportable cases	185
Major complications	
Nonunion	0
Thrombophlebitis	1 (0.5%)
Infection	3 (1.5%)
Hospital deaths	5 (2.5%)
Minor loss of position (varus)	5 (2.3%)
Bursitis requiring removal	25 (12%)
Time to union	
Average	3.6 mo.
Shortest	2 mo.
Longest	7 mo.

This did not interfere with the healing process. There was no case of pulmonary embolism or of nonunion; there was one case of avascular necrosis at 8 years (Table 14–5).

Loss of Position

In view of the vigorous impaction at surgery necessary to gain stability between the proximal and distal fragments, there is very little movement of the pins following surgery. In those few cases in which a pin backed out, it indicated that the fracture had settled somewhat even after impaction at surgery. This occurred in a relatively small number of patients and did not affect the end result.

Removal of Plate and Pins

Removal of plate and pins is done on the same basis for neck fractures and intertrochanteric fractures. The plate and pins are removed in approximately 10% of cases because of a painful bursa, although usually not before 1 year.

REFERENCES

1. Deyerle W.M.: Absolute fixation of fracture of the hip with contact compression: A new fixation device. *Clin. Orthop.* 13:279, 1959.
2. Deyerle W.M.: Impacted fixation over resistant multiple pins. *Clin. Orthop.* 152:102, 1980.
3. *Campbell's Operative Orthopaedics,* ed. 5. St. Louis, C.V. Mosby Co., 1970, vol. 1, p. 586.
4. *Campbell's Operative Orthopaedics,* ed. 6. St. Louis, C.V. Mosby Co., 1980, vol. 1, p. 647.
5. Baril J.D., Sontegard D.A., Mathews L.S.: Rotational control of unstable subcapital fractures. *J. Bone Joint Surg.* 72A:613, 1975.
6. Frankel V.H.: *The Femoral Neck: Function, Fracture Mechanisms, Internal Fixation.* Springfield, Charles C Thomas, Publisher, 1960.
7. Frankel V., Burstein A.H.: *Orthopaedic Biomechanics.* Philadelphia, Lea & Febiger, 1970, p. 69.
8. Cotton F.J.: Artificial impaction hip fractures. *Surg. Gynecol. Obstet.* 45:307, 1927.
9. Anderson L.D.: Compression plate fixation and effect of different types of internal fixation on fracture healing. *J. Bone Joint Surg.* 47A:191, 1965.

10. Brindley H.H.: Avascular necrosis of the head of the femur. *Am. J. Orthop.* 52:50-52, 1963.
11. Eggers G.W., Shindler T.O., Pomerat C.M.: The influence of contact compression factor on osteogenesis in surgical fracture. *J. Bone Joint Surg.* 31A:693, 1949.
12. Frankel C.J., Strider D.V., Pole W.C.: The development of circulation in the femurs of dogs after fracture of the femoral necks. *Surg. Forum* 7:608-610, 1957.
13. Watson-Jones R.: *Fractures and Joint Injuries.* Baltimore, Williams & Wilkins Co., 1952, 1955.
14. Scheck M.: Unstable internal fixation of intracapsular fractures of the neck of the femur of the adduction type. *J. Bone Joint Surg.* 41:558-559, 1959.
15. Rydell N.W.: Forces acting on the femoral head prosthesis: A study on strain gauge supplied prosthesis in living persons. *Acta Orthop. Scand.* 37:88, 1966.
16. Ceder L., Thorngren K.: Prognostic indications and early home rehabilitation in elderly patients with hip fractures. *Clin. Orthop.* 152:173, 1980.
17. Garden R.S., Preston B.V.: Low angle fixation of the femoral neck. *J. Bone Joint Surg.* 93B:647, 1961.
18. Garden R.S.: Malreduction and avascular necrosis in subcapital fractures of the femur. *J. Bone Joint Surg.* 53B:183, 1971.
19. Thorling J., Edholm P.: Methods for assessing fixation and residual angulation in intracapsular hip fractures. *Acta Radiol. Diagn.* 22:441-447, 1981.
20. Thorling J.: Intracapsular hip fractures treated with the Deyerle device: Incidence of non-unions, in Thorling J.: *Intracapsular Hip Fractures Treated With the Deyerle Device.* Linkoping, Linkoping University Medical Dissertations, No. 94, 1980.
21. Thorling J.: Intracapsular fractures treated with the Deyerle device results of the two-year follow-up: Incidence of segmented collapse, in Thorling J.: *Intracapsular Hip Fractures Treated With the Deyerle Device.* Linkoping, Linkoping University Medical Dissertation, No. 94, p. 103.
22. Edholm P., Thorling J.: Measurement of the shortening of the femur following immobilization of intracapsular hip fractures with the Deyerle device. *Acta Radiol. Diagn.* 22:89-95, 1981.
23. McCutchen J.W., Carnesale P.G.: Comparison of fixation in the treatment of femoral neck fractures. *Clin. Orthop.* 171:44, 1982.
24. Meyers M.H., Harry J.P. Jr., Moore T.M.: Treatment of displaced subcapital and transcervical fractures of the femoral neck by muscle pedicle bone graft and internal fixation: A preliminary report of 150 cases. *J. Bone Joint Surg.* 55A:257, 1973.
25. Schwab J.P., Karr R.K.: Subtrochanteric fractures as a complication of proximal femoral pinning with Knowles and Neufeld pins. Unpublished manuscript.
26. Calandruccio R.A., Anderson W.E.: Post-fracture avascular necrosis of the femoral head: Correlation of experimental and clinical studies. *Clin. Orthop.* 152:49, 1980.
27. Ferguson A.B.: Personal communication, 1953.
28. Soto Hall R., Johnson L.H., Johnson R.: Alterations in the intra-articular pressures in transcervical fracture of the hip. *J. Bone Joint Surg.* 46A:622, 1963.
29. Brown J.T., Abrami G.: Transcervical femoral fracture: A review of 195 patients with sliding nail plate fixation. *J. Bone Joint Surg.* 46B:648, 1964.
30. Deyerle W.M.: Multiple pin peripheral fixation in fractures of the neck of the femur: Immediate weight-bearing. *Clin. Orthop.* 39:135, 1965.
31. Crawford H.B.: Conservative treatment of impacted fractures of the femoral neck. *J. Bone Joint Surg.* 42A:471-479, 1960.
32. Deyerle W.M.: Absolute fixation of hip fractures. *Am. J. Orthop.* 9:206, 1967.
33. Deyerle W.M.: Etiology and treatment of nonunion of the femoral neck by grafting and rigid fixation. *Am. J. Orthop.* 10:18, 1965.
34. Deyerle W.M.: Fracture of the neck of the femur: Whither? Union or coexistence? *Am. J. Orthop.* 2:217, 1960.
35. Deyerle W.M.: Plate and peripheral pins in hip fractures, two plane reduction: Total impaction and absolute fixation. *Curr. Pract. Orthop. Surg.* 3:173, 1966.

36. Deyerle W.M.: Surgical impaction over a plate and multiple pins for intertrochanteric fractures. *Orthop. Clin. North Am.* 5:615, 1974.
37. Fielding J.A.: The telescoping Pugh nail in the surgical management of the displaced intracapsular fracture of the femoral neck. *Clin. Orthop.* 152:123, 1980.
38. Sherman M.S., Phemister D.B.: The pathology of ununited fracture of the neck of the femur. *J. Bone Joint Surg.* 29:19-40, 1947.
39. Johnson L.: Personal communication.
40. Metz C.W. Jr., Sellers T.D., Feagin J.A., et al.: The displaced intracapsular fracture of the neck of the femur: Experience with the Dyerele method of fixation in sixty-three cases. *J. Bone Joint Surg.* 52A:113, 1970.
41. Phemister D.B.: Fracture of neck of femur: Dislocation of hip and obscure vascular disturbances producing aseptic necrosis of head of femur. *Surg. Gynecol. Obstet.* 59:415, 1934.
42. Phemister D.B.: Changes in bones and joints resulting from interruption of circulation: General considerations and changes resulting from injuries. *Arch. Surg.* 41:436-472, 1940.
43. Tovee E.B., Gendron E.: The use of radioactive phosphorus in the determination of the viability of the femoral head in dogs after subcapital fractures. *J. Bone Joint Surg.* 36A:185, 1954.
44. Baker B.I., Barrick E.F.: Follow-up notes on article previously published in the *Journal:* Deyerle treatment for femoral neck fractures. *J. Bone Joint Surg.* 60A:2:269, 1978.
45. Chapman M.W., Stahr J.H., Eberle C.F., et al.: Treatment of intercapsular hip fractures by the Deyerle method. *J. Bone Joint Surg.* 57A:735, 1975.
46. Pauwels F.: *Der Schenkelhalsbruch: Ein mechanisches Problem.* Stuttgart, Ferdinand Enke, 1935.
47. Bunata R.E., Fahey J.J., Drennan D.B.: Factors influencing stability and necrosis of impacted neck fractures. *JAMA* 223:41, 1973.
48. Smith F.B.: Effects of rotary and valgus malposition on blood supply to the femoral head. *J. Bone Joint Surg.* 41A:800, 1959.
49. Montgomery W.: Personal communication.
50. Boyd H.B., George I.L.: Complications of fractures of the neck of the femur. *J. Bone Joint Surg.* 29:13-18, 1947.
51. Boyd H.B., Salvatore J.E.: Acute fractures of the femoral neck: Internal fixation or prosthesis. *J. Bone Joint Surg.* 46A:1066, 1964.
52. Bonfiglio M.: Aseptic necrosis of the femoral head in dogs: Effect of drilling and bone grafting. *Surg. Gynecol. Obstet.* 98:591, 1954.

Chapter 15

One-Piece Nail Plate for Treatment of Intertrochanteric Fractures

Alonzo J. Neufeld, M.D.

In 1937 Thornton suggested that a side bar attached to a triflanged nail would be useful for treating intertrochanteric fractures.[1] However, this was a two-piece nail plate and was not as rigid a system as the single-piece nail.

Preston in 1915 introduced a one-piece nail plate.[2] The nail was threaded, and a smooth portion that fitted along the femoral shaft was fixed with a screw. In 1940 I introduced a "V" nail with a plate extension to fix the femoral shaft; experience with this device was reported in 1944.[3] It had the same angular shape as the Preston device but was forged and heavier. The Jewett one-piece nail plate, introduced in 1941, was heavier than the Neufeld device and was popular in orthopedic surgery until the advent of the sliding devices.[4] To reduce the frequency of nail breakage, Holt in 1963 introduced a very stout, rigid nail plate, which was cast.[5] The Neufeld device was later redesigned and made heavier. All of these nail plate combinations are shown in Fig 15–1.

More recently, I designed a one-piece nail plate that can be introduced percutaneously through a small stab wound (see Fig 15–1). It has the added feature of a spring on a screw to reduce the stress shielding of the stiff hip nail.

One-piece nail devices work best when the fracture is stable. The unstable intertrochanteric fracture must be converted to a stable situation by establishing continuity of the bone along the medial aspect of the femoral neck, trochanter, and upper shaft. Reduction and impaction permit the bone to share most of the load and stress applied to the hip.[6] Otherwise, settling and impaction of the fragments on the nail can be of great magnitude. Penetration or pullout of the nail from the head fragment may follow. The stability of reduction and the rigidity of fixation must be maximal. The surgeon should not depend on the fixation device to achieve impaction and settling of the fracture fragments.

Collapsible nails were designed to reduce the frequency of femoral head penetration by the nail on settling or collapse of the unstable intertrochanteric fracture. Their use, however, has encouraged a degree of carelessness on the part of some surgeons, resulting in less than vigorous attempts at compaction of the fragments

172

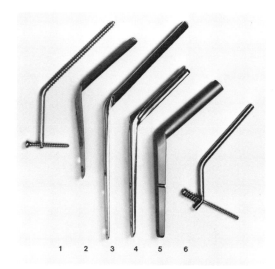

Fig 15–1—Various one-piece nail plate combinations: 1, Preston nail plate; 2, Neufeld nail plate; 3, second-generation Neufeld nail plate; 4, Jewett nail plate; 5, Holt nail plate; 6, percutaneous Neufeld nail plate (experimental design).

at surgery. This violates the principles of internal fixation, in that stability of reduction and rigidity of fixation must be maximal.

One-piece nail plate devices provide a great deal of stress shielding, which weakens the bone. The first Neufeld device is springy and there is a greater danger of stress failure because it is lighter. Because of the stress shielding of this light device, nail breakage has sometimes taken place in 1–2 months. When the nail fails, pain recurs and the patient must return to external support in the form of a walker or crutches until the pain subsides after fracture healing. Removal of the nail fragments may be necessary if they cause irritation or pain on pressure over the lateral aspect of the hip.

Single-nail plate devices for the treatment of intertrochanteric fractures are indicated for stable fractures. Use of these nails in unstable, comminuted, or osteoporotic fractures may be problematic. Additional fixation with screws, wire, or both is often necessary.

SURGICAL TECHNIQUE

In the early period fluoroscopy was used to check fracture reduction and placement of the guide wire. The lateral position was checked radiographically with the leg in the frogleg position. The experienced surgeon often was able to use an index finger to direct the insertion of the guide pin (Fig 15–2).

The technique changed when the rotating fluoroscope became available. The patient is placed on a fracture table. The fracture is then reduced by traction and rotation of the distal fragment while the thigh is held in 20° of flexion and 20° of abduction. After reduction of the fracture, the limb is fixed to the footplate with the limb held in the reduced position. Reduction is achieved while the patient is on the operating table. The accuracy of reduction, as well as the nail insertion, is monitored by fluoroscopy, in planes 90° apart, with the patient secured to the operating table. The actual guide pin or nail can be inserted in a more precise fashion.

Placement of the nail is simplified if the vastus lateralis is cut near its origin and retracted anteriorly. The surgeon then grasps the trochanteric region between thumb and fingers to support the fragments and prevent posterior displacement. A guide pin is inserted and the lateral cortex drilled for nail insertion 3 cm below the

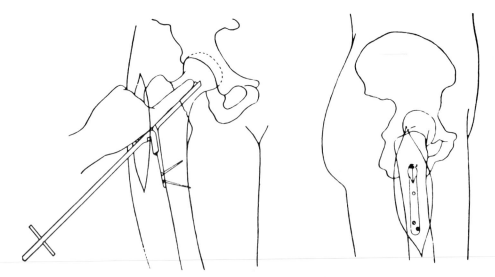

Fig 15–2—Guide pin insertion.

flare of the trochanter. Drilling must be done carefully to avoid fracture of the cortex. A guide pin is inserted and checked for position and nail length. The appropriate nail plate is selected and driven into place. The fracture is further impacted and the plate fixed to the shaft with screws.

Insertion of the nail should proceed with ease. If a mallet is required for insertion, in all probability the nail is penetrating the neck.

Multiple insertions of the nail must be avoided at all costs, since bone is destroyed and firm nail placement is impaired. The ideal position of the nail is in the inferior and posterior halves of the femoral neck and 1–1½ cm from the articular surface of the femoral head. Nail position must be checked in both the anteroposterior and the lateral planes.

In some cases it may be necessary to increase the stability of the fracture by fixing the lesser trochanter with a long screw or cerclage wire.

A very important feature of technique is the nail hole, which should be about 1 cm deeper in the lateral femoral cortex than the nail length. This permits loading of the fracture as healing progresses. The screws that hold the plate to the femoral shaft should be angled and not parallel to each other. This spreads the loading forces and lessens bone or screw breakage.

When there is a large amount of comminution or osteoporosis, we must seek as much bone contact and stability as possible. This may require wire or screws. Closure of the lateral incision by layers is usually not a problem.

The most important part of postoperative care is to have the patient up and sitting in a wheelchair. The second is to have the leg joints, hip, knee, and foot exercise in the painless range. This may require special care to avoid loading to the point of pain. By using pendulum motion, the hip joint can be exercised with little energy expenditure, and the stress at the fracture site will be slight. Pendulum exercises can be carried out by the patient in bed or standing on the floor with a walker. The patient should be conscious of possible harm if he loads the foot and leg too much. It is much easier to retain function than to regain it once it is lost.

Pain on weight-bearing is usually a contraindication to unprotected weight-bearing. The elderly patient is rarely strong enough to use crutches and must depend on other means of support to begin weight-bearing. Walking should be started with the aid of attendants and preferably a physical therapist. Protection should not be abandoned too soon. Pain in the hip with each step means that the fracture is not healed.

COMPLICATIONS

There are several complications that can be prevented.

Late Penetration of the Acetabulum

Penetration of the nail into the acetabulum occurs frequently if the nail is too long or placed improperly. Once the fracture has been reduced and vigorously impacted, the tip of the nail should lie no further than 1–1½ cm from the surface of the femoral head and in the posteroinferior portion of the femoral head, as noted on both anteroposterior and lateral x-ray films. This position will allow further settling after firm impaction at surgery. Should penetration into the acetabulum occur on settling, a shorter nail can be inserted at a second operation. The surgeon may leave the penetrated nail in place until union has occurred, provided that the level of pain does not dictate a change. The nail can then be removed after osseous union.

Disruption of Internal Fixation and Loss of Reduction

This complication arises when there is a severe degree of osteoporosis and the nail selected is short or improperly placed. Displacement of the fragments will occur when the nail is short, since there are few trabeculae in the femoral neck or head for anchoring the nail. The forces exerted on the head fragment will produce movement of the fragment, causing displacement, loss of reduction, and penetration of the nail.

The proper nail length (1–1½ cm from the articular surface of the femoral head) and correct placement in the inferior and posterior halves of the femoral head will reduce the amount of displacement. Although the head fragment may move to a varus position, penetration will not follow. Osseous union with some varus angulation is acceptable in elderly patients with intertrochanteric fractures. The position of the nail in the posterior and inferior halves of the femoral head permits impaction of the trabeculae ahead of the nail while the fragment settles into varus angulation. Frequently, this leads to nail stability prior to penetration.

If osteoporosis is excessive so that the bone is very soft, some form of external fixation or traction is advisable, in addition to internal fixation. If the surgeon anticipates severe osteoporosis, he or she should consider treating the patient with external fixation or preferably traction and avoid an attempt at internal fixation. The nail plate acts only as an internal splint and must secure the fragments. A nail plate with too short a plate will not permit secure screw fixation of the plate to an osteoporotic shaft. The number of screws should be increased, and they should be angled and not parallel.

Inadequate Reduction

Deformities that are a consequence of inadequate reduction are coxa vara, external rotation of the distal fragment, and occasionally coxa valga.

Coxa vara is the most frequent deformity following an inadequate reduction. It is characterized by pain, abductor weakness, and shortening of the extremity. With a severe external rotational deformity the patient finds it difficult to place the foot in a normal position when walking. This can be very disabling for the aged patient. The surgeon must keep in mind that it is essential to manually lift and rotate the distal fragment into the anatomical position during surgery to prevent this complication.

Medial Migration of the Femoral Shaft With Penetration of the Nail

This complication can occur when the fracture is unstable (loss of the medial cortical buttress) or the lateral cortex of the greater trochanter is fractured by rough handling when the fragment is drilled for insertion of the nail, or during insertion of the nail. Some have suggested the addition of an auxiliary plate extending above the plate and abutting the greater trochanter to prevent this complication. The medial displacement procedure (see chapter 23) has been recommended for the severe unstable intertrochanteric fracture in osteoporotic bone.

Delayed Union With Nail Deformity or Breakage

Fracture of the nail usually follows prolonged cyclic loading in the setting of delayed union. Failure to impact the fracture fragments may permit separation of the fragments by the nail. Internal fixation also slows the rate of osseous healing. If these two features are present, unprotected weight-bearing may begin too early. After nail breakage impaction of the fragments can take place, and osseous union follows in a few weeks. When nail breakage occurs the patient should be returned to protected weight-bearing. The surgeon may choose to renail the fracture and add autogenous bone grafts to hasten the healing process.

Failure to Complete Internal Fixation

Occasionally the surgeon may not be able to reduce and securely fix a comminuted intertrochanteric fracture. This is frequently the case when the bone is markedly osteoporotic or the nail has been inserted multiple times. The nail should then be removed and a cast or traction method selected for treatment. Multiple insertions of the nail increase the amount of bone destruction, making fixation impossible.

Others

Fear, anxiety, and pain may result in the patient's refusal to bear weight on the affected extremity. Osteoporosis and contractures are late sequelae that increase the rehabilitation time or result in a permanently disabled nonwalker.

REFERENCES

1. Thornton L.: The treatment of trochanteric fractures: 2 new methods. *Piedmont Hosp. Bull.* 10:21, 1937.
2. Preston M. E.: New appliance for internal fixation of fractures of the femoral neck. *Surg. Gynecol. Obstet.* 18:260, 1914.
3. Taylor G. M., Neufeld A. J., Janzen J: Internal fixation for intertrochanteric fractures. *J. Bone Joint Surg.* 26:707-712, 1944.
4. Jewett E. L.: One piece angle nail for trochanteric fractures. *J. Bone Joint Surg.* 23:803-810, 1941.
5. Holt E.P. Jr.: Hip fracture in the trochanteric region: Treatment with a strong nail and early weight bearing. A report of one hundred cases. *J. Bone Joint Surg.* 45A:687, 1963.
6. Deyerle W.M.: Absolute fixation with contact compression in hip fractures (a new fixation device). *Clin. Orthop.* 13:279, 1959.

Chapter 16

Sliding and Compression Fixation

Edwin T. Wyman, Jr., M.D.

To gain a proper perspective on the use of sliding and compression devices in the considerable fixation armamentarium used in treatment of fractures about the hip, a few historical words may be helpful.

After Smith-Petersen demonstrated in 1931 that fixation of the femoral neck fracture greatly reduced mortality and improved function over that achieved with traction treatment, other devices gradually came into use, either to extend fixation principles to other hip fractures or to make the fixation more solid. With the use of a side plate attached to an intramedullary device fixing the proximal fragment of the femoral neck or intertrochanteric fracture, intertrochanteric fractures could be reduced and held firm and the strength of the device holding the distal fragment of femoral neck fractures could be increased. But such a procedure was not without certain hazards. In femoral neck fractures, gaining fixation on the shaft with such a device (Thornton, Jewett) also meant preventing impaction of the fracture line in fractures that were known not to be exactly reduced by closed manipulation in any case. Thus, nonunion rates after treatment with these devices remained in the vicinity of 25%. In addition, if bone was especially osteopenic, the incompletely reduced and slightly distracted fracture would tend to lose position even after fixation.

Problems developed in intertrochanteric fractures that were not stable, that is, did not have good bone contact throughout the fracture site, particularly at the points of greatest bending moment posteromedially. Solid nail plate devices often failed, either at the nail-plate junction (the screws holding the plate to the femoral shaft), or at the junction between nail and bone in the proximal fragment, which allowed the fractures to deform into varus angulation and external rotation. This problem was even more severe in comminuted intertrochanteric-subtrochanteric fractures.

In 1955 Pugh, and later Massie, advocated fixation devices that allowed impaction of the fracture by shortening the "nail" length—sliding the nail inside a barrel extension of the plate either at the time of fixation or through patient activity in the first few weeks postoperatively, or both. Since better bone contact was achieved by this fixation method, the rate of nonunion of femoral neck fractures fell to about 10% and the position loss and appliance breakage problem in intertrochanteric fracture treatment greatly lessened, although it was not eliminated. These devices had no effect on the incidence of avascular necrosis in intracapsular hip fractures, which remains at about 25% and is more dependent on the type of injury and accuracy of reduction than on the fixation device used.

DESCRIPTION

At present, the sliding or compression devices are widely used and have become standard in the treatment of intracapsular, basicervical, intertrochanteric, and intertrochanteric-subtrochanteric fractures of the femur. The common types are the sliding nail and the compression screw.

The sliding nail is a one-piece apparatus with a strong side plate and a nail with a tip that is flanged with either three or four fins and a proximal end that slides within the barrel attached to the plate. The nail tip is inserted into the femoral head by driving, and impaction is achieved by driving the barrel over the nail after insertion (Fig 16–1).

The compression screw is similar except that the apparatus is in two parts. The tip of the "nail" is a screw which is considerably larger than the flanged tip of the sliding nail and is inserted by turning it in after cutting a track with a tap. Impaction is also achieved by a screw inserted through the lateral end of the barrel into the larger screw to draw it back (Fig 16–2).

Both devices come in a variety of barrel plate angles so that the "nail" can be placed in more or less valgus angulation, depending on the anatomical requirements or the preference of the surgeon.

INDICATIONS
Intracapsular Fractures

Both sliding nails and compression screws may be used to fix this fracture (see Fig 16–2,A). The larger bulk of the compression screw, however, may be a relative contraindication to use in an area where one would like to interfere as little

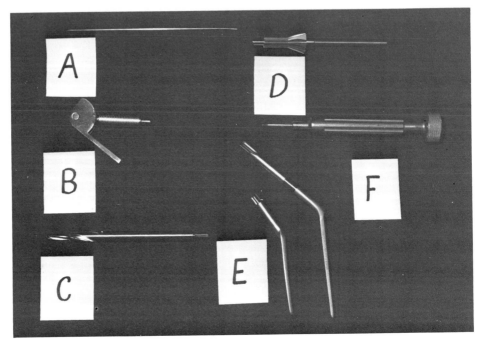

Fig 16–1—Instruments for sliding nail insertion: A, guide pin; B, angle guide; C, step drill; D, chamfering tool; E, sliding nails (note different plate lengths, barrel plate angles, and nails in collapsed and extended positions); F, calibrated driving and impacting tool. See text for further details.

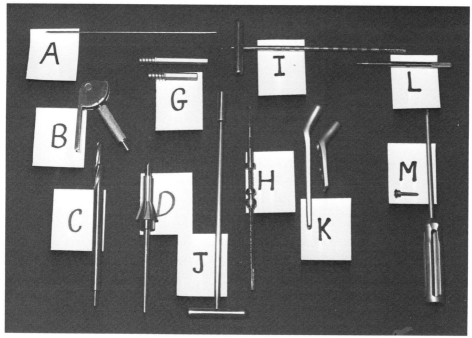

Fig 16–2—Instruments for compression screw insertion: A, guide pin; B, angle guide; C, step drill; D, chamfering tool; G, compression screws (note different lengths); H, calibrated reamer; I, tap; J, inserting tool; K, barrel plates (note different plate lengths and barrel plate angles); L, locator guide; M, compressing screw and screwdriver. See text for further details.

as possible with the remaining vascular supply to the femoral head. Another relative contraindication to use of the compression screw in this fracture relates to the fact that the screw is turned in rather than driven in. Since one of the major deformities of the intracapsular fracture itself involves a flexion-extension movement of the prox-imal fragment on the distal fragment, any excessive torque used in tapping the track for the screw will tend to accentuate this deformity. To prevent this, prior to tapping and placing the screw, it is mandatory to place one or two stout Kirschner wires across the fracture site away from the path of the screw to try to minimize movement. This is especially helpful in younger patients, in whom the bone in the femoral head is much more solid. These relative contraindications are not encountered with the sliding nail, although care must be taken that a low-lying nail does not drive the femoral head into excessive valgus angulation.

It should be noted that in fixing intracapsular fractures that are impacted in the valgus position, maintaining the impaction is the most important part of the fixation. For this reason, sliding nails should not be used in these cases. Compression screws may be utilized, but their tendency to torque the fracture is undesirable. Multiple pin fixation, with pins inserted by drilling rather than by driving, is probably the best fixation method.

Basicervical Fractures

As with intracapsular fractures, both sliding nails and compression screws may be used for fixation. One might say their use is more indicated here simply because some of the other fixation methods are not indicated. Multiple pin fixation, except for devices containing a lateral side plate such as the Deyerle apparatus, does not allow enough fixation on the distal fragment, and condylocephalic nails do not allow enough fixation on the proximal fragment.

Intertrochanteric Fractures

Stable, two-part intertrochanteric fractures, once reduced, require little inherent strength in the fixation device to maintain the reduction position. Thus several fixation methods work equally well and allow early ambulation, including weight-bearing. Both sliding nails and compression screws work well in this situation, but if there is a special need not to open the fracture site or to provide less surgical trauma, then condylocephalic fixation also works well. It must be remembered that the technique of this method is much more demanding than the relatively simple instrumentation would imply. For those who have mastered the technique, however, condylocephalic fixation may be the fixation method of choice in stable intertrochanteric fractures, particularly in patients who are especially poor surgical risks.

Unstable intertrochanteric fractures pose a different problem entirely. The comminution involved requires that either the fracture be converted into a stable configuration (as with displacement fixation) or that the device used be able to shorten as the fracture settles into a position of stability. It is in these fractures that use of the compression screw and sliding nail is most indicated, since other fixation methods are less effective in this regard. While sliding nails are commonly used in unstable intertrochanteric fractures, the compression screw (with its greater surface area holding onto the proximal fragment) seems to provide more resistance to angular deformity (varus and external rotation), at the cost of a slightly increased time of insertion because of the necessity for tapping. The strength of these devices is enough to allow early mobilization of the patient postoperatively without much risk of the fracture displacing, as long as the technical demands of insertion are obeyed. Settling of the fracture always occurs and averages 1½ cm. This takes place within the first 6 weeks after fixation and occurs to the same degree, whether or not ambulation is allowed (Figs 16–3 and 16–4). Therefore there is no advantage to an extended period of bed rest or bed/chair limitations unless osteopenia is so extreme that the bone–fixation device interface is especially weak. Any fixation device is prone to fail in these cases and more consideration should be given to nonoperative treatment methods.

Mention should be made of the intertrochanteric fracture with a reversed obliquity running from proximal medially to distal laterally. These fractures will not achieve a position of stability by displacing in the manner allowed by compression screws or sliding nails. Thus the particular advantage of these devices may actually become a disadvantage, as the device may allow unacceptable displacement of the fracture. In these cases, then, other devices that do not allow any sliding or compression may be indicated.

Intertrochanteric-Subtrochanteric Fractures

These fractures usually are comminuted and often present the most difficult management problems. While large subtrochanteric comminuted fragments may be attached to the main distal femoral fragment by extra screws or circumferential wires to increase stability, the fracture often remains deficient in bony contact medially at the intertrochanteric-subtrochanteric junction, where bone contact to resist the strong varus bending moment is most needed. Both the compression screw and sliding nail are mechanically most susceptible to stresses of this type because of the lateral position of the plate portion of the device. If possible, then, fixation devices that bring more support medially, such as the Zickel or condylocephalic nail, should be used. Still, the compression screw is technically often easier to use and, because of its strength, many times will succeed (Fig 16–5). When a compression screw is utilized in these fractures, it is essential that supplemental bone graft be used to reinforce any bone defect medially in the subtrochanteric area.

Table 16–1 summarizes the principal indications for use of a compression screw or a sliding nail.

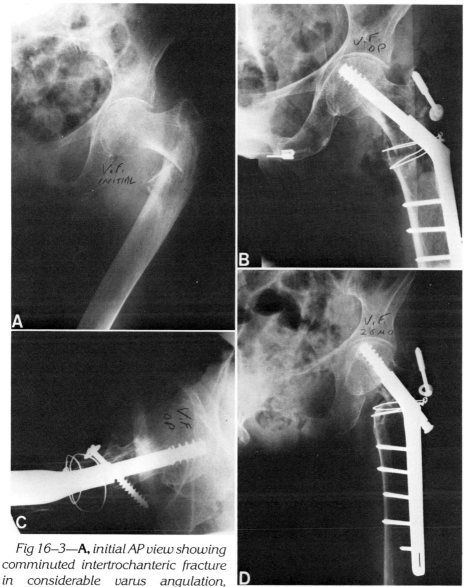

*Fig 16–3—**A,** initial AP view showing comminuted intertrochanteric fracture in considerable varus angulation, indicating instability. **B** and **C,** attempted anatomical fixation (incomplete) with compression screw, circumferential wires, and greater trochanteric screw. **D,** film made 26 months after fracture showing compression of 26 mm in spite of the patient being limited to bed/chair for 3 months. Patient was fully ambulatory.*

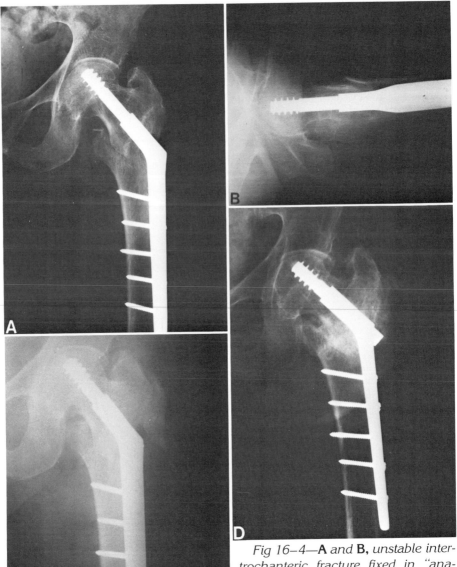

Fig 16–4—**A** and **B**, *unstable inter-trochanteric fracture fixed in "anatomical" position with central screw placement and good head penetration. **C,** position 1 month postoperatively showing 17 mm of compression (patient was on bed rest). **D,** full healing at 4 months with total compression of 22 mm. Patient was ambulatory 2 months postoperatively.*

TABLE 16–1.—Summary of Indications by Fracture Type		
	Compression Screw	**Sliding Nail**
Strong indications	Basicervical	Intracapsular
	Stable intertrochanteric	Basicervical
	Unstable intertrochanteric	Stable intertrochanteric
Relative indications	Intracapsular	Unstable intertrochanteric
	Reversed intertrochanteric	Reversed intertrochanteric
	Inter-subtrochanteric	
Not indicated	Intracapsular impacted in valgus	Intracapsular impacted in valgus
		Inter-subtrochanteric

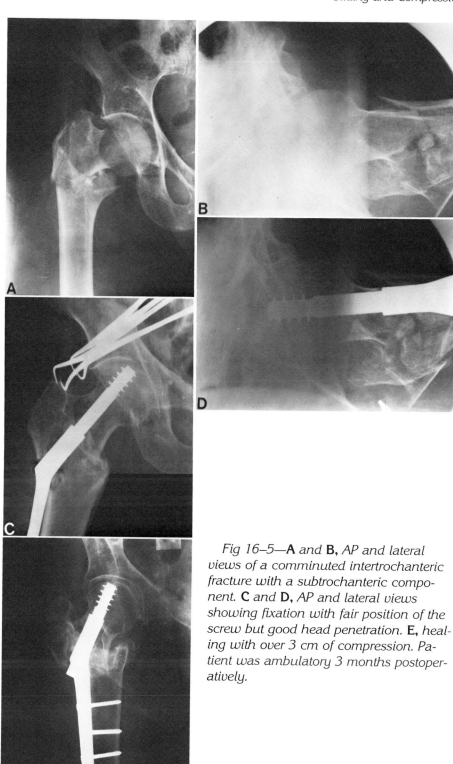

*Fig 16–5—**A** and **B,** AP and lateral views of a comminuted intertrochanteric fracture with a subtrochanteric component. **C** and **D,** AP and lateral views showing fixation with fair position of the screw but good head penetration. **E,** healing with over 3 cm of compression. Patient was ambulatory 3 months postoperatively.*

SURGICAL TECHNIQUE

Both sliding nails and compression screws can be inserted using either regular two-plane x-ray machines and a regular operating table or a C-arm fluoroscope and a fracture table that will accommodate this machine. The latter setup usually is preferred because of the significant saving in time. If a regular operating table is used to treat patients with subcapital fractures, the leg is fixed after closed reduction in hip extension, slight abduction, and full internal rotation, with the knee flexed 90° over the side of the operating table and the foot strapped to a stool to further stabilize the fracture by tightening the rectus femoris. Intertrochanteric fractures are best managed with the patient on a fracture table in traction, in slight flexion, abduction, and internal rotation.

After the x-ray equipment has been positioned and tested to document reductions and to make sure the machines are functioning properly, a lateral exposure of the upper femoral shaft is made. With all intertrochanteric fractures, it is a good policy to place one's forefinger behind the upper portion of the vastus lateralis muscle and gently insert it blindly through the external rotator muscles to palpate the back of the intertrochanteric area. This allows one not only to check reduction in this area but also to find comminution indicating instability, which often is not apparent on x-ray films because the fragments are not large enough. In intertrochanteric-subtrochanteric fractures, large comminuted medial pieces should be reduced to the main distal fragments and held there by circumferential wires or screws placed so as not to interfere with later nail plate placement (see Fig 16–3). These screws may be lagged, if desired, for some compression effect. This may require division of the iliopsoas tendon, which should cause no alarm, and the tendon need not be reattached.

One may decide to reduce more than one of these fragments in comminuted intertrochanteric and intertrochanteric-subtrochanteric fractures, but unless *all* fragments can be anatomically reduced and held well by screws or circumferential wires, the resulting fixation will be unstable and will redisplace later as the fixation device allows settling (see Fig 16–4). Usually, if only the largest fragments are reduced, the remaining smaller fragments may be completely ignored.

Next, the surgeon must decide where the nail or screw is to go in the femoral head. Many advocate a valgus position since the forces on the appliance will be more compressive than bending. This, however, requires that the large lateral hole in the femoral shaft be made through much harder cortical bone and that the end of the nail or screw be in final placement rather high in the head. Others believe that a low-lying nail (on the calcar femorale) will aid in decreasing bending stresses on the device. Certainly it is true that the screw or nail is better in the posterior position of the femoral head rather than the anterior, and inferior rather than superior (Fig 16–6). If the fracture starts to angle after fixation, the screw or nail will be in a position to remain in bone longer since the distal fragment and the device always move into external rotation and the femoral head always moves into a varus position. As a general rule, I feel that one should try to place the nail or screw as close to the center of the femoral neck and head as possible, since this allows maximum penetration and thus fixation on the femoral head.

Once these decisions have been made, a Kirschner guide wire is selected which is the stoutest that will fit in the cannulated instruments and device to be used. If a C-arm machine is being used, the entry point for the hole in the lateral femoral cortex can be determined by placing the guide wire (using an angle guide to determine the barrel plate angle) in the soft tissues just anterior to the femoral neck (see Fig

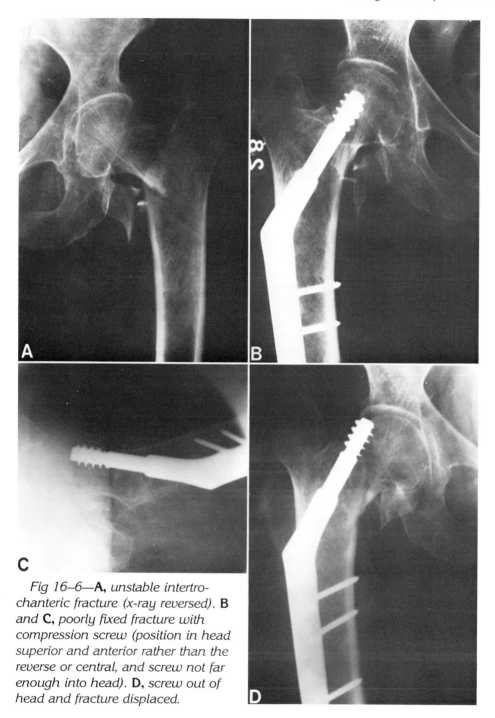

*Fig 16–6—**A**, unstable intertro-chanteric fracture (x-ray reversed). **B** and **C**, poorly fixed fracture with compression screw (position in head superior and anterior rather than the reverse or central, and screw not far enough into head). **D**, screw out of head and fracture displaced.*

16–1,*A* and *B*). A one-eighth inch drill hole is then made and the guide wire is inserted (again using the angle guide) in the proper position, as verified by AP and lateral films. The distance from the lateral cortex to the tip of the guide wire is then measured. A cannulated step drill (see Figs 16–1,*C* and 16–2,*C*) is then placed over the guide wire to cut a path for part of the nail or screw and for all of the barrel. Care must be taken not to vary the angle determined by the angle guide, since this will bend and may jam the wire and the plate eventually will not fit well on the shaft. A chamfering tool (see Figs 16–1,*D* and 16–2,*D*) must then be used to reduce the sharp bone edges of the hole for the barrel inferiorly to allow room for the reinforced material of the device, which can be noted at this spot. At this point, the procedure differs somewhat, depending on whether a sliding nail or compression screw is being used, and so each will be discussed separately.

Sliding Nails

The proper sliding nail is selected, with the surgeon noting carefully the proper maximum and minimum length of the nail, length of the barrel, length of the plate, and plate barrel angle (see Fig 16–1,*E*). The nail is inserted collapsed and with the plate clamped to the femoral shaft. The guide wire is then removed. The nail is then advanced to its proper position using the calibrated driver (see Fig 16–1,*F*) and its position is confirmed by x-ray or C-arm fluoroscopy in both AP and lateral planes. Care should be taken not to insert the nail beyond the point desired (within 1 cm of the articular surface). Since the nail length was selected so that it would be near its full extended length when in proper position, a full potential for collapse of the nail is available. Traction is then released from the leg and the driver adjusted so that impaction can be carried out (see Fig 16–1,*F*). After this has been done, the plate is fixed to the femoral shaft with screws. The length of the plate should allow both cortices of two screws to be within the distal fragment of intracapsular fractures, three for basicervical fractures, and four for intertrochanteric and subtrochanteric fractures.

Special Points

If other than a central position of the proximal end of the sliding nail within the femoral head is selected in intracapsular fractures, one must carefully watch radiographically during driving that the head is not driven into a varus (if the nail is superior) or valgus (if the nail is inferior) position.

If a nail plate angle is selected so the sliding nail is in relative valgus to the femoral neck and head, care must be taken not to leave the nail too superior in the femoral head in the final position (see Fig 16–6).

Since the nail, barrel, and plate are all inserted at one time, special care must be taken to keep the step drill and the nail itself exactly in line with the guide wire. Failure to do so will result in the plate not fitting exactly to the femoral shaft, or in bending the guide wire and possibly driving it into the acetabulum or pelvis. Checking the position of the guide pin radiographically and measuring the length of the protruding portion of the guide pin during insertion of the sliding nail should prevent this complication.

As the sliding nail is inserted, the plate must be carefully lined up with the shaft so that they meet exactly when the nail has been fully inserted. The nail must not be driven too far into the femoral head (within 1 cm of the articular surface is adequate), since slight withdrawal will significantly weaken head fixation.

Compression Screw

A screw (see Fig 16–2,*G*) is selected which is one-half inch shorter than the measured length of the guide pin from the lateral femoral cortex to the tip of the pin to ensure that at least that much compression is available within the device before the screw will protrude from the barrel laterally. One or two Kirschner wires of the same size as the guide wire are then inserted into the femoral head. (They may be carried into the acetabulum for extra stability.) These wires should be placed so that they will not interfere with the tapping or screw placement. The guide wires are to prevent the proximal fragment from displacing in a rotatory manner during tapping. The extra wires need not be used if the bone seems very osteoporotic or in inter-trochanteric fractures (a finger placed on the distal end of the proximal fragment anteriorly during tapping and screw placement will sense excessive torque and frag-ment rotation) but are essential in younger patients and in patients with intracapsular fractures. A cannulated and calibrated reamer (see Fig 16–2, *H*), the diameter of the shaft of the screw, is then used to cut a path along the guide wire, with great care taken to keep the reamer exactly in line with the guide pin. Since this will release the guide pin throughout its length, one should drive the pin farther into the femoral head before reaming. The proper position of the reamer is checked radiographically. (It should be within 1 cm of the articular surface also.) The reamer is removed and the same track followed with the tap (see Fig 16–2, *I*). The point of insertion of the tap in the femoral head is the point of maximum torquing effect. The position of the tap also is checked radiographically. The tap and guide wire are then removed and the selected screw is inserted with the inserting tool (see Fig 16–2, *J*). Since the screw is one-half inch shorter than the length of the guide pin, the lateral end of the screw will be one-half inch deep to the lateral femoral cortex. A barrel plate unit is then selected with the desired length of plate (the same number of screws are needed in the distal fragment as with sliding nails), the proper barrel plate angle, and barrel length (see Fig 16–2, *K*). In some systems, a keyless barrel may be selected that allows free rotation of the screw in the barrel, but I have not found this to be of great practical advantage or disadvantage. A locator guide (see Fig 16–2, *L*) is placed in the recessed lateral end of the screw and the barrel is inserted on the screw and impacted gently into place. The plate is clamped to the shaft, traction released, and the fracture impacted using the handle of the screw inserter (see Fig 16–2, *J*). Further compression is obtained by inserting a small compressing screw (see Fig 16–2, *M*) into the barrel and drawing down on the larger compression screw. This screw may then be removed or left in place. The plate is then fixed to the femoral shaft with screws.

Special Points

Depending on the expected amount of settling of the fracture, the length of the compression screw may be shorter than the one-half inch difference between the length of the guide pin, but it should not be longer.

The barrel length selected should not be so long as to prevent the fracture from settling into a stable position, since this will negate the advantage of the compres-sion screw and cause the apparatus to cut out.

In very osteoporotic bone, tapping may be eliminated to increase the holding power of the screw, but care must be taken in any case not to tighten the screw with more than "three-finger" strength to avoid stripping the threads within the bone.

If a low-lying track is selected, remember that the compression screw is quite large and the tap must not impinge on the calcar as it passes by, since it will not easily tap this hard bone.

There is really only one chance to get a compression screw fixed firmly in the femoral head. Trying to change the path of the compression screw after the reamer has been passed is usually fruitless.

Special care must be taken to keep the reamer and tap exactly lined up with the guide wire during passage. Failure to do so will result in bending the guide wire (and thus advancing the wire into the acetabulum as the reamer or tap is passed), cutting a different path so that the final barrel plate angle will not fit, or occasionally even bending the reamer or tap (if one is trying to hold a certain reduction position with this instrument during use). Frequent use of C-arm fluoroscopy or radiography and measuring the barrel length of the protruding guide pin will help prevent this. The surgeon must be extremely careful not to insert the reamer or tap farther than desired, since this will decrease the holding power of the screw (Fig 16–7).

The plate must be lined up with the femoral shaft during insertion of the barrel so that the fit will be exact.

In using this device for unstable intertrochanteric fractures, the surgeon must make sure that the screw is in the center of the femoral neck and head in both AP and lateral views, that the tip of the compression screw is within 1 cm of the articular surface of the femoral head, that the length of the screw is not so long that it will protrude laterally when the fracture is fully settled, and that the barrel length is not so long as to prevent full settling of the fracture. Very unstable intertrochanteric fractures may settle as much as 3 cm. The small compressing screw should be left in place since cases have been described in which the screw has become disconnected from the barrel proximally. The small compressing screw must not be overtightened, in osteoporotic bone, as it is possible to pull the screw out of the femoral head by overzealous compression.

When using C-arm fluoroscopy, the surgeon should document the final fixation with permanent films.

AFTER TREATMENT

In general, mobilization of the patient is not specifically limited after either a satisfactory sliding nail or compression screw fixation, since the apparatus affords excellent strength and encourages settling of the fracture into a stable position. The leg is supported in a suspension device for comfort in bed, but mobilization to a chair may be begun on the first or second postoperative day, and supported weight-bearing (even though in most elderly patients this amounts to full weight-bearing) as soon as the patient is able. In unstable intertrochanteric and intertrochanteric-subtrochanteric fractures, one should expect to see an additional 1.5–3 cm of settling of the fracture over the first 6 weeks (see Figs 16–3, 16–4, 16–5, and 16–7). One should not be alarmed by this. During the early postoperative period in these fractures, care should be taken during transfer not to lift the patient by pulling on the affected leg, since one may distract the fracture by this maneuver.

COMPLICATIONS

In spite of careful anticipation of the pitfalls of these procedures as outlined above, occasional complications will occur.

NAIL OR SCREW CUTS OUT OR SCREWS IN FEMORAL SHAFT BREAK AND FRACTURE DISPLACES.—This complication usually occurs because the nail or screw was not placed deeply enough in the femoral head (see Fig 16–6), the nail or screw was not centrally placed in the femoral neck and head (except for those deliberately placed in valgus to make the stresses on the apparatus more compressive), the nail or screw fully collapsed before the fracture reached a stable position, the screw pulled out of the barrel proximally, or too long a barrel has been used and it is keeping the fracture

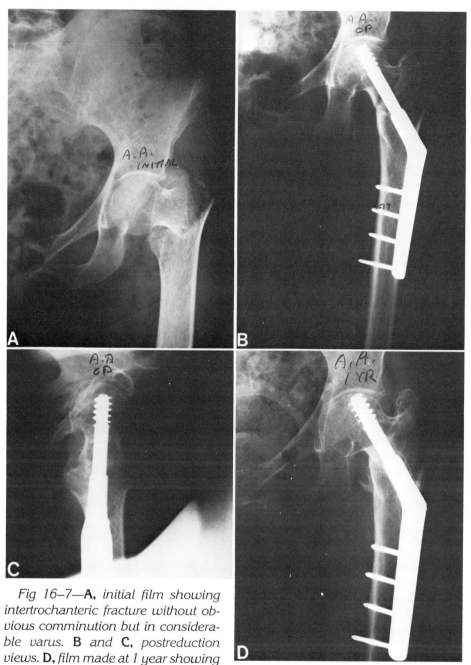

*Fig 16–7—**A,** initial film showing intertrochanteric fracture without obvious comminution but in considerable varus. **B** and **C,** postreduction views. **D,** film made at 1 year showing full healing, screw compression of 13 mm, and slight varus displacement of proximal fragment.*

from settling into a stable position. If one of these complications occurs several weeks postoperatively and the position of the fracture fragments is still satisfactory, it may be that nothing need be done because the fracture (after the fixation apparatus has failed) has now reached a stable position and will progress to union with limited activity only. If the complication occurs earlier and the position is not satisfactory, there are several treatment options. The patient may be placed in traction and treatment instituted as if operative treatment had never been attempted. The fracture may be reoperated on under certain conditions. The screw usually cannot be replaced in a new position because there is not enough good bone remaining in the femoral head to allow adequate fixation. Also, a sliding nail usually cannot be replaced by a compression screw—nor can a fixation device such as a condylocephalic nail be replaced by either a sliding nail or a compression screw. One can replace a compression screw *in the same track* with a longer or shorter one, or replace the barrel plate component of a compression screw with a longer or shorter component, if that will solve the technical problem that gave rise to the complication in the first place. Usually, however, another fixation device and an entirely new track (such as a blade plate with a right angle) must be used to refix the fracture. Consideration can also be given in some fractures to conversion to a prosthetic replacement or total hip replacement with or without calcar substitution. Since severe osteopenia is often partly to blame for the failure of fixation, prosthetic replacement may not be an ideal answer. These severe displacements are more easily prevented by careful preoperative evaluation and operative technique than they are treated once they occur.

GUIDE PIN DRIVEN INTO THE ACETABULUM OR PELVIS.—If the pin is in the acetabulum only, it can be removed and replaced without significant consequence. If the pin is bent, it should be removed without twisting, since that may break the pin at the point of angulation. If the pin has broken and violates the hip joint, it must be removed by separate hip arthrotomy. If the pin has been driven intrapelvically, it should be removed and the patient observed very carefully postoperatively for intrapelvic bleeding, urinary extravasation, or urinary bleeding. These complications must be handled by separate surgical and nonsurgical methods, as needed. It has been my experience that usually no significant damage results from intrapelvic pin protrusion, but very careful postoperative observation is nonetheless mandatory.

THE SMALL COMPRESSING SCREW BECOMES LOOSE IN THE SOFT TISSUE.—This commonly occurs in compression screw fixation and usually produces no symptoms. It can be ignored since the screw has not been needed after initial use, except in very unstable intertrochanteric fractures (where it prevents the main compression screw from moving proximally in the barrel), and is commonly removed by some surgeons at that point. If this loose screw is symptomatic, it may be removed easily under local anesthesia.

SUMMARY

Sliding nails and compression screws have a major role in fixation of fractures of the upper femur. They are strong and their inherent collapsibility make them ideal for intracapsular fractures to minimize the problem of nonunion, and for unstable intertrochanteric fractures to achieve fracture stability. They are not a panacea, however, and strict attention to operative detail is necessary to avoid complications.

The knowledgeable trauma surgeon must be able to use all the fixation techniques discussed in this and other chapters, since there are always individual cases for which one technique is superior to others.

BIBLIOGRAPHY
1. Cameron H.U., Graham J.D.: Retention of the compression screw in sliding screw plate devices. *Clin. Orthop.* 146:219, 1980.
2. Chapman M.W., Stahl J.H., Eberle C., et al.: Treatment of intracapsular hip fractures by the Deyerle method. *J. Bone Joint Surg.* 57A:735, 1975.

3. Clawson D.L.: Trochanteric fractures treated by the sliding screw plate fixation method. *J. Trauma* 4:736, 1964.
4. Dimon J.H., Hughston J.C.: Unstable intertrochanteric fractures of the hip. *J. Bone Joint Surg.* 49A:440, 1967.
5. Evans E.M.: Treatment of trochanteric fractures of the hip. *J. Bone Joint Surg.* 31B:190, 1949.
6. Fielding J.W.: The telescoping Pugh nail in the surgical management of the displaced intracapsular fractures of the femoral neck. *Clin. Orthop.* 152:123, 1980.
7. Garden R.S.: Low angle fixation in fractures of the femoral neck. *J. Bone Joint Surg.* 43B:647, 1961.
8. Jacobs R.R., McClain O., Armstrong H.J.: Internal fixation of intertrochanteric fractures: A clinical and biomechanical study. *Clin. Orthop.* 146:62, 1980.
9. Jewett E.L.: One piece angle nail for trochanteric fractures. *J. Bone Joint Surg.* 23:803, 1941.
10. Kyle R.F., Gustilo R.G., Premer R.F.: Analysis of six hundred and twenty-two intertrochanteric hip fractures: A retrospective and prospective study. *J. Bone Joint Surg.* 61A:216, 1979.
11. Massie W.K.: Extracapsular fractures of the hip treated by impaction using a sliding nail-plate fixation. *Clin. Orthop.* 22:180, 1962.
12. Mulholland R.C., Gunn D.R.: Sliding screw plate fixation of intertrochanteric femoral fractures. *J. Trauma* 12:581, 1972.
13. Pugh W.L.: A self adjusting nail plate for fractures about the hip joint. *J. Bone Joint Surg.* 37A:1005, 1955.
14. Sarmiento A.: Intertrochanteric fractures of the femur: 150 degree angle nail plate fixation and early rehabilitation. A preliminary report of 100 cases. *J. Bone Joint Surg.* 45A:706, 1963.
15. Schrumpelnich W., Jantzen P.U.: A new principle in the operative treatment of trochanteric fractures of the femur. *J. Bone Joint Surg.* 37A:693, 1955.
16. Smith-Petersen M.N., Cave E.F., Van Gorder G.: Intracapsular fractures of the neck of the femur: Treatment by internal fixation. *Arch. Surg.* 23:715, 1931.
17. Taylor G.M., Neufeld A.J., Nickel V.L.: Complications and failures in the operative treatment of intertrochanteric fractures of the femur. *J. Bone Joint Surg.* 37A:306, 1955.
18. Thornton L.: Treatment of trochanteric fractures: Two new methods. *Piedmont Hosp. Bull.* 10:21, 1937.
19. Wolfgang G.L., Bryant M.H., O'Neill J.P.: Treatment of intertrochanteric fractures of the femur using sliding screw plate fixation. *Clin. Orthop.* 163:148, 1982.

Chapter 17

Quadratus Femoris Muscle Pedicle Graft

Marvin H. Meyers, M.D.

T he **quadratus femoris** muscle pedicle graft with internal fixation of displaced femoral neck fractures was developed to improve the rate of osseous union and to decrease the incidence of late segmental collapse of the femoral head.[1] Reports of a 10%–15% incidence of nonunion and a 30% late segmental collapse of the femoral head in united fractures continued unabated following the introduction of the Smith-Peterson nail, despite subsequent changes in technique and innovations in the design of metallic fixative devices.

In 1962, Judet reported the use of a muscle pedicle graft of the quadratus femoris muscle in displaced femoral neck fractures.[1] Earlier and contemporary reports indicated that muscle pedicle bone grafts could provide a significant capillary blood supply to bone in humans[2-8] and animals.[9-13] In 1962 and 1963 the blood supply was successfully restored in experimentally induced avascular femoral heads of dogs.[11, 14] In 1974, my colleagues and I reported on the first large series of patients treated with the muscle pedicle technique and major modifications in the Judet surgical procedure.[15]

INDICATIONS

The quadratus femoris muscle pedicle graft is indicated in displaced femoral neck fractures after closure of the proximal femoral epiphyseal growth plate. I also utilize the pedicle graft in impacted or undisplaced femoral neck fractures with an avascular femoral head fragment (see chapter 6).[16] Avascularity is determined by a technetium 99m sulfur colloid scan of the pelvis prior to surgery.[17]

CONTRAINDICATIONS

Patients who are unable to cooperate in the postoperative rehabilitation program because of serious concurrent medical or mental illnesses are not candidates for this procedure. Parkinsonism, concomitant ipsilateral hemiplegia, or spasticity would prevent the patient from complying with the postoperative regimen. Patients who have minimal or no ambulatory ability, a short life expectancy, or a severe debility likewise are not candidates. Patients with pathologic fractures or severe concomitant ipsilateral arthritis of the involved hip should be treated by other methods.

ADVANTAGES

There are several advantages to this procedure over alternative methods. Most fracture surgeons agree that the patient is better off with his own femoral head and a healed femoral neck fracture as long as the proximal end of the femur remains in a normal anatomical configuration and the head does not collapse. The muscle pedicle graft provides a source of blood supply to an avascular femoral head that has lost its blood supply as a consequence of the fracture, and it provides, by capillary ingrowth, an additional source of blood to a subtotally avascular head fragment.

A more anatomical reduction of the fracture is possible under direct vision since the capsule is opened. Iliac bone chips can be added to fill any defect that may be present in the posterior neck of the femur. A defect has been reported in 70% of all displaced femoral neck fractures.[18]

The pedicle graft acts as a neutralization force and provides an additional stabilizing factor for the fracture.

DISADVANTAGES

The operating time is approximately 30 minutes longer than the time required for conventional closed reduction and internal fixation. There is more soft tissue dissection, and the hip joint is invaded, which increases the risk of infection. The operation is technically more demanding than conventional procedures.

SURGICAL TECHNIQUE

The patient is anesthetized and placed in a prone position on the fracture table. Traction is applied to the fractured leg. The leg is internally rotated 30° and abducted 15°.

Two x-ray machines are positioned to obtain anteroposterior and lateral views (Fig 17–1,A). An image intensifier fluoroscope is preferred if one is available (Fig 17–1,B). The reduction is checked by radiography or fluoroscopy. Traction can be adjusted if the reduction is not acceptable. Minor adjustments to achieve reduction of the fracture can be made later under direct vision when the capsule is opened and the fracture has been exposed.

Preparation of the skin and draping of the limb are left to the surgeon's preference. The surgical field should include an area cephalad to the trochanter, caudally to the midthigh, and posteriorly to include the posteroinferior iliac spine.

The skin incision begins 8 cm cephalad and 8 cm posterior to the postero-superior margin of the greater trochanter (Fig 17–2). The incision is made in a curvilinear fashion between those points and then along the posterolateral aspect of the femur for a distance of 20 cm.

The layers of soft tissue below the skin, which include subcutaneous fat, deep fascia, fascia lata, and the greater trochanteric bursa, are incised in order and retracted, exposing the quadratus femoris muscle (Fig 17–3).

The caudal and cephalad borders of the quadratus femoris muscle are defined. The graft is outlined with a small osteotome (Fig 17–4). It includes the trochanteric crest, beginning 4 mm from the tip of the greater trochanter to a point approximately 1.5 cm distal to the caudal edge of the quadratus femoris muscle. The width of the graft should be about 1.5 cm from the posterior edge of the trochanteric crest. It ends medial to the linea aspera at the distal portion (Fig 17–5).

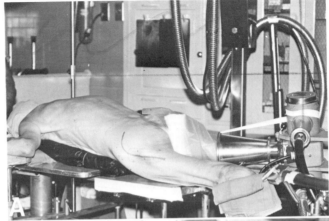

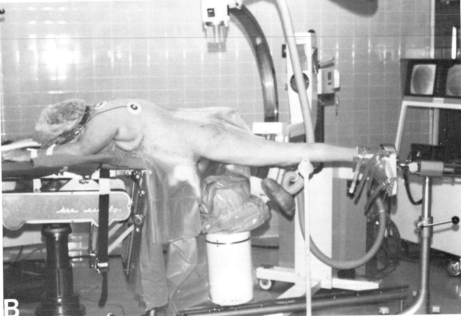

*Fig 17–1—**A,** patient in prone position on fracture table. Skeletal traction is being applied on the fracture side in an amputee. **B,** a patient positioned for fluoroscopic intensifier.*

Marking the dimensions of the graft and cutting the pedicle graft must be done carefully to avoid fracturing the graft. The insertion of the quadratus femoris muscle must not be encroached on so that the muscle is not detached from the graft.

The following precautions will prevent a fracture of the graft. The distal end of the graft (the portion distal to the muscle) should be outlined with drill holes, which are then connected by using a small osteotome. The entire graft should be undermined with a 1.5-cm curved osteotome. The curved osteotome should be inserted at right angles to the cortex to a depth of 1.5 cm. Insertion beyond this point usually cuts into the cortex of the posterior aspect of the femoral neck. The entire graft is then elevated with a large straight osteotome by lifting the end of the instrument and wedging the graft upward from its bed.

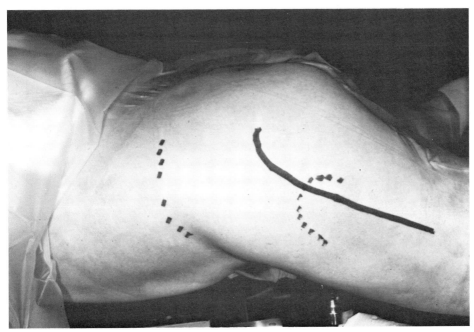

Fig 17–2—Incision line for surgery. Dotted lines *outline superior crest of the ilium and superior border of the greater trochanter. The* uninterrupted line *outlines the incision. (From Meyers et al.*[15] *Reproduced by permission.)*

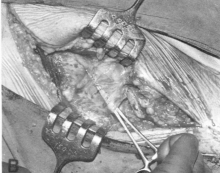

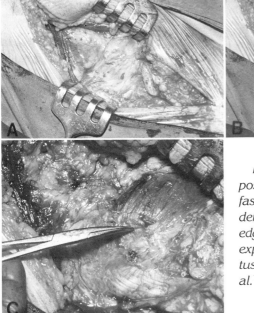

*Fig 17–3—**A**, trochanteric bursa exposed by retraction of cut edges of fascia lata. **B**, trochanteric bursa undermined prior to incising. **C**, cut edges of trochanteric bursa retracted, exposing the insertion of the quadratus femoris muscle. (From Meyers et al.*[15] *Reproduced by permission.)*

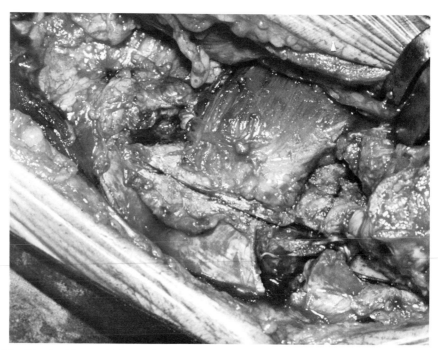

Fig 17–4—The pedicle graft has been outlined with an osteotome. The cephalad tip of the greater trochanter is to the left and the lesser trochanter is to the right at the caudal edge of the quadratus femoris muscle. (From Meyers et al.[15] Reproduced by permission.)

The pedicle graft is elevated from the posterior aspect of the hip joint capsule by blunt dissection and retracted (Fig 17–6). A small cobra retractor is placed between the graft and the inferior aspect of the neck of the femur. The sciatic nerve is protected by the retracted pedicle graft (Fig 17–7).

An inverted T incision is made in the posterior part of the capsule. The stem of the T commences at the acetabulum midway between the inferior and superior aspects of the femoral neck and proceeds to the base of the neck. The posterior femoral capsular attachment is incised to complete the T, and the flaps are retracted with two small cobra retractors, one between the capsule and inferior neck and one between the capsule and the superior aspect of the femoral neck. The entire posterior aspect of the femoral neck can now be seen. The fracture is in view and the degree of comminution of the neck can be ascertained (see Fig 17–7). Frequently the small rotators must be severed to complete the capsular incision.

Final reduction of the fracture can now be accomplished under direct vision. I strive for an anatomical reduction, or fracture reduction with the inferior edge of the head fragment within the intramedullary portion of the distal fragment and resting on the inferior aspect of the neck.

The tendinous origin of the vastus lateralis is cut and elevated to permit insertion of the metal fixative device of choice (Fig 17–8). The preferred fixation method is with four pins of 0.4-cm shank length and 0.45-cm cancellous thread width. Holes 0.45 cm in diameter are drilled in the lateral cortex of the femur, 2 cm distal to the base of the trochanter, to permit insertion of the pins. The pins should traverse the posteroinferior intramedullary position of the neck into the head and rest approximately 3 mm from the subchondral surface of the femoral head. The surgeon should attempt to place the pins in a rectangular pattern. The reduction and first pin placement are checked by x-ray after placement of the first pin. Recently, we have used Asnis or 6.5 AO cancellous screw pins for fixation. The other pins (total of four) are inserted after the cavity in the posterior neck is packed with iliac bone chips (see below) (Fig 17–9).

If a cavity is present in the posterior neck, it is packed with iliac bone chips prior to placement of the remaining pins (Fig 17–10). If supplemental bone is inserted into the cavity after placement of the pins, it may not be possible to obliterate the cavity because of interference by the pins. Iliac bone chips are obtained through a separate small incision over the posterior superior iliac spine.

Should the head fragment spin or roll during insertion of the first two pins, the following maneuver will prevent this event. The head fragment is impaled with two Steinmann pins, which are then held by an assistant to secure the fragment while the pins are driven into position.

The cephalad end of the pedicle graft is trimmed with a rongeur, and all soft tissue beyond the muscle is scraped from the bone with a scalpel. The graft should be 1.5 cm wide and approximately 0.5 cm deep. The length depends on the available bone and varies from patient to patient.

A mortising chisel is placed flat on the posterior aspect of the femoral neck and is then driven into the femoral head fragment for 1–2 cm, depending on the cephalad length of the pedicle graft available beyond the quadratus femoris muscle

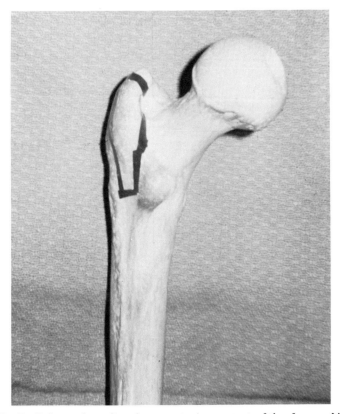

Fig 17–5—Pedicle graft outlined on posterior aspect of the femur. Note that the lesser trochanter is not included and the end of graft is cut medial to the linea aspera.

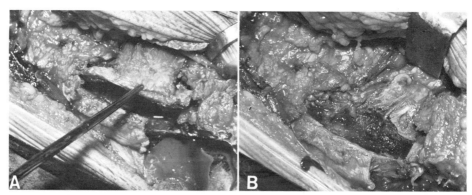

Fig 17–6—**A,** *pedicle graft has been cut and undermined with straight and curved osteotomes.* **B,** *pedicle graft retracted, exposing posterior capsule and short rotators of the hip at upper end of defect created in posterior shaft of the femur by retraction of the graft. (From Meyers et al.[15] Reproduced by permission.)*

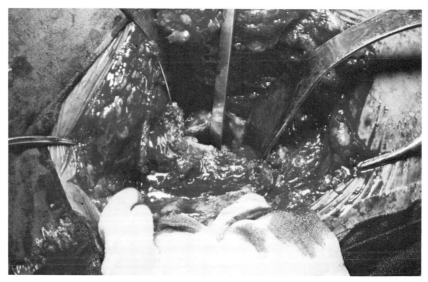

Fig 17–7—*Pedicle graft and cut edges of capsule are retracted by cobra retractors placed between the capsule and the femoral neck. The osteotome is in a large posterior neck defect. (From Meyers et al.[15] Reproduced by permission.)*

(Figs 17–11 and 17–12). A 1.4-cm (1/2-inch) osteotome can be used for this step in place of a mortising chisel.

The proximal end of the graft is inserted through the prepared opening into the head (Fig 17–13), lightly impacted, and fixed with a screw through the caudal end of the graft into the femoral neck (Fig 17–14). If modified Hagie pins are used, the nuts are tightened on the washers with a wrench, as one would tighten the lugs on an automobile wheel. The excess portion of each pin is cut away. The Asnis pins or AO cancellous screws do not require cutting since there is a selection of pin lengths available. The wound is then closed in layers over two suction tubes and dressed.

The patient can be turned frequently and is allowed to sit up in a wheelchair as tolerated within 24 hours. Non-weight-bearing ambulation is started after the first day, as the strength and agility of the patient permit. Active exercises are encouraged

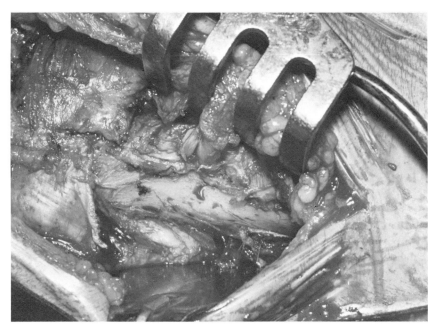

Fig 17–8—Origin of vastus lateralis muscle cut and retracted to expose the shaft of the femur. This step can be carried out before or after elevation of the pedicle graft.

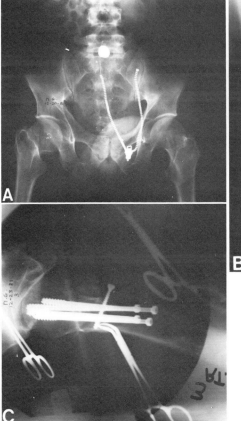

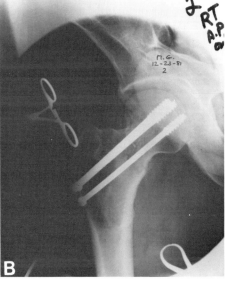

*Fig 17–9—**A,** AP x-ray film of pelvis with displaced intracapsular fracture. **B,** AP view showing fracture reduced and fixed with four Asnis pins. **C,** lateral x-ray film. Fracture has been reduced and fixed with four Asnis screws and the pedicle graft has been fixed with one screw.*

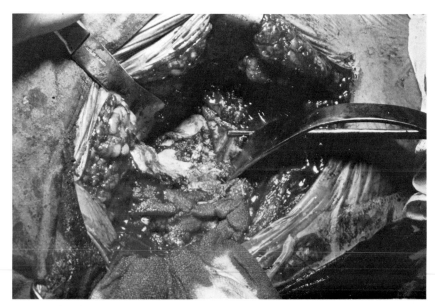

Fig 17–10—*Cavity shown in Figure 17–7 has been packed with iliac bone chips. (From Meyers et al.[15] Reproduced by permission.)*

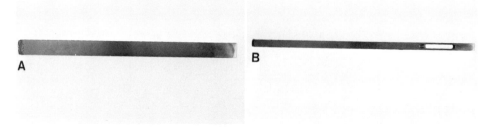

A B

Fig 17–11—*Two views of mortising chisel:* **A,** *front;* **B,** *side.*

soon after surgery. Weight-bearing is contraindicated for 4–8 weeks and is permitted only when an x-ray examination demonstrates fracture healing. The average time to beginning partial weight-bearing is about 6 weeks.

Maneuvers to Forestall Complications

Several steps in the procedure should be clarified and certain precautionary measures emphasized in order to avoid errors.

The reduction is gentle. Vigorous manipulation, as with a Leadbetter maneuver, is not necessary. Excessive force could cause more damage to the circulation in the head fragment and further comminution at the fracture site. Final reduction of the fracture under direct vision is possible after the capsule has been opened. Traction can be increased and the position of the distal fragment can be changed by manipulating the fracture table. In some cases a large bone clamp can be applied to the distal fragment and additional internal rotation obtained by forcing the handle of the clamp downward. On occasion the patient's skin may not tolerate traction. Skeletal traction can be utilized to manipulate the distal fracture fragment during

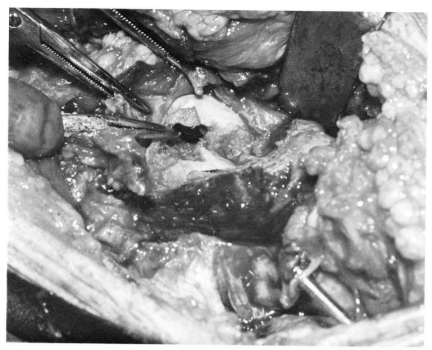

Fig 17–12—Opening in femoral head created by mortising chisel. (From Meyers et al.[15] Reproduced by permission.)

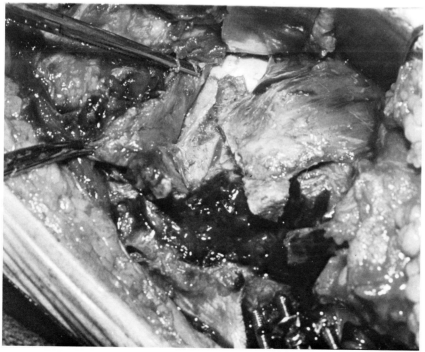

Fig 17–13—Cephalad end of pedicle graft is inserted into opening in the femoral head. (From Meyers et al.[15] Reproduced by permission.)

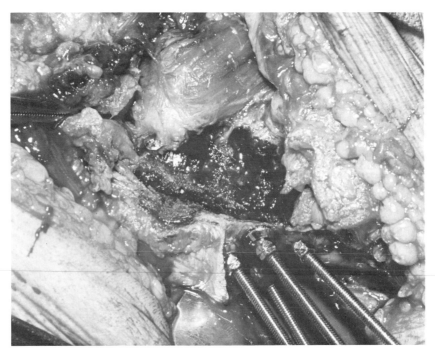

Fig 17–14—Graft in place and fixed with a single screw. Hagie pins are placed and held with washers prior to removing excess portion of pins. (From Meyers et al.[15] Reproduced by permission.)

surgery. This modification can also be utilized in the amputee with an intracapsular hip fracture in the amputated extremity (see Fig 17–1,A).

Overzealous traction should be avoided. Pudendal nerve neuropraxia has been reported in males as a result of traction against the perineal post of the fracture table.[7] Impotency can be the consequence. The patient should be placed on the table with the perineal post between the genitalia and the uninjured limb in order to minimize the chances of damage to the pudendal nerve.

The pedicle graft can be fractured by rough handling. The chance of the graft fracturing is minimized by outlining the graft with drill holes and then connecting them by means of a small osteotome.

It must be emphasized that obliteration of the cavity in the posterior neck, when such a cavity is present, requires iliac bone chips. These must be impacted into the cavity after fracture reduction has been achieved and the fracture fragments have been fixed with a guide pin. The remaining pins or nails are inserted after the cavity has been packed with iliac bone. Placement of the pins prior to filling the cavity will not permit complete obliteration of the cavity with additional bone. Sufficient bone is available in the greater trochanter to pack small defects.

If the surgeon encounters a femoral head that spins during insertion of the fixation nails, two smooth Steinmann pins can be drilled into the head fragment. An assistant holds the pins to prevent rotation while the hip nails are inserted.

The bone may be very hard in young adults so that insertion of metal pins and nails is difficult. Predrilling with a drill that has a slightly smaller diameter than the metallic fixation device will make it easier to insert the device.

The surgeon must make certain that the threads of the hip pins do not bridge the fracture line, especially in patients with good bone stock. Bridging can interfere with impaction of the fragments and lead to delayed union or nonunion of the fracture.

SPECIAL INTRAOPERATIVE COMPLICATIONS

The possibility that the pedicle graft may fracture has been mentioned. In the event that the graft fractures, more than one screw may be required to fix the distal end of the graft. A screw can be inserted through the insertion of the muscle without serious damage to the circulation.

In rare instances, the quadratus femoris muscle may be inadvertently avulsed from its insertion. Gray states that the quadratus femoris muscle is absent in 1% or 2% of humans.[19] However, I have found it present in each of the 300 patients who underwent this surgical procedure. Absence or avulsion of the insertion reduces the chances of successfully restoring the circulation to an avascular head fragment.

Fracture of the lesser trochanter may occur if the distal end of the graft is cut too large. This complication does not have an effect on the final result.

Cutting the distal end of the graft so that it involves a large area of the linea aspera may weaken the subtrochanteric area and result in a fracture intraoperatively or in the postoperative period. A subtrochanteric fracture that is recognized intra-operatively can be managed with a sliding nail plate. Postoperatively the patient can be treated in traction or reoperated on and a sliding plate inserted.

Rarely, internal fixation may be inachievable because of marked bone atrophy, or when fracture reduction is impossible. When internal fixation is not feasible, excision of the femoral head and prosthetic replacement is possible through the recommended operative approach.

SPECIAL POSTOPERATIVE COMPLICATIONS

Nonunion, avascular necrosis, and infection are addressed in other chapters. Subtrochanteric fractures were mentioned previously. Up to 20% of varus deformity due to shifting of the fragments is acceptable. When there is a greater degree of deformity a subtrochanteric valgus osteotomy should be considered so that the shearing force at the fracture site will be converted to a compression force. This will improve the opportunity for osseous union. In some cases a second attempt at reduction and renailing should be considered.

Penetration of the head fragment by the pins due to absorption at the fracture site followed by compression occurs infrequently. In many cases the pins can be removed after osseous union occurs. In some cases a second operation may be necessary to retract and shorten the pins by removing the excess length with a pin cutter.

Absorption of bone at the fracture site, resulting in a short femoral neck and backing out the pins, may cause an irritative bursa on the lateral aspect of the upper thigh. The pins can be removed after fracture union has taken place.

REFERENCES

1. Judet R.: Traitement des fractures du col du femur par greffe pediculee. *Acta Orthop. Scand.* 32:421, 1962.
2. Cole P.P.: Pathological fracture of the mandible: Nonunion treated with pedicled bone graft. *Lancet* 1:1044, 1940.
3. Cuneo M.M.B., Block J.C.: Technique d'osteoplastic et plus specialement de celle du femur. *J. Chir.* 23:113, 1924.

4. Farmer A.W.: The use of a composite pedicle graft for pseudarthrosis of the tibia. *J. Bone Joint Surg.* 34A:591, 1952.

5. Hibbs R.A.: An operation for stiffening the knee joint. *Ann. Surg.* 53:404, 1941.

6. Hibbs R.A.: A preliminary report of twenty cases of hip joint tuberculosis. *J. Bone Joint Surg.* 8:522, 1926.

7. Hofmann A., Jones R.E., Schoenvogel R.: Pudendal-nerve neuraproxia as a result of traction on the fracture table. *J. Bone Joint Surg.* 64A:1136-1141, 1982.

8. Venable O.S., Stuck W.G.: Muscle flap transplant for the relief of painful monarticular arthritis (aseptic necrosis) of the hip. *Ann. Surg.* 123:641, 1946.

9. Baadsgaard K., Medgyesi S.: Muscle-pedicle bone grafts. *Acta Orthop. Scand.* 35:279, 1965.

10. Davis J.B., Taylor N.A.: Muscle-pedicle bone grafts: Experimental study. *Arch. Surg.* 65:330, 1958.

11. Frankel C.J., Derian P.S.: The introduction of subcapital femoral circulation by means of an autogenous muscle pedicle. *Surg. Gynecol. Obstet.* 115:473, 1962.

12. Hartley J., Silver N.: Muscle-pedicle bone grafts. *J. Bone Joint Surg.* 36A:800, 1954.

13. Stuck W.G., Hinchey J.J.: Experimentally increased blood supply to the head and neck of the femur. *Surg. Gynecol. Obstet.* 78:160, 1944.

14. Launois B., Judet R.: *Epaule: Fractures du Col du Femur.* Paris, Masson, 1963.

15. Meyers M.H., Harvey J.P. Jr., Moore T.M.: The muscle-pedicle bone graft in the treatment of displaced fractures of the femoral neck: Indications, operative technique, and results. *Orthop. Clin. North Am.* 5:779, 1974.

16. Meyers M.H.: Impacted and undisplaced femoral neck fractures, in *The Hip: Proceedings of the Tenth Open Scientific Meeting of the Hip Society.* St. Louis, C.V. Mosby Co., 1982, pp. 239-246.

17. Meyers M.H., Telfer N., Moore T.M.: Determination of the vascularity of the femoral head with technetium-99m-sulphur colloid: Diagnostic and prognostic significance. *J. Bone Joint Surg.* 59A:658, 1977.

18. Meyers M.H., Harvey J.P. Jr., Moore T.M.: Treatment of displaced subcapital and trans-cervical fractures of the femoral neck by muscle-pedicle bone graft and internal fixation. *J. Bone Joint Surg.* 55A:257, 1973.

19. Goss C.M. (ed.): *Gray's Anatomy of the Human Body.* Philadelphia, Lea & Febiger, 1966.

Chapter 18

The Use of Ender Nail Fixation for Extracapsular Fractures About the Hip

Timothy J. Bray, M.D.
Michael W. Chapman, M.D.

The **superior** results achieved with operative treatment of peritrochanteric fractures, in terms of both survival and function, are now universally accepted by the majority of fracture surgeons. When modern concepts of internal fixation are applied, most patients are fully weight-bearing in the immediate post-operative period. Ambulation, in turn, aids in the prevention of the deleterious effects of prolonged bed rest, including pulmonary complications, urinary tract infections, and pressure sores.

It is estimated that more than 200,000 hip fractures occur in the United States each year, at an annual expense of nearly 1 billion dollars.[1] Nearly 30% of all patients hospitalized for the treatment of fractures have fractures related to the hip.[2] The socioeconomic effects are felt by all members of the health care team, including the family, patient, and hospital administrators. However, no less is the concern of the surgeon responsible for the fixation decisions.

HISTORY

In the early 1940s the innovative German surgeon Gerhardt Kuntscher revolutionized the care of long bone fractures by introducing the concept of "intramedullary fixation devices."[3] He thought this type of internal fixation device had great benefits. If the nail were placed in the center of the bone, the rod would be in a position of maximum load sharing and thereby, would provide greater stability for immediate weight-bearing. Kuntscher also thought that percutaneous placement of the rod would decrease the risk of infection, since the fracture could remain operatively unviolated; this was the origin of the term, "closed intramedullary nailing."

In 1942 Kuntschner first described the use of closed intramedullary nails for treating fractures of the femoral shaft.[3] At that time, intertrochanteric fractures were generally treated by open reduction and internal fixation with fixed-angle devices, similar to the Smith-Peterson nail.[4] The sharp nail was driven into the head-neck fragment and the plate was secured to the shaft fragment by screws. Therefore, the majority of stress was exerted on the plate-nail interface, and fixation failures were quite common. Fractures with loss of medial bone stock were at especially high risk of failure when this type of fixation system was used.

Because of these problems, Kuntscher in 1966 described the use of a condylocephalic nail, which was introduced over a guide pin placed in the medial condyle of the femur.[5] This nail was then driven into the intramedullary canal and passed superiorly to stabilize the intertrochanteric fracture. Using the same reasoning he applied to fractures of the femoral shaft, Kuntscher described the advantages in the treatment of hip fractures: stresses shared along axial loads, a small operative incision, and percutaneous placement of the fixation device.

Following this revolutionary concept, Hans Ender described in the German literature an intramedullary fixation device with a prebent round elastic nail.[6] This new fixation system consisted of multiple flexible pins introduced percutaneously from the knee and passed proximally into the femoral head. The pins were designed to fan out in the femoral head and provide stable rotational control of the proximal fragment, allowing axial compression to occur at the fracture site. On weight-bearing, the load would be distributed along the entire length of the pins within the intramedullary canal. This technique allowed impaction of the fracture and gave a high degree of stability, with few reported complications. This procedure was truly a percutaneous operative approach.

Over the next 5 years this technique grew in popularity in Western Europe, and many reports became available for review in the literature.[1-3, 7-18] In 1978, Ender described this technique and reported results in 1,258 patients." Some 13.2% of patients sustained complications, including hematomas, infections, loss of fixation, loss of stability, and reoperation. There was very little objective documentation as to the long-term functional results in this large series.

Bohler described the use of this technique in 353 patients at the Lorenz Bohler Hospital from 1971 to 1974.[19] There was a 10.3% hospital mortality and a 3.9% infection rate. Once again, there were no long-term patient follow-up reports and therefore functional results remained questionable. Kuderna et al. then reported in the American literature in 1976 on this same series with an average follow-up of 131 days.[20] According to a scheme of grading infrequently used in the United States, the results were reported as 52% very good, 32% good, 13% satisfactory, and 3% unsatisfactory. Of interest, 33% of patients had knee pain.

As the experience with Ender pins expanded into American orthopedic practice, many authors reported the frequent occurrence of knee pain, distal pin migration, residual external rotational deformity, and pin penetration of the femoral head.[12, 13, 21] Many authors have compared Ender pins with nail plate devices and have concluded that the use of Ender pins offers advantages over the nail plate devices.[14, 15, 22] The advantages include a decrease in surgical morbidity, less operating time, less blood loss, and a decreased incidence of operative infection. However, because of the external rotation deformity and high incidence of problems about the knee, the use of Ender pins in a younger, more active patient population is probably less desirable than the compression screw. A recent report from San Francisco General Hospital, presented at the American Academy of Orthopedic Surgeons in Atlanta in 1984, substantiated this concern.[23]

Therefore, the initial enthusiasm recorded in the literature dwindled as experience was gained with the procedure. The complications of knee pain with pin backout and external rotation deformity, as well as the late occurrence of supracondylar femoral fractures, have remained as a persistent criticism of the procedure. Currently, other fixation devices are more appealing than Ender pins in the treatment of extracapsular fractures about the hip. Nevertheless, the unique features of Ender pins have made them a useful adjunct in the fixation armamentarium of the orthopedist dealing with complex problems of the lower extremity.

Although Ender pins are most commonly relied on for stability in the severely debilitated, elderly nonambulatory patient with a hip fracture, there are definite indications for their use in other problematic conditions.

INDICATIONS

As with all new operative procedures, fixation methods, or treatment modalities, the initial spectrum of fractures treated by Ender pinning included almost every bone in the body. The pendulum now has swung in the opposite direction, and the technique is seldom considered the fixation method of choice, except in the circumstances described below.

Elderly, Debilitated, Nonambulatory Patients With Extracapsular Hip Fractures

Many nursing home ambulators or nonambulators are brought to the orthopedist's attention with an extracapsular hip fracture (Fig 18–1). These patients inevitably have severe medical problems, at times contraindicating general anesthesia, prolonged blood loss, and extensive surgical procedures. We believe such patients

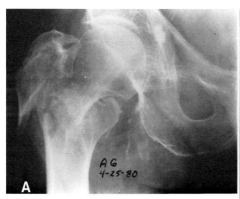
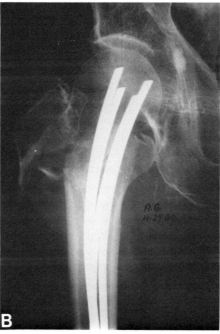

*Fig 18–1—**A** and **B**, unstable intertrochanteric fracture in a debilitated 75-year-old woman. This Kyle type III fracture is stable and can be managed with Ender pinning, with special considerations. Postoperatively, four Ender pins were fanned into adequate position, ignoring the greater trochanter. Note that the femoral canal is not stacked with Ender pins **(B)**. Note also the relative varus position of the head. This patient was managed with a derotation splint while in bed and was permitted to move about with a walker. Great caution should be used in the management of these fractures with Ender pins.*

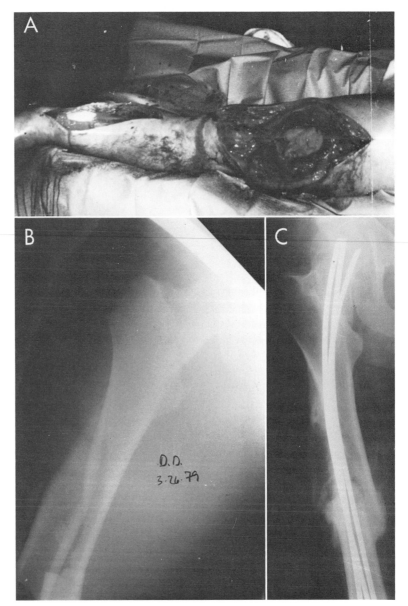

*Fig 18–2—**A** and **B**, 25-year-old polytraumatized motorcycle accident victim with type III fracture of the femur and base of neck hip, and an open tibia. The fracture was internally splinted with three Ender pins. Because of this patient's compromised pulmonary status, he was nursed in Neufeld roller traction, with bed to wheelchair transfers allowed. **C**, roentgenogram obtained 1 year postoperative demonstrating union of the neck and diaphyseal fractures. The patient was left with one-half inch shortening and 10° of external rotation.*

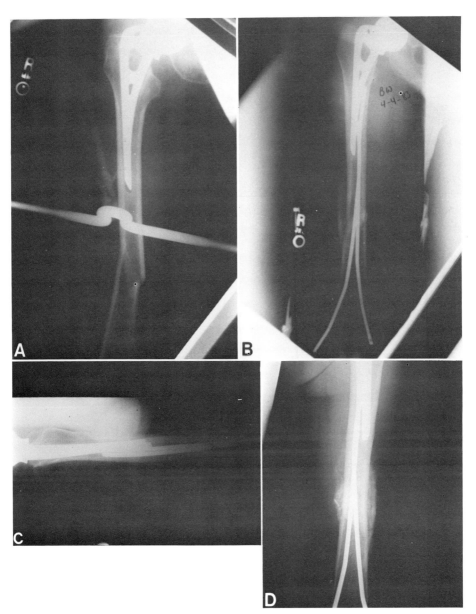

*Fig 18–3—***A,** *65-year-old woman with a midshaft diaphyseal fracture. An endoprosthesis is in position.* **B** *and* **C,** *two Ender pins have been placed medially and laterally between the medial cortex of the femoral shaft and the endoprosthetic stem. As is evident from the lateral view* **(C),** *it is quite easy to perforate the cortex near the endoprosthetic stem in the osteoporotic patient. Therefore, frequent fluoroscopic views should be taken and care should be exercised when resistance is met as the nails are driven in.* **D,** *at 12-week follow-up there was abundant callus. Removal of the cast brace was possible at this time.*

should be seriously considered for Ender pinning. The low infection rate with Ender pinning[12, 16, 17, 20, 21] continues to be an appealing aspect of the procedure and is an additional advantage in elderly debilitated patients, who are more susceptible to infections. However, the question still remains whether the advantages of less blood loss, reduced operating time, and decreased rate of infection offset the increased incidence of pin penetration, knee pain, and reoperation rates commonly found with Ender pinning.

Skin Problems About the Hip

Frequently the polytraumatized elderly or indigent patient with a hip fracture must be mobilized for lifesaving pulmonary reasons. There may be abrasions, old cutaneous lesions, or dermatologic bacterial conditions that ordinarily would contraindicate nail plate fixation via the lateral approach. In this situation, use of Ender pins is a temporizing measure for achieving immediate stability via the knee approach. When the life-threatening condition has passed and/or the skin lesions have healed, the Ender pins can be removed electively at the time of definitive treatment by nail plate fixation. This two-step approach has worked particularly well for the polytraumatized patient with multiple fractures when time is short and many stabilizing procedures must be carried out simultaneously. These patients usually return to the operating room for other reasons, and elective hip stabilization can then be carried out under optimum conditions.

Ipsilateral Femoral Shaft and Hip Fractures

Polytraumatized patients occasionally have combinations of hip fractures and femoral shaft fractures (Fig 18–2).[18] In major open fractures with massive soft tissue wounds, Ender pinning has provided fracture stability without the pin tract complications of external fixators. External fixation is equally unattractive, as fixation across the hip joint is associated with poor biomechanical frame configuration. Certainly traction is a poor alternative in this situation, as the extensive nursing care, difficulty in wound management, and patient discomfort are major reasons for fracture fixation.

Femoral Diaphyseal Fractures Below Prosthetic Devices or Nail Plate

The stresses delivered to the tip of an endoprosthesis or femoral side plate are enough to initiate a fracture below the implant (Fig 18–3). In the elderly debilitated patient who cannot withstand a major reconstructive procedure, it may be possible to pass Ender pins across the fracture site and achieve stability thereby. Of course, if the femoral implant is cemented into position, passage of the pins is more difficult and open reduction may be indicated.

Stable Intertrochanteric Fractures

Although not our fixation method of choice, Ender pins can be used in stable intertrochanteric fractures[12] if the surgeon and patient are willing to accept the known potential complications. Even more critical is understanding the fracture pattern and the biomechanical shortcomings of the unstable fracture configuration treated by this method.[12]

RADIOGRAPHIC EVALUATION

Based on radiographic appearances, hip fractures may easily be classified according to the criteria of Kyle et al.[24] Figure 18–4 illustrates a type I intertrochanteric hip fracture which is intrinsically stable and exquisitely suited for Ender pinning. These fractures can be pinned in the percutaneous fashion, and no postoperative protection in traction is necessary.

The type II intertrochanteric fracture is shown in Figure 18–5. It is displaced and usually associated with a varus deformity. A small fracture fragment of the lesser trochanter is evident. This is also a stable fracture pattern and suitable for Ender pinning without specific postoperative modification.

The Kyle type III fracture (Fig 18–6) is extremely unstable, displaced, and involves the greater trochanter with severe comminution of the posterior medial wall. It is usually associated with a varus deformity. This fracture type was initially classified by Ender as a "gaping" fracture and can be managed with Ender pinning. However, it does require special postoperative considerations.

The type IV intertrochanteric fracture (Fig 18–7) described by Kyle is unstable, displaced, and severely comminuted. The use of Ender pins is definitely contraindicated for this challenging fracture.

Although not described specifically by Kyle, short transverse or short oblique subtrochanteric fractures are stable fracture patterns and occasionally can be treated with Ender nails (Fig 18–8).[12] Treatment entails the use of medial and lateral pins, postoperative protection, and close follow-up to prevent rotational deformities. Long oblique subtrochanteric fractures are very unstable and difficult to nail using the Ender method (Fig 18–9). These fractures frequently shorten and rotate and are poor candidates for Ender pinning.[12]

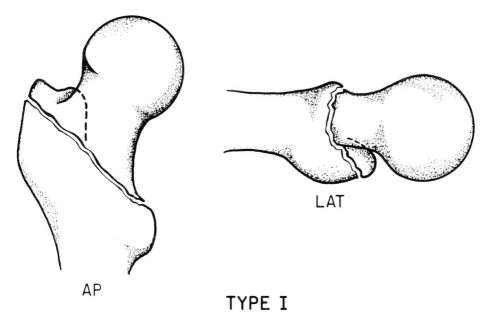

LAT

AP

TYPE I

Fig 18–4—Kyle type I intertrochanteric fracture. This two-part fracture is intrinsically stable and suitable for Ender pinning. (From Chapman M.W.: The use of Ender's pins in extracapsular fractures of the hip. J. Bone Joint Surg. 63A:14-28, 1981. Reproduced by permission.)

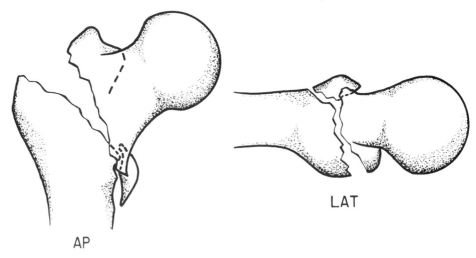

AP

LAT

TYPE II

Fig 18–5—Kyle type II intertrochanteric fracture. The fracture is generally displaced, with a small avulsion of the lesser tuberosity. It is intrinsically stable and therefore suitable for Ender pinning. (From Chapman M.W.: The use of Ender's pins in extracapsular fractures of the hip. J. Bone Joint Surg. 63A:14-28, 1981. Reproduced by permission.)

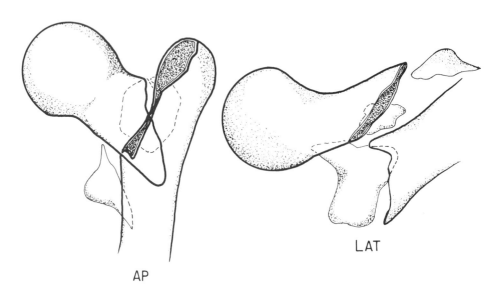

AP

LAT

TYPE III

Fig 18–6—Kyle type III intertrochanteric fracture. This fracture is grossly unstable, with comminution of the posterior medial wall. In general Ender pinning is contraindicated for these fractures. (From Chapman M.W.: The use of Ender's pins in extracapsular fractures of the hip. J. Bone Joint Surg. 63A:14-28, 1981. Reproduced by permission.)

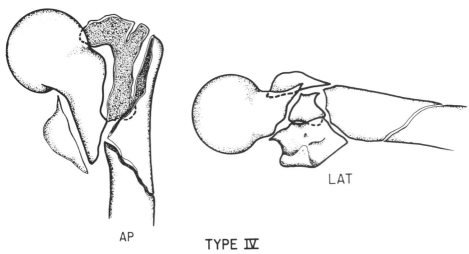

TYPE IV

Fig 18–7—Kyle type IV intertrochanteric fracture. This fracture is grossly un-stable and severely comminuted. There is posterior medial wall comminution and subtrochanteric extension. This fracture pattern precludes the use of Ender nails. (From Chapman M.W.: The use of Ender's pins in extracapsular fractures of the hip. J. Bone Joint Surg. 63A:14-28, 1981. Reproduced by permission.)

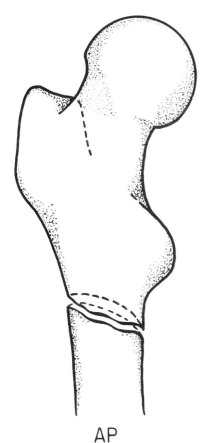

Fig 18–8—Short oblique subtrochanteric fractures can be treated with postoperative rotational protection.

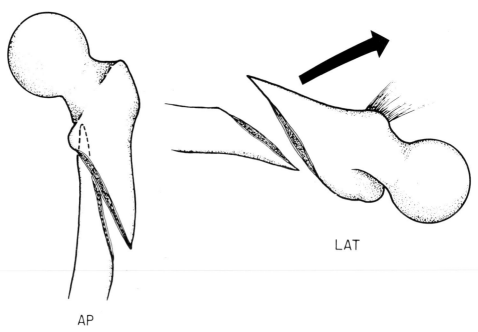

AP

Fig 18–9—A long oblique subtrochanteric fracture, intrinsically unstable because of its propensity to shorten. Ender nails will not adequately control rotation or length and therefore are not suitable for use in the treatment of this fracture. (From Chapman M.W.: The use of Ender's pins in extracapsular fractures of the hip. J. Bone Joint Surg. *63A:14-28, 1981. Reproduced by permission.)*

Understanding these various fracture patterns allows the surgeon to choose Ender pins when indicated and to recognize danger patterns that preclude adequate fixation with Ender pins.

TECHNIQUES OF PREOPERATIVE CARE

Preoperative splinting of the extremity serves a dual purpose: (1) to prevent further capsular injury and soft tissue damage, and (2) to decrease the muscle spasm and pain associated with the unstable fracture patterns.[25] The type of splint is usually dependent on the patient's preoperative medical condition. The majority of patients are operated on within 24 hours, and a soft foam Buck-type splint is used for the interim traction period. All traditional forms of skin traction have been discontinued because of the very thin atrophic skin along the tibial border, which is prone to traction slough.

Skeletal pin traction by a modified Russell technique is preferred for patients who will require a long period of preoperative traction or for patients who are unable to undergo immediate open reduction and internal fixation. It is less confining to the patient, more comfortable, and allows the patient to move more freely in bed.

Nutritionally, many patients are catabolic on admission and show evidence of protein depletion and negative nitrogen balance. Since wound healing and fracture healing are directly proportional to good nutritional standards, patients should be placed on high caloric diets, multiple vitamins, and vitamin C. Additionally, aspirin should be used as embolic prophylaxis in a dose of 10 grains twice daily.

TABLE 18–1.—Recommended Instruments for Ender Pinning

C-arm fluoroscopy unit and disk recorder
Major orthopedic instrument tray
Sharp-tipped awl
Duckbill ronguer
Double-action bolt cutter (Harrington rod cutter or Zimmer model 1270)
Insertion driver (guiding tool)
Seating driver
Bending instrument
Ender extractor
Ender pins, 34 cm to 49 cm
Ender compactor

Many of these patients have severe life-threatening medical problems which contraindicate general anesthesia. In these cases, general anesthesia can be substituted, with spinal anesthesia and a narcotic infusion technique. An inadequate or partial spinal block may preserve hip muscle tone and therefore create forces strong enough to prevent a reduction. This results in a difficult reduction and makes the operation technically challenging. It is the surgeon's responsibility to ensure that muscle relaxation is adequate for reduction prior to making the skin incision. Operating room conversation must be kept to a minimum when these patients are awake. Finally, the surgeon must be familiar with the fluoroscopic unit and be able to supervise its use. The surgeon must be certain that all instrumentation is available for each operative case, as the blame for faulty instruments lies with the surgeon, not the assistants (Table 18–1).

PITFALLS OF PREOPERATIVE PLANNING

Since Ender prescribed a period of postoperative bed rest in nearly 40% of his patients,[26] it is imperative that each case be planned preoperatively to allow immediate mobilization of the patient postoperatively. As previously described,[24] the configuration of the fracture is a major determinant of postoperative mobility. Good quality anteroposterior (AP) and lateral films of the involved hip must be obtained prior to operative intervention. Kyle type I and II fractures are most suitable for Ender pin fixation and immediate mobilization is possible. If the patient can tolerate anti-rotation splints and bed rest with protected weight-bearing, then the Kyle type III and IV fractures can be considered for Ender nails. However, serious consideration should be given to alternative fixation methods in patients with these unstable fracture patterns.

Anatomical variability of the femoral shaft[12] must be closely examined on the preoperative AP and lateral views. Since most patients considered for Ender nails are elderly, the incidence of osteoporosis is high. With large-diameter femoral canals it is often difficult to obtain adequate purchase on the femoral head and entry site. Therefore, the pins have a tendency to back out, causing the well-known problem of knee pain. On the other hand, a very narrow femoral canal will permit passage of only one or two pins into the femoral head, which results in minimal purchase, poor fixation, and a high probability of failure.

Certain ethnic groups such as Orientals may also present technical problems as their femora can be quite short, curved, and foreshortened in the AP dimension distally where the pins are inserted.[12] In these patients it can be difficult to position the pins at the knee. A large entryhole is required, and there is the possibility of a late supracondylar fracture. Most frequently, a proximal tibial skeletal pin has been placed for traction. This pin *must* be removed prior to placing the patient on the fracture table, as otherwise it will interfere with the Ender driving instruments. Appropriate arrangements should be made to remove these pins preoperatively, as extra procedures in the debilitated patient may result in a prolonged anesthesia time.

PATIENT POSITIONING*

After adequate anesthesia, the patient is placed in the supine position on the fracture table with both legs in 45° of abduction (Fig 18–10).[12] The feet are padded well and tied to the fracture table, as skeletal traction is usually unnecessary. This allows adequate space both for the operating surgeon to perform the procedure on the medial aspect of the involved extremity and for rotation of the fluoroscopy unit in the AP and lateral planes. It is imperative that the fracture be adequately visualized on AP and lateral views before the procedure is begun and that the fluoroscopy unit not interfere with the sterile, draped field. Permanent films are sometimes required if the adequacy of the reduction is in question prior to operative fixation. If the patient has limited hip abduction which limits the space available for the operating surgeon, the uninvolved lower extremity can be placed in the leg-holder with the hip and knee flexed at right angles (Fig 18–11). It cannot be overemphasized that the use of the fluoroscopic disk recorder is very useful in reducing radiation exposure during the procedure. All personnel in the operating room should wear lead aprons, including the unscrubbed surgeon.

The leg is then prepared and draped in sterile fashion, with allowance made for the rare necessity of a lateral approach to the hip should closed Ender nailing be unsuccessful. The use of a tourniquet is discouraged, as the greater trochanteric area is important for the reduction maneuver.

The unscrubbed surgeon is responsible for the manipulative aspects of the reduction and management of the orthopedic table and the fluoroscopy unit. The Ender procedure should not be attempted without the use of a C-arm fluoroscopy unit and two trained surgeons.

REDUCTION

It is extremely important to obtain an accurate reduction prior to pin insertion as most intraoperative difficulties originate from the inability to reduce the fracture. Most rotational problems arise from delayed external rotation. Therefore, the limb should be placed in slight internal rotation for nailing. Internal rotation of 20°–30° will provide adequate alignment to prevent postoperative complications.

In general, it is not necessary to attempt a formal reduction maneuver in the operating room. Placing the extremity in slight abduction and internal rotation with axial distraction will reduce the fracture in the majority of cases. If the fracture tends to sag posteriorly on the lateral fluoroscopic view, a crutch placed posterior with an anteriorly directed force will help reduce the fracture fragments (see Fig 18–11,A).[12] The crutch can be angled so that it does not interfere with the fluoroscopic control or sterile draping. As previously described for femoral neck fractures,[25] the head and neck fragment should align itself with the shaft at 10° of anteversion. On

---

*The following steps in surgery were reported by Chapman et al. in 1981.[12]

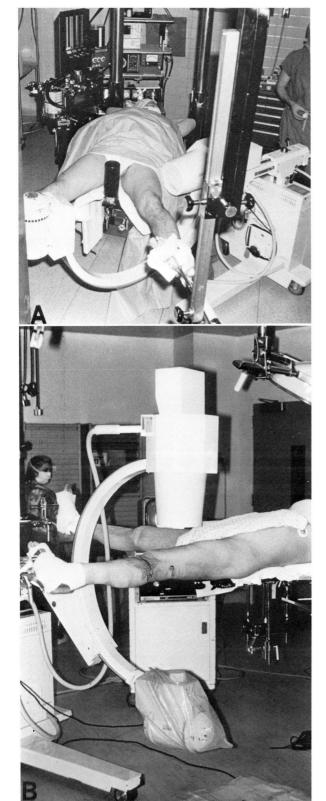

*Fig 18–10—**A,** patient positioning for routine Ender nailing. Legs are abducted 45°, feet are well padded, and the involved extremity (here, the left) is internally rotated 30°. This allows easy access to the medial aspect of the left thigh for the surgeon and unobstructed fluoroscopic control in the lateral plane. **B,** standard fluoroscopic position in AP plane. Note the well-padded, internally rotated left foot. Tibial traction pin was removed preoperatively. Tibial pins will interfere with Ender driving instruments if left in place intraoperatively. (From Chapman M.W.: The use of Ender's pins in extracapsular fractures of the hip. J. Bone Joint Surg. 63A:14-28, 1981. Reproduced by permission.)*

the AP view, an anatomical reduction or slight valgus position is preferred, as this position will facilitate pin insertion. Instead of towel clips, which obstruct fluoroscopic visualization, routine skin staplers have been used to hold drapes. This method is quick, easy, and never produces the skin necrosis seen so frequently with improperly placed towel clips (see Fig 18–11,B).

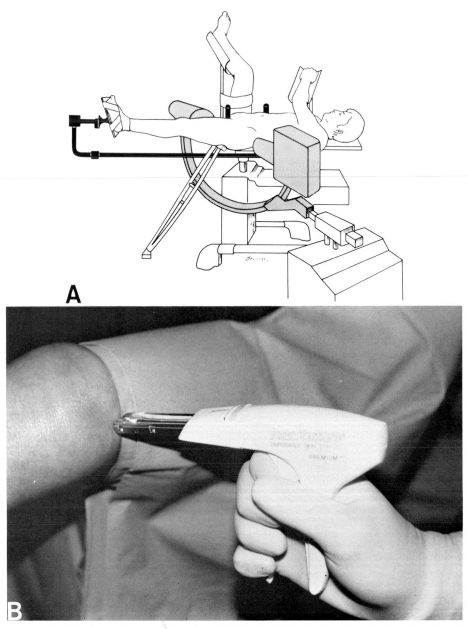

A

B

*Fig 18–11—***A,** *in elderly patients with limited hip abduction, the fractured limb is positioned in abduction and internal rotation, while the uninvolved extremity is placed in a 90–90 well leg holder. This facilitates medial exposure and allows C-arm fluoroscopy to be carried out in the AP and lateral planes. The crutch helps prevent posterior sag of fracture fragments.* **B,** *use of a skin stapler decreases draping time and prevents obstruction of fluoroscopic visualization by bulky towel clips.*

INCISION

The medial supracondylar area is approached via a 9-cm incision begun at the adductor tubercle and carried proximally (Fig 18–12,A).[12] The interval between the vastus medialis and the medial intermuscular septum is then entered. It is important to remain anterior to the medial intermuscular septum and posterior to the vastus medialis, as an approach too far posterior could result in injury to the femoral artery. An entryhole is then contoured, initially with an awl, and then with a duckbill rongeur to enlarge the hole (Fig 18–12,B). The most distal end of the hole should

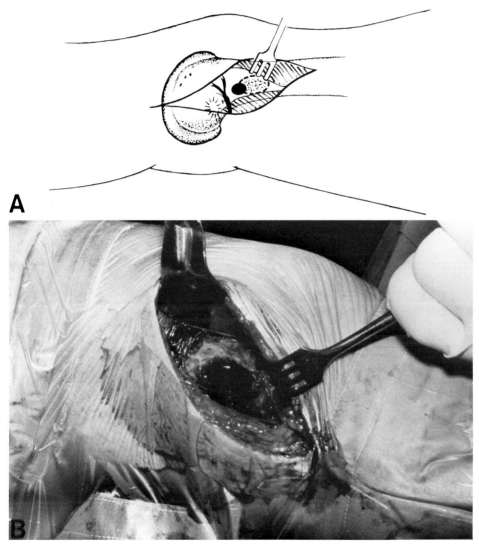

Fig 18–12—**A,** *medial approach to the supracondylar area of the femur. The vastus medialis is retracted anteriorly and the geniculate artery is identified. The entryhole should be made with an awl one to two fingerbreadths above the artery and expanded with the duckbill rongeur to produce a smooth-edged oval hole, as demonstrated in the stippled area.* **B,** *appropriate entryhole in the medial aspect of the left distal femur. (From Chapman M.W.: The use of Ender's pins in extracapsular fractures of the hip.* J. Bone Joint Surg. *63A:14-28, 1981. Reproduced by permission.)*

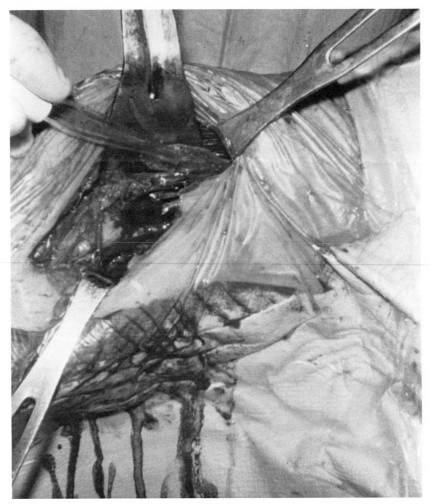

Fig 18–13—Fracture of the anterior cortex of the femur as noted at the tip of the sucker. This complication is relatively frequent and can be minimized by enlarging the entryhole. (From Chapman M.W.: The use of Ender's pins in extra-capsular fractures of the hip. J. Bone Joint Surg. 63A:14-28, 1981. Reproduced by permission.)

lie approximately two fingerbreadths above the geniculate artery and should be approximately 3 cm in length by 1½ cm in width. The entryhole is enlarged with a duckbill rongeur to produce a smooth-edged oval hole, with the posterior border of the hole abutting the flat posterior surface of the femur. A fracture of the proximal cortex of the hole is frequently encountered when the pins are driven in, and usually an enlarged hole size can decrease this complication (Fig 18–13). Occasionally, a small branch of the medial superior geniculate artery is encountered. This can be clamped, ligated, and tied off in the routine fashion.

OPERATIVE TECHNIQUE

The appropriate nail length is selected by superimposing the nail over the femur and checking the length with the image intensifier. The appropriate-length nail is one whose proximal tip projects to the level of the subchondral bone of the femoral head and which distally abuts the cortex at the level of the entryhole. The nail is then inserted into the Ender driving guide. Its proximal tip is inserted into the hole by means of light, quick taps of a mallett. The nail is then directed anteriorly until it reaches the fracture site. Under image intensification the nail is driven past the fracture site and externally rotated to make contact with the femoral calcar. Once the nail tip is on the calcar it will seek its own path for appropriate insertion into the femoral head. The nail should be left short of the subchondral bone, as subsequent placement of nails will force previously inserted nails more proximally. Nails should be placed in the head are in a fan position for better fracture stability.

Technically, pins should never be driven against substantial resistance unless their position has been verified fluoroscopically. In the osteoporotic patient, it is extremely easy to penetrate the diaphysis of the femur and cause a subsequent iatrogenic fracture.

To avoid excessive radiation, the disk recorder rather than continuous fluoroscopy should be used. One should be cautious in pin placement and crossing the fracture site. Frequent image verification of proper pin position at these two crucial stages of the operation is advised.

When three pins have been successfully placed into the head and neck fragment, the distal traction can be released and impaction of the fracture attempted. Additional pins can then be inserted despite the often difficult nature of passing a final pin through a relatively full canal. Occasionally, as the final pins are driven in, the entire pin group will slip proximally. Slippage can usually be prevented by holding the already placed pins with the pin extractor while driving the final pin into position. According to Nelson et al.,[27] the criteria for a good nailing are the following: (1) the

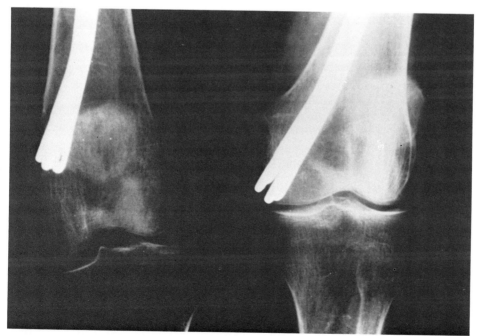

Fig 18–14—In the early experience with pin placement at the knee, pins were positioned far too distally. Although pins were stacked in appropriate position close to the cortex (left), 6 weeks later they backed out, causing severe knee pain (right).

reduction of the fracture must be adequate, (2) the nail tips should be fanned within the head and neck segment, (3) the nail tips should lie approximately 5 mm from subchondral cortex, (4) the femoral canal should be filled with the nails, (5) the insertion hole should not be too proximal, and (6) the flat distal tips should lie like "shingles on a roof" on the femoral cortex (Fig 18–14).

POSTOPERATIVE TREATMENT

Patients with stable fractures are permitted immediate weight-bearing as soon as their wounds are healed. Patients can be up at the bedside on the first postoperative day and can begin ambulation as their medical condition progresses. As the Ender pins do not provide absolute fracture stability, rotational control is extremely important. Legs treated by this method have a tendency to rotate externally while the patient is lying in bed. For these reasons, an antirotation splint should be used while the patient is in bed. The splints can be disregarded during ambulation.

Unstable fractures require protection, and occasionally skeletal traction must be used for a minimum of 3 weeks and sometimes (rarely) as long as 5–6 weeks. The unstable fracture patterns are more frequently treated with a compression screw[23] and side plate, while the subtrochanteric fractures are more often treated with locked intramedullary nailing. Pain at the knee is a frequent complaint, and after the fracture has healed, the Ender pins are usually removed. Younger, active patients will inevitably have knee symptoms and require pin removal for relief of the pain.

RESULTS

One of the most extensive series in the literature is that reported by Hult and Nilsson.[16] They reviewed more than 900 patients who underwent Ender pinning between 1971 and 1976. Of the 900 patients, 208 were evaluated prospectively and 712 retrospectively; 70% of fractures had healed within 3 months and more than 90% within 6 months. Hult and Nilsson also noted an external rotation deformity of more than 20° in 10% of patients, a mortality of 9.5%, and an infection rate of 0.76%. Their conclusions suggest that the elderly patient who requires a limited procedure for an intertrochanteric fracture benefits most from this operation.

We reviewed, prospectively and retrospectively, 77 cases of Ender pinnings of fractures about the hip and femur treated at the University of California, Davis, Medical Center between October 1978 and January 1983. The mean follow-up period was 8.4 months. The average age of the patient was 72 years, and 69% of the intertrochanteric fractures were unstable in nature. Forty percent of the patients had subsequent knee pain, 40% of patients required reoperation, and five patients sustained late supracondylar fractures through the entryhole (Fig 18–15). Because of these findings, Ender pins are no longer our method of choice of internal fixation for most unstable extracapsular hip fractures. Their versatility, however, continues to be a valuable asset in treating selected patients with stable extracapsular fractures of the hip, patients with hip fractures in whom soft tissue injuries preclude a proximal approach to the intertrochanteric area, and patients with special problems, including ipsilateral neck and femoral shaft fractures, fractures with internal fixation devices in place, and some polytraumatized patients.

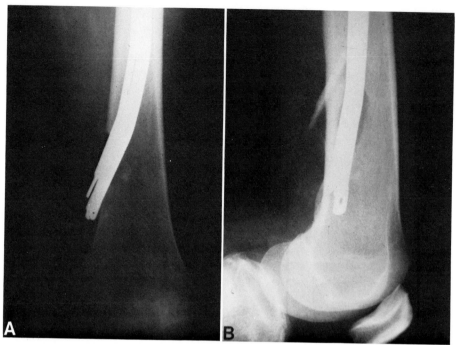

*Fig 18–15—**A** and **B**, AP and lateral roentgenograms of the distal pin insertion sites in the left femur. The entryhole on the AP roentgenograph is approximately 1 cm to the proximal aspect. Although the pins lie flush against the femur and are ideally stacked, the risk of fracture of the femur through the entryhole is extremely high when pins are placed too far proximally. A small cortical fragment that has split off the proximal rim of the entryhole is seen. However, this rarely causes problems.*

CONCLUSIONS

Ender nails provide an additional fixation method for the orthopedic surgeon who routinely treats complex unstable intertrochanteric fractures in the elderly debilitated patient (Fig 18–16). Although Ender and others have suggested that most intertrochanteric fractures can be treated by this method,[7-10, 28-38] some surgeons have reported more favorable results with the compression hip screw and sliding nail plate device.[39-46] With modern anesthesia techniques, improved blood bank products, and better postoperative care, the slightly lower operating time, reduced blood loss, and lower infection rate may not offset the problems that have been associated with the Ender pins.[12, 13, 21]

Unquestionably, the infection rate is less with Ender pinning than with other techniques,[12, 16, 17, 20, 21] and for this reason alone it has a significant advantage over other fixation methods. Although the technique is not overly demanding for the experienced fracture surgeon, the indications for its use are best learned with experience and preoperative interpretation of the fracture classification. Stable fracture patterns usually do well with Ender fixation.[12] However, rotational deformities are best treated by compulsive prevention. In most series, knee pain is quite frequent, and patients should be warned preoperatively that knee discomfort can occur. Most symptoms are usually alleviated by eventual removal of the pins. In the selected

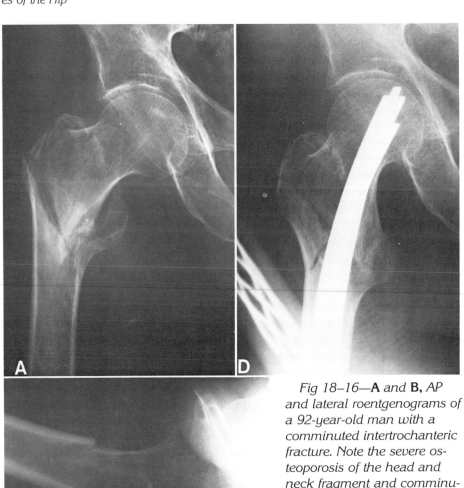

*Fig 18–16—**A** and **B**, AP and lateral roentgenograms of a 92-year-old man with a comminuted intertrochanteric fracture. Note the severe osteoporosis of the head and neck fragment and comminution of the greater and lesser trochanters. The osteoporosis and wide femoral canal with severe comminution are relative contraindications to the use of Ender nails. **C** and **D**, postoperative roentgenograms demonstrating anatomical reduction in the AP and lateral planes. Because of the patient's elderly and debilitated status, Ender pins were selected. Ideally, the pins should have fanned into the femoral head for better fixation. However, the subchondral pin placement along the medial calcar and the bridge position of the AP walls of the canal improve their purchase.*

patient, Ender nails contribute to the treatment of complex fractures about the hip and are a useful addition to the armamentarium of the orthopedic surgeon.

REFERENCES

1. Lewinnek G.E., et al.: The significance and a comparative analysis of the epidemiology of hip fractures. *Clin. Orthop.* 152:35, 1980.
2. Alffram P.A.: An epidemiologic study of cervical and trochanteric fractures of the femur in an urban population. *Acta Orthop. Scand. Suppl.* 65:1, 1964.
3. Kuntscher G.: Die stabile Osteosynthese bei der Osteotomie. *Chirurg* 14:161, 1942.
4. Smith-Peterson M.N., et al.: Intracapsular fractures of the neck of the femur treated by internal fixation. *Arch. Surg.* 23(2):715, 1931.
5. Kuntscher G.: Zur operativen Behandlung der pertrochanteren Frakturen. *Zentralbl. Chir.* 91:281, 1966.
6. Ender H.: Probleme bei frischen per und subtrochanteren Oberschenkelbruche. *Unfallheilkunde* 106:2, 1970.
7. Bohler J., Ender H.G., Bohler N.: Erfahrungen mit der percutanen intramedullaren Fixation pertrochanterer Frakturen mit elastischen Rundnageln nach Ender. *Monatschr. Unfallheilkunde* 78:361-370, 1975.
8. Ender J., Simon-Weidner R.: Die Fixierung der trochanteren Bruche mit runden elastischen Condylennagel. *Acta Chir. Austr.* 1:40-42, 1970.
9. Kuderna H., Bohler N., Collon D.: Treatment of intertrochanteric and subtrochanteric fractures of the hip by the Ender method. *J. Bone Joint Surg.* 58A:604-616, 1976.
10. Thomas B., et al.: Use of Ender pins in the fixation of intertrochanteric hip fractures. Read before the annual meeting of The American Academy of Orthopaedic Surgeons, Dallas, February 1978.
11. Ender H.: Treatment of pertrochanteric and subtrochanteric fractures of the femur with Ender pins, in *The Hip: Proceedings of the Sixth Open Scientific Meeting of the Hip Society.* St. Louis, C.V. Mosby Co., 1978, pp. 187-206.
12. Chapman M., et al.: The use of Ender's pins in extracapsular fractures of the hip. *J. Bone Joint Surg.* 63A:14, 1981.
13. Kuderna H., et al.: Treatment of intertrochanteric and subtrochanteric fractures of the hip by the Ender Method. *J. Bone Joint Surg.* 58A:604-611, 1976.
14. Poigenfurst J.: Änderung der Behandlingsergebnisse bei pertrochanteren Bruchen durch Stabilisierung mit elastischen Rundnageln. *Wien. Med. Wochenschr.* 123:155-160, 1973.
15. Wynn Jones C., et al.: A comparison of the treatment of trochanteric fractures of the femur by internal fixation with a nail plate and the Ender technique. *Injury* 9:35-42, 1977.
16. Hult L., Nilsson M.: Ender spikning ar trokantara femur frakturer. *Lakartidningen* 75:4603, 1978.
17. Hugh J., Lund B.: Ender eller McLaughin I Behandlingen at laterale collum femoris frakturer. Read at the Nordic Orthopaedic Association 40th Congress, Helsingfors, June 11–14, 1980.
18. Casey M., Chapman M.: Ipsilateral concomitant fractures of the hip and femoral shaft. *J. Bone Joint Surg.* 61A:503-509, 1979.
19. Bohler J.: Percutaneous intramedullary nailing of intertrochanteric fractures, in *The Hip: Proceedings of the Third Open Scientific Meeting of the Hip Society.* St. Louis, C.V. Mosby Co., 1975, pp. 167-179.
20. Kuderna H., et al.: Treatment of intertrochanteric and subtrochanteric fractures of the hip by the Ender method. *J. Bone Joint Surg.* 58A:604-611, 1976.
21. Raugstad T., et al.: Treatment of pertrochanteric and subtrochanteric fractures of the femur by the Ender method. *Clin. Orthop.* 138:231, 1979.
22. Thomas B., et al.: Use of Ender pins in the fixation of intertrochanteric hip fractures. Read before the annual meeting of The American Academy of Orthopaedic Surgeons, Dallas, February 1978.
23. Trafton P., et al.: Harris nail versus compression hip screw for intertrochanteric femur

fractures: A prospective randomized comparison. Read before the annual meeting of The American Academy of Orthopaedic Surgeons, Atlanta, Feb. 12, 1984.

24. Kyle R., et al.: Analysis of six hundred and twenty-two intertrochanteric hip fractures. *J. Bone Joint Surg.* 61A:216-221, 1979.

25. Bray T., Chapman M.: Percutaneous pinning of intracapsular hip fractures. *Instr. Course Lect.* 33:168–179, 1984.

26. Ender H.: Treatment of pertrochanteric and subtrochateric fractures of the femur with Ender pins, in *The Hip: Proceedings of the Sixth Open Scientific Meeting of the Hip Society.* St. Louis, C.V. Mosby Co., 1978, pp. 187-206.

27. Nelson C., et al.: Ender nailing of intertrochanteric fractures, in *Controversies in Orthopaedic Surgery.* Philadelphia, W.B. Saunders Co., 1982, pp. 139-153.

28. Bohler J.: Percutane Trochanterosteotomie bei der Nagelung intertrochanter Oberschenkelbruche. *Monatschr. Unfallheilkunde* 75:480-484, 1972.

29. Bohler J.: Percutaneous intramedullary nailing of intertrochanteric fractures, in *The Hip: Proceedings of the Third Open Scientific Meeting of the Hip Society.* St. Louis, C.V. Mosby Co., 1975, pp. 166-179.

30. Ender H.G.: Treatment of pertrochanteric and subtrochanteric fractures of the femur with Ender pins, in *The Hip: Proceedings of the Sixth Open Scientific Meeting of the Hip Society.* St. Louis, C.V. Mosby Co., 1978, pp. 187-206.

31. Frauscher H.: Operative Behandlung trochanternaher Oberschenkelbruche mit Ender-Nageln. *Monatschr. Unfallheilkunde* 78:1-9, 1975.

32. Laskin R., Gruber M., Zimmerman A.: Intertrochanteric fractures of the hip in the elderly. *Orthop. Trans.* 2:195-196, 1978.

33. Persch W.F., Birkner H.: Frühergebnisse der operativen Behandlung trochanterer Oberschenkelbruche und lateraler Schenkelhalsbruche mit den Kondylennageln nach Simon-Weidner und Ender. *Monatschr. Unfallheilkunde* 78:49-57, 1975.

34. Poigenfurst J.: Änderung der Behandlingsergebnisse bei pertrochanteren Bruchen durch Stabilisierung mit elastischen Rundnageln. *Wien. Med. Wochenschr.* 123:155-160, 1973.

35. Ruedi T.: Indication: Pro and contra of Ender nail. Read at the Twenty-fifth AO Course, Davos, Switzerland, December 1978.

36. Simon-Weidner R.: Die Fixierung trochanterer Bruche mit multiplen elastischen Rundnagelen nach Simon-Weidner. *Unfallheilkunde* 106:60-62, 1970.

37. Waddell J., Czitrom A.: The treatment of intertrochanteric and subtrochanteric fractures of the hip by the Ender method. Read before the annual meeting of the American Academy of Orthopaedic Surgeons, San Francisco, Feb. 23, 1979.

38. Wynn Jones C., et al.: A comparison of the treatment of trochanteric fractures of the femur by internal fixation with a nail plate and the Ender technique. *Injury* 9:35-42, 1977.

39. Callender G. Jr.: Callender hip assembly, in *Proceedings of The American Academy of Orthopaedic Surgeons. J. Bone Joint Surg.* 49A:1235, 1967.

40. Clawson D.: Trochanteric fractures treated by the sliding screw plate fixation method. *J. Trauma* 4:737-752, 1964.

41. Ecker M., et al.: The treatment of trochanteric hip fractures using a compression screw. *J. Bone Joint Surg.* 57A:23-27, 1975.

42. Harrington K., Johnston J.: The management of comminuted unstable intertrochanteric fractures. *J. Bone Joint Surg.* 55A:1367-1376, 1973.

43. Kyle R., et al.: Analysis of six hundred and twenty-two intertrochanteric hip fractures. *J. Bone Joint Surg.* 61A:216-221, 1979.

44. Laskin R., et al.: Intertrochanteric fractures of the hip in the elderly. *Orthop. Trans.* 2:195-196, 1978.

45. Schumpelick W., Jantzen P.: A new principle in the operative treatment of trochanteric fractures of the femur. *J. Bone Joint Surg.* 37A:693-698, 1955.

46. Thomas, B., et al.: Use of Ender's pins in the fixation of intertrochanteric hip fractures. Read before the annual meeting of the American Academy of Orthopaedic Surgeons, Dallas, February 1978.

Chapter 19

Condylocephalic Nailing of Intertrochanteric and Subtrochanteric Fractures

Leslie J. Harris, M.D.

Patients with intertrochanteric fractures are often elderly and debilitated and have a high incidence of cardiovascular disease, pulmonary disease, diabetes, and organic brain syndrome.[1-3] Approximately 75% of patients have significant functional loss 6 months following hip fracture, and 20%–40% die within a year.[1, 2, 4-9] The surgical procedure required for placement of fixed or sliding nail plate devices typically entails a large operative exposure, 2 or more units of blood loss, and 2 hours of anesthesia time, and carries a definite risk of infection. Closed nailing techniques offer the potential advantage of reducing the operative trauma to medically fragile patients.

In contrast, subtrochanteric fractures occur in a younger age group and are often the result of major trauma. Because of the better physiologic condition of these patients, they are better able to withstand bed rest without experiencing the degree of morbidity and mortality seen in patients with intertrochanteric fractures. However, when nail or screw plate fixation is used, mechanical failures occur in as many as 44% of cases[10] and are commonly associated with nonunion. The advantages of an intramedullary device for treating subtrochanteric fractures have been well shown by Zickel[11] and confirmed by our own experience with the condylocephalic nail.

History and Design Considerations

The closed nailing of intertrochanteric and subtrochanteric fractures was an outgrowth of the closed nailing of femoral shaft fractures. Kuntscher, Rush, Street, and others have demonstrated the advantages of closed nailing procedures, which include minimal blood loss, reduced anesthesia time, a low nonunion rate, and a negligible infection rate. In 1970 Kuntscher introduced the concept of condylocephalic nailing, i.e., retrograde nailing of hip fractures, to extend the advantages of the closed technique used for femoral shaft fractures to the upper femoral region.[12] The Kuntscher nail curved into the head and neck of the femur at an angle of 160° to the shaft, approximately parallel to weight-bearing forces. The Kuntscher procedure illustrated the technical feasibility of condylocephalic nailing, but there also emerged a unique set of complications: proximal or distal migration of the nail with or without loss of fracture reduction, external rotation deformity, knee pain, and limitation of knee motion.[13,14]

In 1973, my colleagues and I began an investigation into condylocephalic nailing. In particular, we addressed the complications of Kuntscher's procedure with changes in instrumentation and technique. A relatively new orthopedic material, titanium-aluminum-vanadium, was used to take advantage of its 50% lower modulus of elasticity than that of stainless steel.[15] The relative elasticity of the nail facilitates passage through the various curves of the femoral canal without jamming. The diamond-shaped cross-section of the Street nail was utilized such that at the isthmus of the femur, the major and minor diameters of the nail are aligned with the major and minor diameters of the femoral canal (Fig 19–1). Experience with intramedullary nailing of femoral shaft fractures as well as experimental data have demonstrated that nails that provide edge control are more effective in controlling rotation than the smooth Kuntscher nail or two clustered Kuntscher nails.[16] Clinically, an accurate rotatory reduction depends in large part on the reduction seen on the lateral view. The nail therefore incorporates an anterior posterior bow and an anteversion curvature, which necessitates left and right nails (Fig 19–2). Intertrochanteric fractures often settle with weight-bearing, with a resultant shortening of up to 2 cm. With shortening at the fracture site, there is relative inferior displacement of the distal end of the nail, which then might project into the soft tissues about the knee. To avoid knee symptoms, the initial nail length selected should allow the distal end of the nail

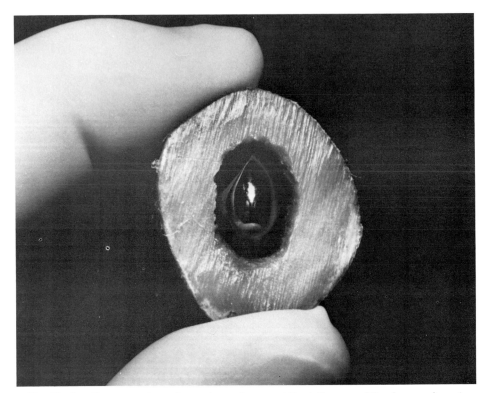

Fig 19–1—Cross-section of a cadaver femur at the isthmus of the femur showing the elliptical shape of the canal and the corresponding diamond cross-section of the condylocephalic nail.

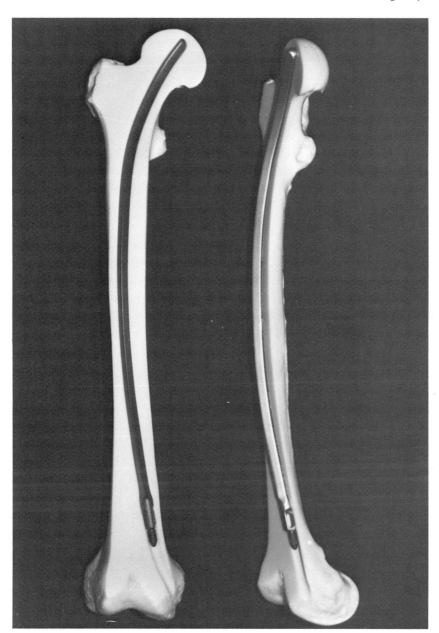

Fig 19–2—Frontal and oblique views of condylocephalic nail in femoral models. In the frontal plane, the proximal portion of the nail is aligned approximately 160° to the femoral shaft. In the lateral plane, the nail incorporates a 10° AP bow and an 8° anteversion angle. The distal end of the nail should lie at least 2 cm within the medullary canal. (From Harris L.J.: Condylocephalic nailing of intertrochanteric and subtrochanteric fractures, in American Academy of Orthopaedic Surgeons: Instructional Course Lectures. *St. Louis, C.V. Mosby Co., 1980, vol. 29. Reproduced by permission.)*

to lie at least 2 cm proximal to the cortical window, i.e., to be countersunk 2 cm proximally. Since it is difficult to estimate precisely the nail length prior to performing the procedure, a set of nail extenders enables the surgeon to alter the nail length during the course of the procedure. The extenders have left-handed threads and are used with a reverse-threaded driver-extractor.

INTERTROCHANTERIC FRACTURES
Operative Technique

The use of the fracture table is strongly recommended for most intertrochanteric and subtrochanteric fractures. Only minimally displaced, stable intertrochanteric fractures are good candidates for "free-hand" procedures. The image intensifier should be positioned lateral to the fractured hip, in contrast to routine hip nailings, in which the image intensifier is positioned between the patient's legs. The insertion site for the nail is two fingerbreadths anterior to the adductor tubercle at the edge of the flare of the medial femoral condyle (Fig 19–3). A skin incision approximately 2.5 cm long is made slightly distal to this site to avoid damage to the skin with passage of the nail. As previously mentioned, a nail length is selected such that its distal end will lie 2 cm proximal to the cortical window when the nail is in its final position. Often a 3-cm extender is used at the start of the procedure and removed after the nail is finally positioned. As the nail is introduced, it is aligned slightly externally rotated to the femur so that it will track anteriorly in the femoral canal and more easily negotiate the fracture site. The nail guide should not be used to forcibly rotate the nail within the femoral canal. (In this respect, the technique differs significantly from the Ender procedure.) The nail is negotiated across the fracture site by the surgeon's manipulating the shaft fragment and the nail as a unit. Adduction of the

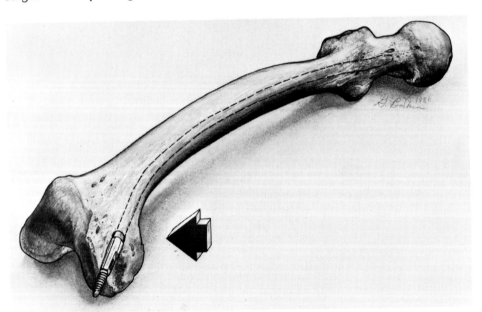

Fig 19–3—The condylocephalic nail is partially inserted to demonstrate the location of the entrance hole in the medial femoral condyle immediately distal to the medial flare of the femur. (From Harris L.J.: Condylocephalic nailing of intertrochanteric fractures. Contemp. Orthop. *3:147-154, 1981. Reproduced by permission.)*

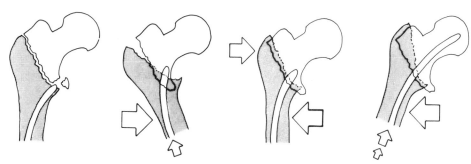

Fig 19–4—If the nail tip threatens to exit the fracture site medially, manipulation of the leg is required to pass the nail into the proximal fragment. If the leg is abducted, the nail tip is directed in a more lateral direction to engage the proximal fragment. Releasing the distal traction facilitates this maneuver. Once the proximal fragment is engaged, the fracture must be reduced in a valgus position before the nail is driven home. (From Harris L.J.: Intramedullary nailing of intertrochanteric and subtrochanteric fractures of the femur, in American Academy of Orthopaedic Surgeons: Instructional Course Lectures. *St. Louis, C.V. Mosby Co., 1982, vol. 32. Reproduced by permission.)*

leg projects the proximal nail tip laterally, external rotation of the leg projects the nail anteriorly, and so on. Often the shaft fragment sags posterior to the proximal fragment in the lateral view. Reduction is achieved by the assistant lifting the thigh anteriorly as the nail is tapped across the fracture site. After the nail is passed across the fracture site, the reduction should be carefully assessed before the nail is driven home. As with other hip nails and techniques, multiple passes into the femoral head should be avoided.

A valgus reduction should be obtained in all unstable intertrochanteric fractures. In most cases, this can be obtained by abducting the leg after the nail is just across the fracture site (Fig 19–4). Occasionally the greater trochanteric spike attached to the femoral shaft prevents the proximal fragment from tilting into a valgus position, and a percutaneous osteotomy is required. The image intensifier is used to localize the position of an osteotome inserted through a small stab incision through the proximal thigh. Only the lateral cortical shell requires an osteotomy (Fig 19–5). The nail tip should be placed centrally in the femoral head in the anteroposterior and lateral views to within 5 mm of the joint line. The traction is then released and the fracture is impacted manually.

Fracture Stability

An analysis of fixation failures that have occurred following condylocephalic nailing emphasizes several important considerations. Fixation failures occurred in 3 of 13 basilar neck fractures (23%), and one nonunion occurred (7.7%), suggesting that basilar neck fractures are a relative contraindication for condylocephalic nailing. In a recent series, Ender pinning of four basicervical fractures led to fixation failure in each case.[17]

Fixation failures have been the major concern in most series of unstable intertrochanteric fractures. In recent years, sliding nail plate and screw plate systems have gained popularity over fixed-angle nail plate devices. In general, the sliding devices offer the advantages of allowing fracture impaction, diminished stress shield-

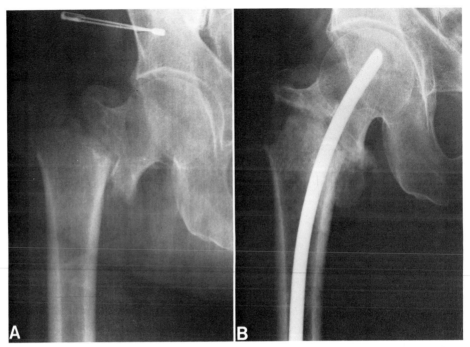

*Fig 19–5—**A,** shearing type of intertrochanteric fracture characterized by a proximal and lateral position of the femoral shaft and a neutral to valgus position of the proximal fragment. **B,** a percutaneous osteotomy facilitates placement of the femoral shaft medially beneath the proximal fragment and also allows a valgus reduction of the fracture. (From Harris L.J.: Condylocephalic nailing of intertrochanteric fractures.* Contemp. Orthop. *3:147-154, 1981. Reproduced by permission.)*

ing, and a lower incidence of implant failures. In the last 20–25 years, failure rates for both stable and unstable intertrochanteric fractures fixed with sliding devices have varied between 5.5% and 10.4%.[2, 6, 18-23] In our own series of condylocephalic fixation of 149 unstable intertrochanteric fractures, there was complete loss of fixation in 4.2%.

An analysis of these fixation failures demonstrates technical considerations common to other implant systems. Varus reductions, shallow placement of the nail tip in the femoral head, and poor centering of the nail tip in AP and lateral views are associated with failures. Anatomical factors include degree of comminution, extension of the fracture into the femoral neck area, and degree of osteoporosis. Although Dimon and Hughston[5] illustrated the posterior and medial fragments typical of unstable intertrochanteric fractures (Fig 19–6), anatomical variables produce a wide spectrum of instability. Figure 19–7 shows an unstable intertrochanteric fracture in a patient with Singh grade II osteoporosis. The proximal fragment is relatively short and the fracture extends intracapsularly in the posterior neck region. Fixation of this fracture with any available fixation device would likely fail. This patient is a candidate for either a sliding screw device with supplemental methylmethacrylate cement, or a primary endoprosthetic replacement. Figure 19–6 shows an unstable intertrochanteric fracture with large posterior and medial fragments. However, the bone quality is good and there is a relatively long proximal fragment, providing much-improved purchase for an intramedullary nail. This patient is a good candidate for condylocephalic nailing.

Fixation failures with the condylocephalic nail have been associated with distal migration of the nail out of the proximal fragment. A similar mechanism occurs with Ender pinning. This phenomenon was studied experimentally with loading tests on the MTS machine with simulated intertrochanteric fractures in cadaver femurs. At clinical loads, the proximal fragment displaces along the oblique fracture line from the superior aspect to the inferomedial aspect. When the load is released, the head and neck fragment springs back to its original position from the recoil of the implanted nail. Cyclic loading in this manner eventually results in the nail working distally, with loss of fixation of the proximal fragment. Experimentally and clinically, the nail does not migrate proximally unless it has been previously driven through the subchondral

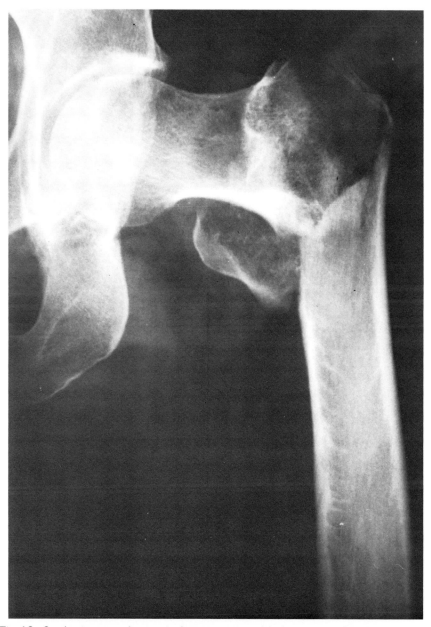

Fig 19–6—An intertrochanteric fracture, unstable by virtue of its large posterior and medial fragments. See text.

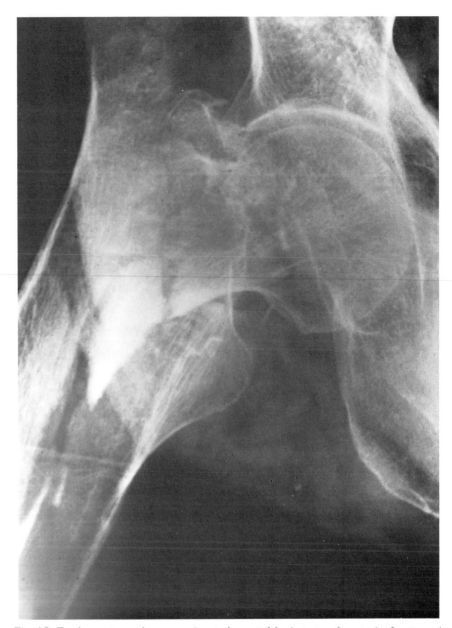

Fig 19–7—An extremely comminuted unstable intertrochanteric fracture in a patient with severe osteoporosis. The fracture extends into the cervical area posteriorly. See text.

cortex of the femoral head. The more vertical the fracture line, the greater the potential displacement of the proximal fragment. A practical solution to this sequence of events is the percutaneous trochanteric osteotomy, which creates a more horizontal fracture configuration. Currently, percutaneous osteotomies are performed for unstable intertrochanteric fractures when a valgus reduction cannot be obtained by manipulation alone.

Two variations of unstable intertrochanteric fractures deserve special comment. Shearing fractures with proximal and lateral displacement of the shaft are unique in that the proximal fragment is aligned in a valgus position rather than the usual varus position (see Fig 19–5). With longitudinal traction, the proximal fragment shifts into a greater valgus angulation as the surgeon attempts to position the shaft medially under the proximal fragment. Ender recommended a solution to this dilemma that consisted of initially externally rotating and adducting the leg, followed by internal rotation and abduction of the lower extremity. Even with this maneuver, in my experience, a percutaneous osteotomy is often required to place the shaft sufficiently medially under the proximal fragment.

The proximal fragment of an unstable fracture may include a long anterior spike. The proximal fragment is in a flexed position with the spike projecting anteriorly such that on the lateral view, the fracture line is quite vertical, extending from the spike anteroinferiorly to posterosuperiorly (Fig 19–8). The fracture line may extend intercapsularly into the posterior neck region, leaving very little support for the nail posteriorly. Reduction of this fracture is facilitated by placing the lower extremity in a flexed position (as one would for a subtrochanteric fracture). The anterior spike must be anatomically "keyed" into the shaft or loss of fixation is quite likely to occur.

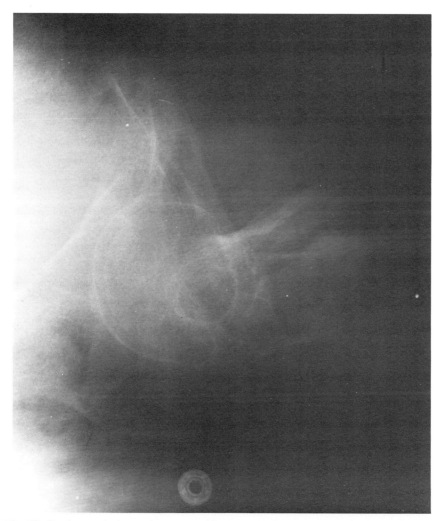

Fig 19–8—Lateral view of an unstable intertrochanteric fracture demonstrating the flexed position of the proximal fragment and the anterior spike. The fracture extends into the cervical area posteriorly. See text.

External Rotation Deformity

External rotation deformities have been reported in 1.2%–71% of patients with Ender pins.[24-29] In our series of 514 patients, 12% of patients had greater than 15% loss of internal rotation compared to the opposite lower extremity. The mechanisms for this deformity include the following: (1) Retroversion of the proximal fragment secondary to posterior comminutation at the fracture site. This is most likely to occur in unstable intertrochanteric fractures. (2) External rotation of the femoral shaft about the nail. (3) Soft tissue contracture (external rotation contractures can be seen following nondisplaced intertrochanteric fractures). The incidence of external rotation deformity can be reduced by obtaining an accurate fracture reduction at the time of surgery and using an antirotation splint for 1–2 weeks postoperatively. For aged patients who are debilitated, institutionalized, disoriented, or nonambulatory, an external rotation deformity is of little concern. However, relatively active and alert patients with unstable intertrochanteric fractures are probably better served with open screw plate fixation and precise control of rotation.

Shortening

Several studies have indicated shortening of 1–2.5 cm of intertrochanteric fractures when various sliding devices as well as remote nailing techniques have been used (Table 19–1). Significant shortening may be seen in stable intertrochanteric fractures, and the amount of shortening is not always predictable by the preoperative

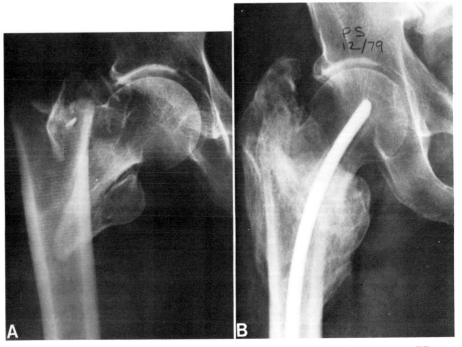

*Fig 19–9—**A,** an extremely comminuted intertrochanteric fracture in a 75-year-old man. **B,** roentgenogram obtained 3 months postoperatively, at which time the patient was fully ambulatory using a cane. The fracture has impacted with a resultant 1.8-cm shortening and considerable new bone formation. (From Harris.[30] Reproduced by permission.)*

TABLE 19–1.—Intertrochanteric Fracture Shortening Following Treatment With Various Devices

Study, Year	Device*	Amount of Shortening
Clawson, 1964[31]	Sliding screw	1.2 cm (av.)
Harrington and Johnston, 1973[32]	Sliding screw	1.5 cm (av.)
Ecker et al., 1975[6]	Sliding screw	2 cm (19.4% av.)
Ganz et al., 1979[33]	AO blade plate	1 cm (13% av.)
Laskin et al., 1978[34]	Sliding screw and MDO	1.5 cm (av.)
Raugstad et al., 1979[27]	Ender pins	>2 cm (20%)
Jacobs et al., 1980[18]	Jewett device	0.99 cm (25% av.)
	Sliding screw	1.57 cm (6% av.)
Siegel et al., 1981[29]	Ender pins	2.5 cm (19% av.)

*MDO, medial displacement osteotomy.

radiographic appearance. The ability of the sliding implant and remote nailing techniques to allow shortening and impaction of fracture fragments appears to be a desirable feature for early fracture union and a low implant failure rate (Fig 19–9).

Mortality

The 6-week postoperative mortality in our primarily county hospital patient population was 4% and the 6-month mortality was 10.2%. Following various open fixation procedures, mortalities of 11%–16% during the early postoperative period and of 20%–42% at 1 year have been reported.[1, 2, 4-9] Closed remote nailing techniques appear to offer improved survival in high-risk patients.

Summary of Relative Indications and Contraindications

Basilar neck fractures are a relative contraindication for condylocephalic nailing. Stable intertrochanteric fractures are excellent candidates for this type of fixation, as are unstable fractures in elderly debilitated patients. Unstable intertrochanteric fractures in active, alert patients, in whom precise control of rotation is essential, are relatively better candidates for open reduction with screw plate devices. The rare patient with an extremely comminuted unstable fracture with a short proximal fragment and a Singh grade I or II osteoporosis is better treated with a screw plate device and supplemental methylmethacrylate cement or primary endoprosthetic replacement. These more drastic measures appear justified when one considers the likely alternative: fixation failure and a salvage procedure under anesthesia.

SUBTROCHANTERIC FRACTURES
Operative Technique

Technically, subtrochanteric fractures are more difficult to nail in a closed manner than trochanteric fractures. The proximal fragment is often extremely flexed and externally rotated. The fracture table must be set up with the lower extremity flexed and externally rotated to match the proximal fragment. The oblique views subsequently obtained using the image intensifier may be difficult to interpret. An alternative method is to drive a large threaded Steinmann pin into the greater trochanter percutaneously. The pin is then used as a lever to internally rotate and extend the proximal fragment until the nail can be driven across the fracture site. The

Steinmann pin is then removed. Medially comminuted fractures present special problems during the nailing procedure. The proximal nail tip tends to exit the femoral canal medial to the proximal fragment. For these fractures, we now prestraighten the nail with the nail bender slightly in the frontal plane to aid in bypassing a medial defect. The proximal tip of the straightened nail will lie more superior in the femoral head, which is acceptable for subtrochanteric fractures (see Fig 19–10,B). Manipulation of the leg is also more often required to bypass medially comminuted areas than with intertrochanteric fractures (see Fig 19–4).

When attempts at closed nailing fail, a small midlateral thigh exposure is required to guide the nail across the fracture site under direct vision. When large fragments or a long oblique fracture line are present, then supplemental cerclage wires or screws are needed to improve stability. Four of sixty-four unstable subtrochanteric fractures in our series required open reduction (Fig 19–10).

Fracture Stability

Several principles that have evolved from the intramedullary nailing of femoral shaft fractures apply directly to condylocephalic nailing of subtrochanteric fractures. (1) Transverse or short oblique fractures impact about the nail with insignificant shortening. (2) Long oblique fractures or fractures with more significant comminution may shorten significantly. Open reduction with supplemental screw or cerclage fixation improves length stability, but postoperatively balanced suspension or traction for 3–6 weeks is also required. For young, healthy patients who can tolerate prolonged bed rest, we favor closed nailing and postoperative traction to avoid shortening (Figs 19–11 and 19–12). For older, debilitated patients with long oblique fractures, I prefer open reduction with cerclage wiring followed by early wheelchair or non-weight-bearing ambulation.

The purchase of the condylocephalic nail in the proximal fragment of a subtrochanteric fracture is far superior to that in an intertrochanteric fracture, since the proximal fragment is much larger and the degree of osteoporosis is often far less. Distal migration of the condylocephalic nail has not been seen in subtrochanteric fractures, and loss of rotational control has been exceedingly rare.

Results

Of 514 fractures, 126 were subtrochanteric (24.5%), 47 were transtrochanteric (Boyd III), 64 were unstable subtrochanteric, and 15 were stable subtrochanteric fractures. Transtrochanteric fractures were anatomically intermediate between intertrochanteric and subtrochanteric fractures.[30] Intramedullary nail fixation appeared superior in this group than in the intertrochanteric group, a finding which has been attributed to the greater area for purchase in the proximal fragment. There were no fixation failures in this group. The intramedullary nail prevents medial migration of the shaft, which is the common mechanism of failure when fixed-angle nail plate devices are used.

There were two fixation failures in 64 unstable subtrochanteric fractures (3.1%). This compares exceedingly well with the 44.5% failure rates recently reported with nail plate devices.[10] Some 55% of the unstable fractures had shortening, averaging 1.1 cm. Loss of rotational control was not documented. One patient who underwent closed nailing had a 30° internal rotation deformity that required reoperation. As opposed to the intertrochanteric group, distal migration of the nail did

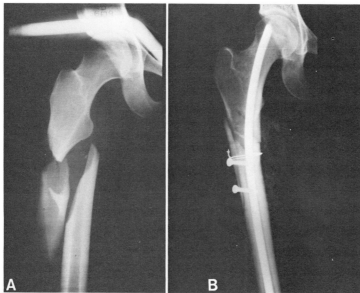

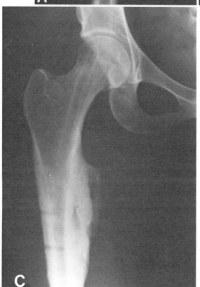

Fig 19–10—**A,** *comminuted subtrochanteric fracture in a 17-year-old girl who has a partial sciatic nerve deficit.* **B,** *roentgenogram obtained 6 weeks postoperatively. The patient had undergone open reduction and internal fixation of the fracture with exploration of the sciatic nerve. The procedure was done in a prone position. The patient was maintained in balanced suspension for 4 weeks postoperatively before partial weight-bearing ambulation was allowed. The nail has been straightened slightly in the frontal plane in the area of the subtrochanteric fracture, with a resultant superior position of the proximal tip in the femoral head.* **C,** *roentgenogram taken shortly after removal of hardware 2 years after injury. There has been complete recovery of sciatic nerve function. There is no detectable shortening and no rotatory deformity.*

not occur. The two fixation failures occurred in elderly patients with long oblique fractures. In both cases, after closed nailing, early weight-bearing was attempted and resulted in telescoping of fracture fragments about the nail and loss of fixation. The important factors here are the vertical angle of the fracture and the large diameter of the femoral canal compared to the diameter of the nail. Packing the canal with pins, as in the Ender procedure, has not been effective in eliminating shortening if weight-bearing is allowed. Therefore, open reduction and supplemental cerclage wiring is required for these patients to be up in a chair soon after their procedure.

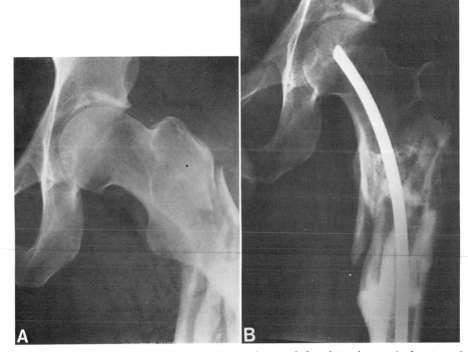

*Fig 19–11—**A,** an extremely comminuted open left subtrochanteric fracture, in a 46-year-old man. The patient was taken to surgery for debridement of wounds and thereafter was maintained in proximal tibial skeletal traction for 10 days, until the wounds were healing well. **B,** patient underwent closed condylocephalic nailing and was maintained in 5 pounds of tibial pin traction for 3 weeks post-operatively. Non-weight-bearing ambulation was started at that time, and weight-bearing was begun 6 weeks following closed nailing. Roentgenogram was obtained 4 months following condylocephalic nailing and demonstrates progressive fracture healing. There was no clinical shortening or rotatory deformity.*

Previously Fused Hips With Subtrochanteric Fractures

Although not a common clinical entity, patients with previously fused hips may sustain subtrochanteric fractures which cannot be approached at the hip for a standard intramedullary nailing procedure. The condylocephalic nail can be passed across the fusion mass into the ilium for improved fixation in the proximal fragments (Fig 19–13).

Pathologic Fractures

The condylocephalic nailing technique has been used for a variety of pathologic lesions of the proximal femur. An osteoblastic lesion such as metastatic prostatic carcinoma may occlude the femoral canal with dense bone that cannot be penetrated by the nail. Using excessive force in an attempt to drive the nail past an occluded area of the femoral canal may cause iatrogenic fracturing of the femoral shaft. Multiple lytic lesions of the femur such as occur with multiple myeloma also present the potential for iatrogenic fracturing of the femur and therefore are a relative contraindication. The condylocephalic nailing technique has proved most useful in patients with impending fractures of the proximal femur who are to undergo radiation therapy. Prophylactic nailing is a minimal procedure that can be accomplished within a few minutes. A fracture occurring through a large osteolytic area may result in considerable shortening. After closed nailing of a fracture (or prophylactic nailing), supplemental methacrylate is used percutaneously. A stab incision is made over the distal aspect of the greater trochanter. A three-eighths inch drill bit is then used to drill from the greater trochanter to the lytic area under image intensification. The lytic area is then curetted or aspirated and cement is injected in a liquid state under image intensification control. Pathologic lesions, which have led to considerable loss of bone stock and ultimately fracture, have been treated on the basis of the patient's medical condition and life expectancy. For patients who have less than a few weeks' life expectancy and who may not survive major surgery, closed condylocephalic nailing is done to stabilize the fracture sufficiently for nursing care, and considerable shortening or rotatory deformity of the extremity is not a major concern. However, for patients with a life expectancy of 6 months or more, open reduction with more rigid intramedullary nail or plate fixation with methylmethacrylate cement has been used.

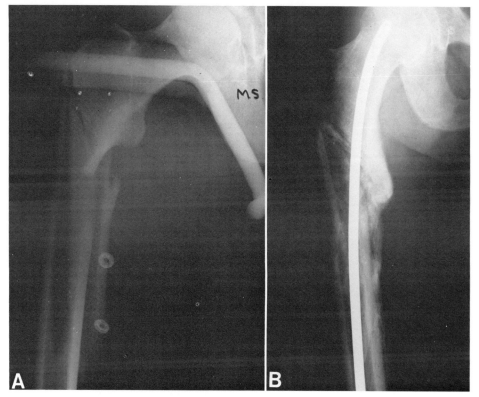

*Fig 19–12—**A,** unstable subtrochanteric fracture. **B,** fracture was nailed in a closed manner and the patient was maintained in balanced suspension with light traction for 3½ weeks before ambulation with limited weight-bearing was allowed. Roentgenogram obtained 4 months postoperatively demonstrates progressive healing of the fracture. The nail has been straightened slightly in the frontal plane to facilitate the surgical technique. See text.*

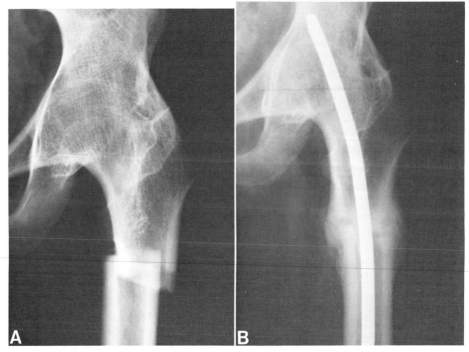

*Fig 19–13—**A,** stable subtrochanteric fracture in a patient who had previously undergone arthrodesis of the left hip. **B,** fracture was nailed in a closed manner and the nail driven across the fused area into the ilium. The patient was maintained in balanced suspension for 1 week postoperatively, at which time progressive weight-bearing was allowed.*

Ipsilateral Basicocervical-Femoral Shaft Fractures

The closed nailing of ipsilateral basicervical and femoral shaft fractures is technically feasible with the condylocephalic nail. However, several factors must be kept in mind. (1) The nail should be straightened in the area of the corresponding location of the shaft fracture to avoid a varus reduction. (2) In addition to the condylocephalic nail, supplemental screw fixation of the basicervical fracture is recommended. For the proximal fracture, we have used percutaneous pinning with three to five threaded pins in addition to the condylocephalic nail. (3) This patient population consists primarily of young patients involved in vehicular accidents. The bone in the femoral head fragment is quite dense. Therefore, as the nail is driven across the femoral neck fracture into the femoral head, distraction of the basicervical fracture often occurs. This distraction must be eliminated before the supplemental pins or screws are driven across the femoral neck fracture. Impaction of the fracture can be achieved by working the condylocephalic nail back and forth several times as well as by manual impaction at the knee. (4) Alternatively, a short condylocephalic nail can be used for fixation of the shaft fracture. The proximal end of the nail is placed just distal to the femoral neck. The canal of the femoral neck is then completely unobstructed so that percutaneous pinning of the neck fracture may be more easily accomplished from the lateral thigh.

SUMMARY

The use of closed condylocephalic nailing for elderly patients with intertrochanteric fractures has resulted in substantially improved mortality. The incidence of fixation failures and the degree of shortening are similar to what is experienced with sliding screw and sliding nail plate systems. Stable intertrochanteric fractures have been routinely managed with the condylocephalic nail. However, since rotational deformities may occur in patients with unstable intertrochanteric fractures, the procedure appears to be most beneficial for unstable fractures in patients who are aged, debilitated, institutionalized, disoriented, or nonambulatory.

Transtrochanteric fractures are ideal for condylocephalic fixation. The more distal fractures afford better fixation in the proximal fragment than intertrochanteric fractures. Medial migration of the shaft is not seen with intramedullary fixation.

In general, subtrochanteric fractures occur in a younger group of patients. Since the proximal fragment is usually larger and the quality of bone superior in this group of patients, the fixation failure rate is extremely low and loss of rotatory reduction has not been significant.

The body of experience gained in recent years with closed nailing techniques for femoral shaft and tibial fractures is directly applicable to the closed nailing of intertrochanteric and subtrochanteric fractures. Extremely comminuted fractures or long oblique fractures are subject to shortening, and rotatory control must always be a matter of concern with intramedullary fixation. These difficulties must be carefully weighed in each case against the advantages of a negligible infection rate and the extremely low nonunion and implant failure rate.

REFERENCES

1. Jensen J.S., Tondevold E.: Mortality after hip fractures. *Acta Orthop. Scand.* 50:161, 1979.
2. Miller C.W.: Survival and ambulation following hip fractures. *J. Bone Joint Surg.* 60A:930, 1978.
3. Nieman K.M.W., Mankin H.J.: Fractures about the hip in an institutionalized patient population. *J. Bone Joint Surg.* 50A:1327, 1968.
4. Cobey J., et al.: Indicators of recovery from fractures of the hip. *Clin. Orthop.* 117:258, 1976.
5. Dimon J.H., Hughston J.C.: Unstable intertrochanteric fractures of the hip. *J. Bone Joint Surg.* 49A:440, 1967.
6. Ecker M.C., Joyce J.J., Kohl E.J.: Treatment of trochanteric hip fractures using a compression screw. *J. Bone Joint Surg.* 57A:23, 1975.
7. Evans E.M.: The treatment of trochanteric fractures of the femur. *J. Bone Joint Surg.* 31B:190, 1949.
8. Holt E.P.: Hip fractures in the trochanteric region: Treatment with a strong nail and early weightbearing. *J. Bone Joint Surg.* 45A:687, 1963.
9. Sarmiento A.: Intertrochanteric fractures of the femur. *J. Bone Joint Surg.* 45A:706, 1963.
10. Seinsheimer F.: Subtrochanteric fractures of the femur. *J. Bone Joint Surg.* 60A:300, 1978.
11. Zickel R.E.: An intramedullary fixation device for the proximal part of the femur: Nine years' experience. *J. Bone Joint Surg.* 58A:866, 1976.
12. Kuntscher G.: A new method of treatment of pertrochanteric fractures. *Proc. R. Soc. Med.* 63:1120, 1970.
13. Herrero F.C., Brichs J.W., Beltran J.E.: Condylocephalic nail fixation for trochanteric fractures of the femur. *Orthop. Clin.* 5:669, 1974.
14. Herrero F.C., Villa J., Beltran J.E.: Condylocephalic nail fixation for trochanteric fractures of the femur. *J. Bone Joint Surg.* 55B:774, 1973.

15. Titanium, a technical report, in *Product Encyclopedia.* Warsaw, Ind., Zimmer-USA, 1978.
16. Allen W.C., et al.: A fluted femoral intermedullary rod. *J. Bone Joint Surg.* 60A:506, 1978.
17. Levy R.N., et al.: Complications of Ender pin fixation in basicervical intertrochanteric and subtrochanteric fractures of the hip. *J. Bone Joint Surg.* 65A:66, 1983.
18. Jacobs R.R., McClain D., Armstrong H.J.: Internal fixation of intertrochanteric hip fractures: A clinical and biomechanical study. *Clin. Orthop.* 146:62, 1980.
19. Jensen J.S., Sonne-Holm S.: Critical analysis of Ender nailing in the treatment of trochanteric fractures. *Acta Orthop. Scand.* 51:817, 1980.
20. Jensen J.S., Sonne-Holm S., Tondevold E.: Unstable trochanteric fractures. *Acta Orthop. Scand.* 51:949, 1980.
21. Jensen J.S., Tondevold E., Sonne-Holm S.: Stable trochanteric fractures. *Acta Orthop. Scand.* 51:811, 1980.
22. Kyle R.F., Gustilo R.B., Premer R.F.: Analysis of six hundred and twenty-two intertrochanteric hip fractures: A retrospective and prospective study. *J. Bone Joint Surg.* 61A:216, 1979.
23. Massie W.K.: Fractures of the hip. *J. Bone Joint Surg.* 46A:658, 1964.
24. Hult L., Nilsson M.H.: Ender-spikning av trokantara femurfrakturer. *Lakartidningen* 75:4603, 1978.
25. Kuderna H., Boshler N., Collon D.: Treatment of intertrochanteric and subtrochanteric fractures of the hip by the Ender method. *J. Bone Joint Surg.* 58A:604, 1976.
26. Pankovich M.A., Traabishy I.E.: Ender nailing of intertrochanteric and subtrochanteric fractures of the femur. *J. Bone Joint Surg.* 62A:635, 1980.
27. Raugstad T.S., et al.: Treatment of pertrochanteric and subtrochanteric fractures of the femur by the Ender method. *Clin. Orthop.* 138:231, 1979.
28. Russin O.A., Sonni A.: Treatment of intertrochanteric and subtrochanteric fractures with Ender's intramedullary rods. *Clin. Orthop.* 148:203, 1980.
29. Siegel M.G., Levy R.N., Sedlin E.: Ender pin experience in patients with hip fractures. *Orthop. Trans.* 5:470, 1981.
30. Harris L.J.: Closed retrograde intramedullary nailing of peritrochanteric fractures of the femur with a new nail. *J. Bone Joint Surg.* 62A:1185, 1980.
31. Clawson D.K.: Trochanteric fractures treated by the sliding screw plate fixation method. *J. Trauma* 4:737, 1964.
32. Harrington K.D., Johnston J.O.: The management of comminuted unstable intertrochanteric fractures. *J. Bone Joint Surg.* 55A:1367, 1973.
33. Ganz R., Thomas R.J., Hammerle C.P.: Trochanteric fractures of the femur. *Clin. Orthop.* 138:30, 1979.
34. Laskin R.S., Gruber M.A., Zimmerman A.J.: Intertrochanteric fractures of the hip in the elderly. *Clin. Orthop.* 141:188, 1979.

Chapter 20

Zickel Nail

Robert E. Zickel, M.D.

In 1963 at St. Luke's Hospital in New York City, work began on the design of a new fixation device for subtrochanteric fractures of the femur. Failure of nail plates, causing nonunion, fostered interest in evaluating other methods of fixation. It became evident that intramedullary fixation of the proximal femoral shaft had definite advantages over extramedullary fixation by creating a load-sharing relationship between the appliance and the bone. In subtrochanteric fractures, however, intramedullary fixation was hampered by poor purchase in the short, wide canal of the femur proximal to the fracture. Frequently the trochanteric mass itself contained fracture lines, which further jeopardized fixation with the standard intramedullary rods then available.[1]

The design concept was to fabricate an intramedullary rod that could be securely fixed to the head and neck of the femur with an anchoring nail. The first prototype had a straight but tapered rod wide enough at its proximal end to have good purchase in the trochanteric canal. The large proximal part also had a round tunnel through which a triflanged nail was to be driven into the head and neck of the femur. Early cadaver work in which subtrochanteric fractures were created with an osteotome revealed problems with the straight rod in aligning the tunnel with the neck of the femur, and allowing varus deformities. These problems were corrected by bowing the rod to match the anterior midshaft bow and the posterior subtrochanteric bow of the femur and by angling the proximal end into slight valgus. This corrected the varus problem and more closely aligned the tunnel with the normal neck shaft angle of the femur.

The design was modified several times between 1963 and 1965, and the first prototype was manufactured in 1966. The appliance consisted of three parts: a contoured and bowed intramedullary rod, a special triflanged nail, and a set screw. The rod, which was 17 mm square at its proximal or trochanteric part, tapered to a bowed stem that matched the medullary canal of the femur. The large proximal part of the rod had an angled tunnel that subtended an angle of 125° with the stem. The special triflanged nail was actually cylindrical and $7/16$ inch in diameter. The distal $1/2$ inch of the nail was triflanged, while the proximal end had three circumferential grooves to receive a set screw. When the appliance was assembled, the nail was passed through the tunnel of the rod until one of the grooves was engaged by the set screw, inserted and tightened through a threaded hole in the top of the rod (Fig 20–1).

A few special tools had to be developed for operative insertion of the appliance. A special instrument, now called a tunnel locator gauge, was a jig that could be applied to the top of the rod with an arm to accept a thin guide pin. This instrument is used to determine the correct position of the tunnel of the rod in relation to the neck of the femur and to determine the proper spot to remove cortical bone from

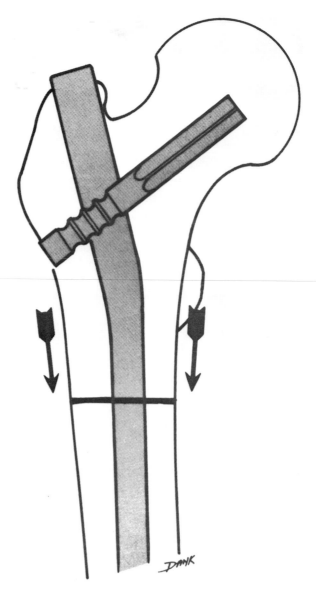

Fig 20–1—Components of the Zickel subtrochanteric nail appliance.

the lateral femoral cortex so that the triflanged nail could be inserted through the tunnel of the rod. It was decided to use an impactor extractor with slight modification of a standard available model (McReynolds driver extractor) with special adapters to fit the threads of both the top of the rod and the triflanged nail. Finally, a standard hexagonal screwdriver was selected to use for the set screw that locks the nail into the rod. The rest of the equipment is standard and the same as that used in any intramedullary nailing. Straight and flexible reamers with power are necessary for performing the procedure. There must be a 17-mm medullary reamer to prepare the trochanteric canal for the proximal part of the rod.

The rod is currently manufactured in two lengths, 35 cm and 40 cm, with four stem diameters, 11 mm, 13 mm, 15 mm, and 17 mm. Because of the bowed design of the rod, separate rods are necessary for right and left femora. Each is

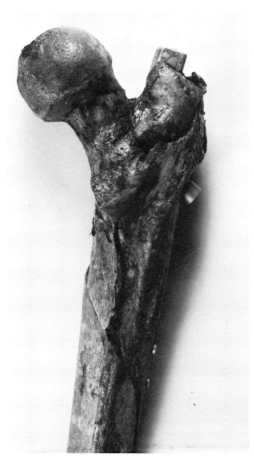

Fig 20–2—Early nailing in a patient who died 2 weeks after operation for pulmonary embolus.

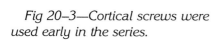

Fig 20–3—Cortical screws were used early in the series.

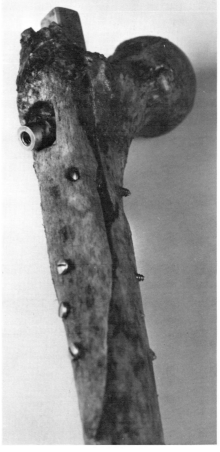

marked to indicate the stem diameter and size (e.g., 13 mm R). The complete set includes 16 rods and 5 triflanged nails of graded lengths.

The first operation utilizing the device was performed in 1966 on an elderly patient with a long oblique subtrochanteric fracture of the femur (Fig 20–2). It became apparent at surgery that because of the length and obliquity of the fracture, additional fixation would be necessary, and several cortical bone screws bypassing the rod were used for this purpose (Fig 20–3). A few years later cerclage wires were used instead of cortical screws because they were easier to apply and less damaging to the cortex. The cerclage technique has remained the preferred method of providing additional fixation when needed and has been extremely satisfactory (Fig 20–4).

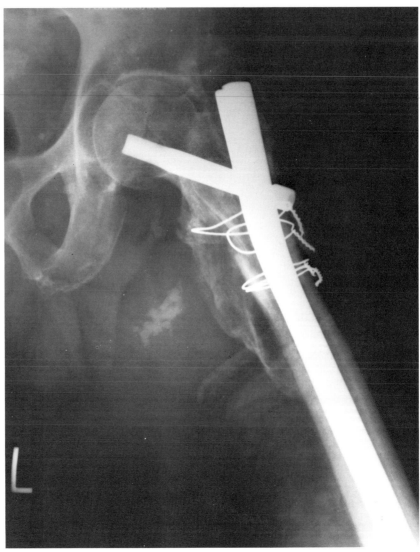

Fig 20–4—Cerclage wires are currently used for accessory fixation.

OPERATIVE TECHNIQUE
1. Positioning the Patient

We prefer to place the patient on a standard operating table in the semisupine position (Fig 20–5). A roll or sandbag is placed beneath the patient, from the superior border of the pelvis to the chest, to elevate the pelvis on the operative side. This permits easier access to the tip of the greater trochanter.

ALTERNATE METHODS OF POSITIONING.—A lateral decubitus position (Fig 20–6) may be used if the surgeon is comfortable with the orientation of the femur in that position. The position is usually chosen for x-ray purposes (the horizontal x-ray giving the anteroposterior view and the vertical x-ray giving the lateral view).

Some surgeons perform the procedure on a fracture table (Fig 20–7). In using a fracture table the surgical team must be able to adduct, abduct, and rotate the leg intraoperatively to permit reduction of the fracture and insertion of the nail.

2. Operative Approach

The skin is incised along the posterior border of the trochanter in a somewhat curved incision that begins at the fracture site distally and extends 6 cm proximally to the tip of the trochanter. The incision must be posterior to the trochanter for easy access to the tip of the trochanter (Fig 20–8). The fascia lata and fascia lata tensor are divided in line with the incision. The vastus lateralis is detached from the vastus ridge, leaving a cuff of tissue at the ridge for reattachment later. It is split posteriorly and retracted anteriorly after mobilization with a periosteal elevator (Fig 20–9). It is important to mobilize the fracture so that an exact reduction may be performed. Simply "lining it up" is not sufficient and can result in technical problems, described later.

3. Preparing the Femur for the Rod

With the fracture mobilized, the leg is adducted so that the medullary canal of the distal shaft is brought into the field (Fig 20–10). A rod appropriate for the side

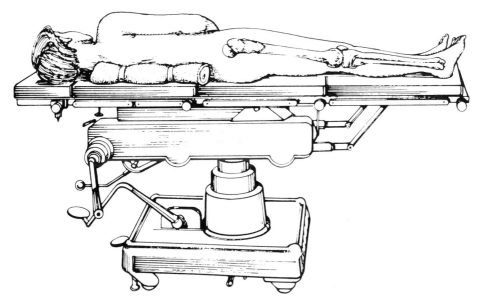

Fig 20–5—Semisupine position on a standard operating table.

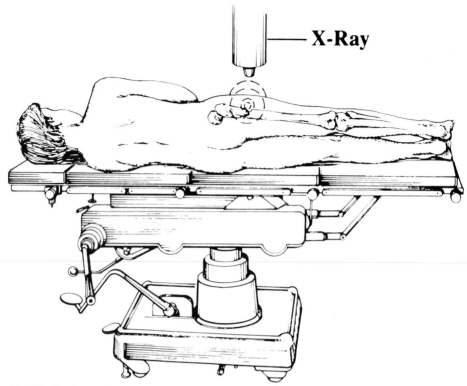

Fig 20–6—Lateral decubitus position used for convenience of x-ray apparatus.

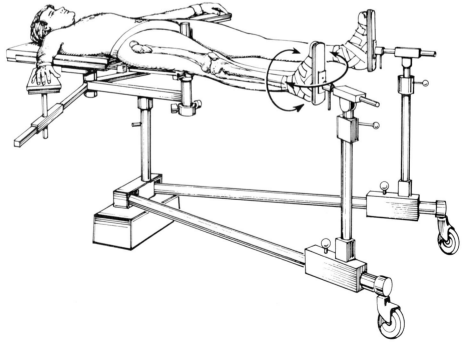

Fig 20–7—Position on a standard fracture table.

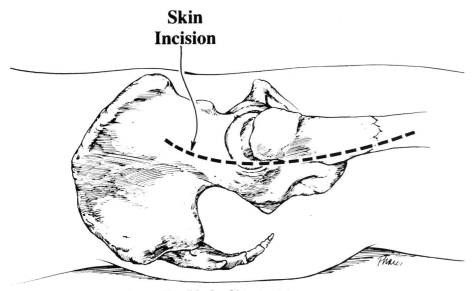

**Skin
Incision**

Fig 20–8—Skin incision.

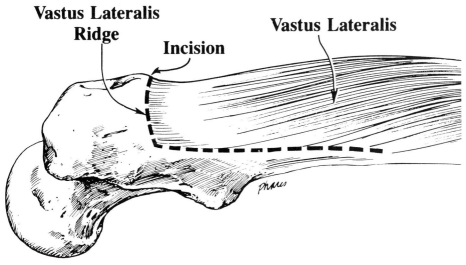

**Vastus Lateralis
Ridge**

Incision

Vastus Lateralis

Fig 20–9—Vastus lateralis is detached at the ridge.

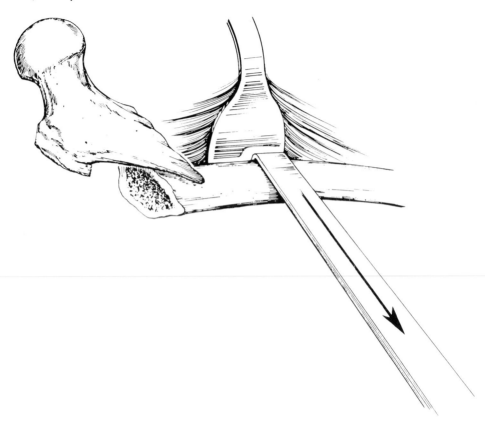

Fig 20–10—Adequate exposure of the fracture.

and of appropriate stem diameter (each rod is clearly marked for side—R or L—and for stem diameter) is selected. During testing of the fit in the distal shaft, the rod must be oriented properly so the anterior bow matches the anterior bow of the femur (Fig 20–11). Reaming the distal canal with femoral reamers is usually necessary to achieve a proper snug fit. The rod is then extracted and the proximal canal prepared. Reaming the proximal or trochanteric canal can be performed retrograde or antegrade (Fig 20–12). Careful assessment of possible fracture lines in the trochanteric area helps to determine the method used. If the trochanteric area is without fractures, then retrograde reaming can safely be performed. If fracture lines are present, then the entire fracture should be reduced and stabilized with bone clamps or cerclage wires. Antegrade reaming is now performed. With either method the trochanteric canal must be reamed to 17 mm with the reamer directed through the tip of the trochanter. Cutting the small proximal tip of the greater trochanter with a ½-inch osteotome after splitting the gluteus muscle ensures proper orientation of the reamer (Fig 20–13).

4. Assembling the Rod for Insertion

The proper side and sized rod is now assembled with the tunnel locator (Fig 20–14). The tunnel locator is secured to the top of the rod by the threaded adapter from the driver extractor. This must be securely tightened so that there is no play between the tunnel locator and the rod. A guide pin is passed through the arm of the tunnel locator, which, if in proper alignment, should pass through the central axis of the round tunnel in the rod. The guide wire is now removed.

5. *Inserting the Rod*

The leg must be adducted to permit insertion through the tip of the trochanter. Before insertion the fracture is inspected to be sure that the proximal and distal portions of the femur move together without loss of reduction (Fig 20–15). The tip of the rod is then passed through the trochanteric canal and driven gently through the fracture site into the distal shaft (Fig 20–16). When the stem has crossed the fracture and entered the distal shaft, rotational alignment of the rod must be determined.

With the leg positioned so the patella points directly anteriorly, the arm of the tunnel locator should be approximately 15° anteverted from the horizontal plane of the body (Fig 20–17). The surgeon must step well back from the operating table to observe the version, while an assistant supports the tunnel locator and rod. Rotational adjustments can be made by gently rotating the tunnel locator, which acts as a handle during impaction of the rod. At all times the impactor and tunnel locator must be kept tightly secured to the rod. As the anterior bow of the rod passes the fracture site, there may be slight displacement of the fracture. This usually reduces when the rod is fully seated. The rod is impacted until the arm of the tunnel locator points to a spot 2.5 cm distal to the vastus lateralis ridge (Fig 20–18). A guide pin

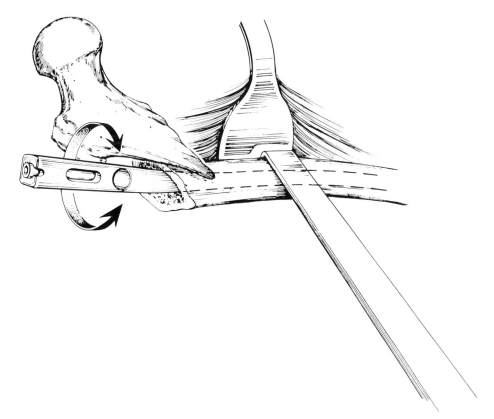

Fig 20–11—Testing stem size in the distal canal.

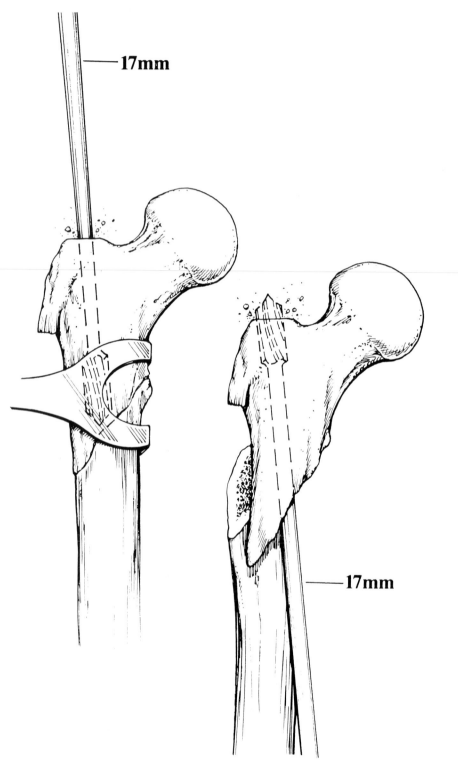

Fig 20–12—Reaming is done retrograde or antegrade, depending on the frac-ture.

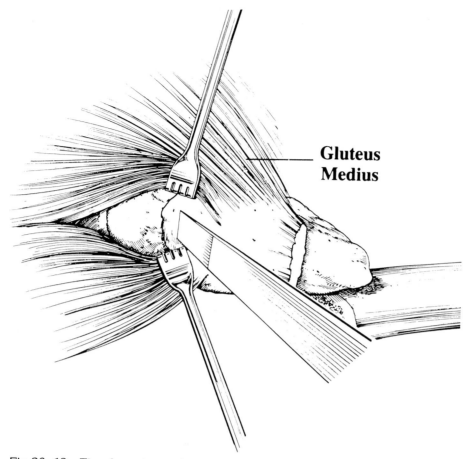

Gluteus Medius

Fig 20–13—Tip of greater trochanter is cut with an osteotome before reaming.

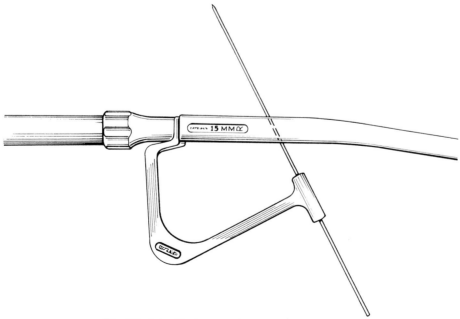

15 MM α

Fig 20–14—Rod assembled with impactor.

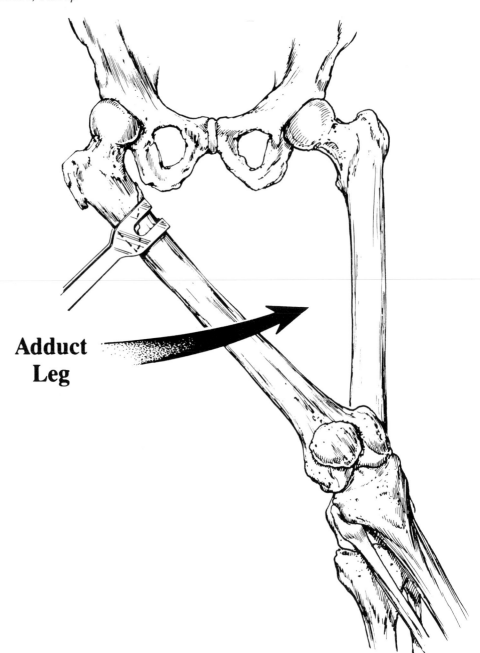

**Adduct
Leg**

Fig 20–15—Leg adducted to test stability of reduction.

is now drilled through the arm of the tunnel locator up into the neck of the femur. X-ray films are made in two planes to determine the correct position of the guide pin (Fig 20–19). If the pin is too superior or too inferior, the rod is simply driven or extracted, as necessary. Anterior or posterior correction requires a change in the rotation of the rod. This is done by extracting the rod halfway out of the bone and redriving it in the correct position.

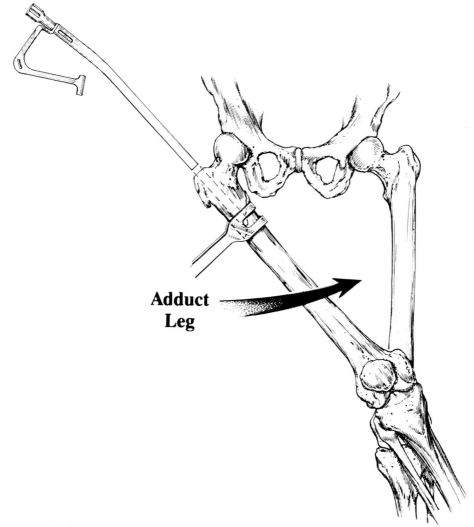

Adduct Leg

Fig 20–16—Rod with tunnel locator gauge inserted into canal with leg adducted.

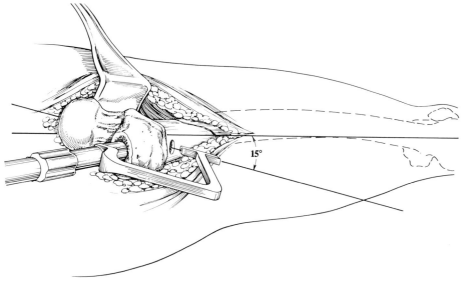

15°

Fig 20–17—Tunnel locator determines 15° anteversion with leg in neutral position.

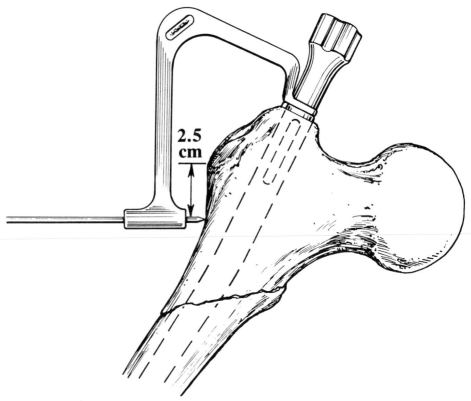

Fig 20–18—Arm of tunnel locator is 2.5 cm distal to vastus ridge.

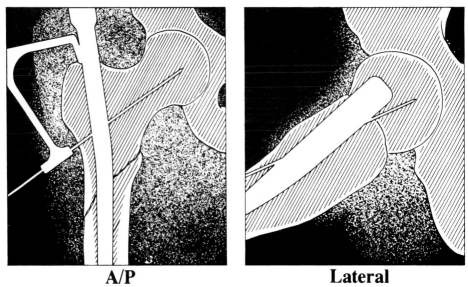

A/P **Lateral**

Fig 20–19—X-ray films are made with the guide pin in place.

6. Inserting the Triflanged Nail

After the driver is disengaged, the tunnel locator can be removed, leaving the guide pin in place. A ½-inch cannulated drill is threaded on the guide pin and a hole is drilled in the lateral cortex (Fig 20–20). Only the cortical bone is removed, as the intramedullary rod is directly beneath the cortex. The bone hole may be enlarged with a curet, permitting easy insertion of the triflanged nail (Fig 20–21). The guide pin is extracted and the tunnel in the rod is visualized. The special triflanged nail is assembled to the driver with its own adapter and is inserted into the tunnel of the nail and driven into the neck and head of the femur. The direction of the nail is determined by the fixed angle of the tunnel in the rod. The nail should pass easily through the tunnel, with the grooves semicircular at the proximal end and facing superiorly (Fig 20–22).

Difficulty encountered in this step is usually due to failure to remove sufficient cortical bone. A triflanged nail of appropriate length is driven to the desired depth and x-ray films are made to verify the correct position. The three grooves permit a range of penetration for each nail. The set screw is now placed through the top of the rod and tightened with a hexagonal screwdriver (Fig 20–23). When the screw is flush with the top of the rod, it has engaged one of the grooves. If two or more threads of the set screw are visible, it has not engaged a groove of the nail. The screw should be loosened, the nail driven or extracted slightly, and the screw retightened. It should then engage the nail properly.

7. Accessory Fixation

In long oblique or comminuted subtrochanteric fractures, accessory fixation may be required. Number 18-gauge wire for cerclage has been successfully used for fixation (Fig 20–24), and problems of bone necrosis beneath the wires have not occurred.

Figure 20–25 shows the appearance of the fracture after nailing has been completed.

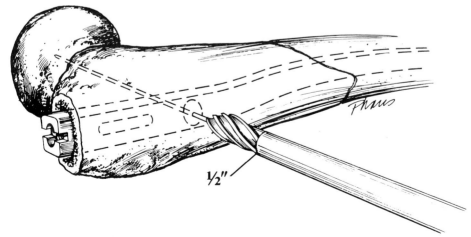

Fig 20–20—Cannulated cortical reamer over guide pin.

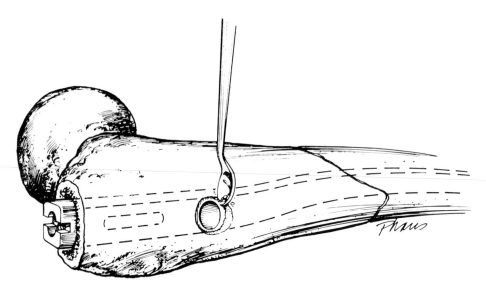

Fig 20–21—Enlarging hole with bone curet.

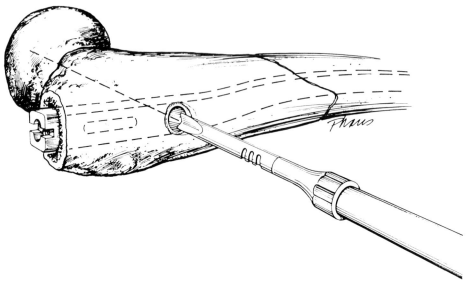

Fig 20–22—Impacting triflanged nail through exposed tunnel in rod.

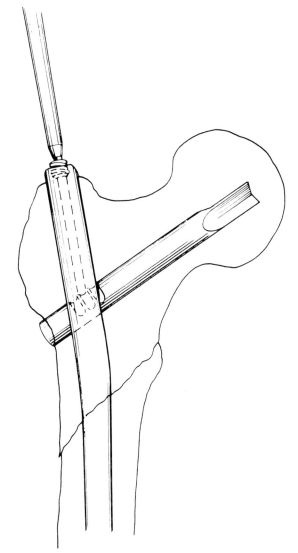

Fig 20–23—Locking triflanged nail with set screw.

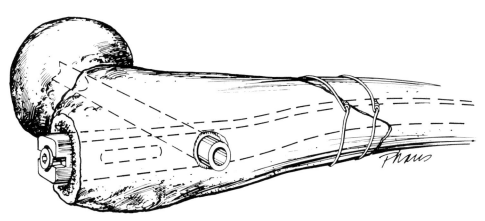

Fig 20–24—Cerclage wires added.

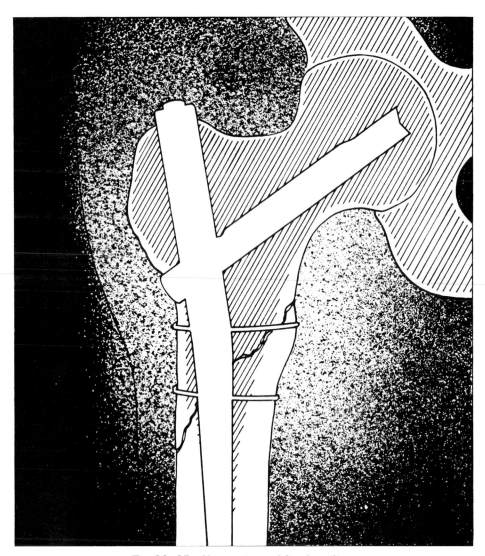

Fig 20–25—X-ray view of final nailing.

PATHOLOGIC LESIONS

Prophylactic fixation of femora with bony metastasis is performed as described but through a somewhat shorter incision than is used for femora with fractures. Reaming is always performed in an antegrade direction and with flexible reamers (Fig 20–26). In femora with cortical lysis, special care must be exercised to prevent the reamer from wandering out of the shaft at points where the cortex is significantly eroded. A special tunnel locator gauge has been designed for use by surgeons who prefer to perform this procedure as a semiclosed nailing. The gauge permits drilling the cortical bone for the triflanged nail without incising the lateral musculature. The triflanged nail itself can also be directed through the rod using this special gauge (Fig 20–27).

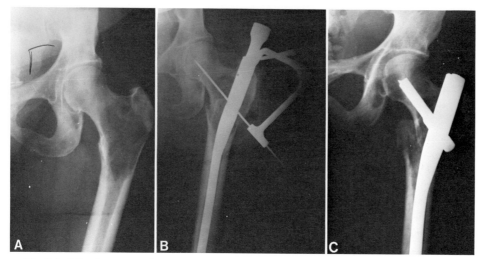

Fig 20–26—**A,** *impending pathologic fracture from lytic lesion.* **B,** *intraoperative film with guide pin in place (note lesion fractured).* **C,** *final nailing.*

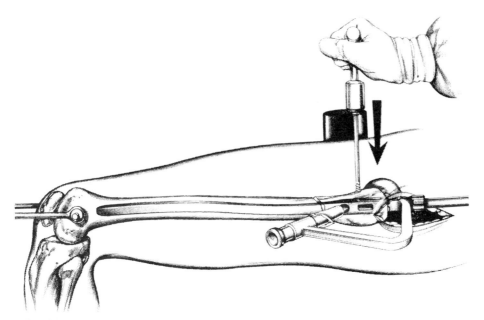

Fig 20–27—*Special tunnel locator guage is used for closed nailing. (Courtesy of B. Browner, M.D.)*

COMMON TECHNICAL PITFALLS
Control of the Leg

Some surgeons in performing the procedure on a fracture table do not provide for adequate control of the leg intraoperatively. It is necessary that the leg can be rotated, adducted, abducted, or flexed as necessary during surgery to achieve proper alignment and to permit insertion of the rod.

Inadequate Exposure

Complex subtrochanteric fractures are difficult to reduce unless there is adequate exposure and mobilization of the fragments to permit accurate reduction. Detaching the vastus lateralis muscle and mobilizing particularly the distal shaft so that the medullary canal can be brought in the operative field are important to achieving a good reduction.

Fit of the Rod in the Distal Shaft

While mobilizing the fracture for reduction, it takes little time to test the stem of the rod in the distal medullary canal. The rod should fit snugly, as a loose-fitting rod can permit rotational deformities later. After the rod is tested, it is extracted and the procedure continues as in the protocol.

Reaming the Trochanteric Canal

The trochanteric canal must be reamed to 17 mm with the channel made through the top of the trochanter and not through the notch medial to the greater trochanter, as is done with many intramedullary rods. Failure to do so may result in the rod being too medially displaced, and the arm of the tunnel locator gauge will not pass around the greater trochanter during impaction. Cutting the top of the trochanter with a ½-inch osteotome after splitting the gluteus muscle ensures proper orientation of the reamer.

Comminution of the Greater Trochanter

If fracture lines are present in the trochanteric mass, reaming the trochanteric canal is best performed antegrade after the fracture is reduced, and with the reduction maintained with bone clamps and cerclage wires. Retrograde reaming can explode the trochanter in these cases.

If part of the initial fracture is a severely comminuted greater trochanter, the operation is technically more difficult. The appliance can be inserted by retracting the comminuted trochanter, inserting the rod into the distal shaft, and completing the nailing under direct visualization. Abducting the leg before driving the triflanged nail avoids varus deformity. After placement of the nail the trochanteric fragments should be wired back to the femoral shaft with an 18-gauge wire (Fig 20–28).

Alignment of the Proximal Femur

Maintaining alignment of the proximal femur with the distal femur during adduction of the leg is essential to avoid intraoperative comminution of the greater trochanter (Fig 20–29). If the reduction cannot be maintained with bone clamps during the maneuver, a bone hook can be used around the superior base of the femoral neck to pull the proximal femur into adduction as the remainder of the leg is adducted.

Rotational Alignment of the Rod

The tunnel locator controls rotation during impaction of the rod. When the rod is fully seated, the arm of the gauge will be slightly anteverted (approximately 10°–15°) with the leg in the neutral position. The surgeon must step well back from

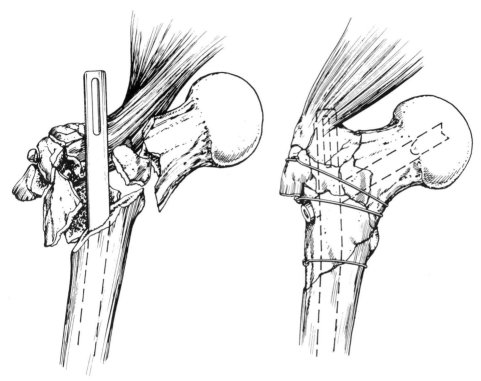

Fig 20–28—Insertion of the nail after exploding the greater trochanter.

the operating table to determine the version of the gauge. The new series of rods have been designed with 6° of anteversion of the proximal part (Fig 20–30). Alternatively, proper version of the neck of the femur can be determined by palpating or placing a guide pin along the anterior capsule of the hip.

Lateral X-ray View

We have used the frogleg lateral x-ray view when performing the procedure on a standard operating table. When obtaining this view, it is important to flex the hip close to 90° and then abduct the leg slightly so that the thigh does not obstruct the x-ray tube. A common error in attempting the frogleg lateral view is flexing the hip only to 45°, which then gives an oblique view of the femoral neck and not a true lateral view. Figure 20–31 shows the correct position.

Driving the Triflanged Nail

Before the triflanged nail is driven through the tunnel in the rod, the tunnel should be clearly visualized and the nail should slide easily in the tunnel. Failure to remove sufficient cortical bone may prevent easy access to the tunnel. Attempts to drive the nail forcibly before it is properly seated can result in displacement of position of the rod and the fracture.

Deformities of the Hip

Fixed deformities of the hip or femur must be recognized before surgery. An obliterated or deformed medullary canal from an old fracture, operation, or bone

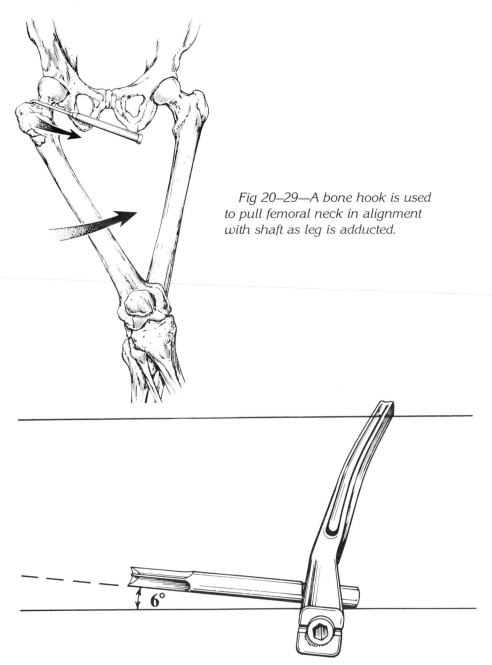

*Fig 20–29—A bone hook is used
to pull femoral neck in alignment
with shaft as leg is adducted.*

Fig 20–30—New series of nails with 6° anteversion in proximal end.

disease can make insertion of this or any medullary rod difficult or impossible. A fixed varus deformity, from an old hip fracture or arthritis, which does not permit sufficient adduction of the leg to allow insertion of the rod can be a contraindication.

INDICATIONS

The Zickel nail appliance has been used for a large variety of fractures of the proximal femur and for pathologic lesions with impending fracture of the proximal

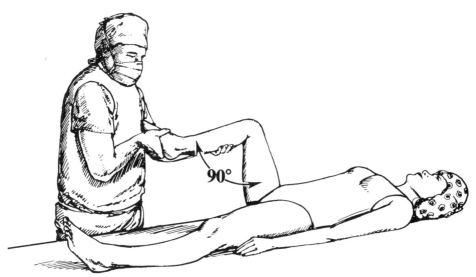

Fig 20–31—Proper flexion for frog-leg lateral x-ray view.

femur. Although the appliance is ideally suited for treating fractures between the midshaft and the lesser trochanter, it has been successfully used to treat fractures extending proximally into the trochanteric mass and the base of the neck of the femur and distally into the midshaft and below.[2] It can be used for the combined trochanteric and midshaft fracture, and experience has been reported with intracapsular and midshaft fractures by other investigators.[3]

In the combined series from St. Luke's Hospital in New York, the nonunion rate was 3%, with mechanical failure of only four appliances in a series that included more than 220 femora. Comminution, obliquity, and segmental fractures have not been contraindications for the use of the Zickel nail. Contraindications included obliteration or marked deformity of the femoral medullary canal from old injuries or bone diseases. For example, the nail cannot be successfully inserted into the femur of a patient with Paget's disease if there is either complete obliteration of the medullary canal or marked varus bowing. Meticulous attention to the operative protocol is essential, and the inexperienced surgeon should practice the technique first on either a cadaver or synthetic femoral bone.

Fractures at the junction of the femoral neck and shaft deserve special consideration. I have classified these as trochanteric-subtrochanteric fractures, if the major fracture involves the intertrochanteric area, or as subtrochanteric-intertrochanteric, if the major portion is subtrochanteric. A device is selected according to its ability to provide intramedullary support of the fracture. A comminuted intertrochanteric fracture with short subtrochanteric extension (trochanteric-subtrochanteric fracture) may often be treated with conventional nail plate or screw plate devices. A high angled nail plate device started distally on the shaft can provide intramedullary support to such fractures.

Conversely, a fracture that is predominantly subtrochanteric but has an intertrochanteric component (subtrochanteric-intertrochanteric fracture) is best treated by the Zickel subtrochanteric nail (Fig 20–32). Several severely comminuted fractures of the proximal femoral shaft due to unusual trauma or gunshot wounds have been treated successfully with this appliance. Such treatment is particularly feasible if the greater or lesser trochanter is well intact (Fig 20–33).[4]

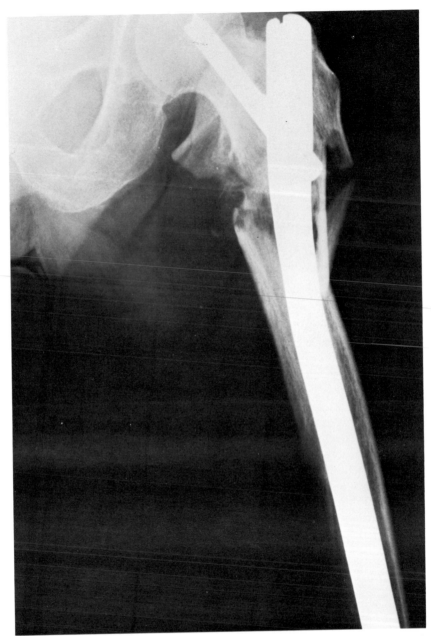

Fig 20–32—Comminuted subtrochanteric-intertrochanteric fracture with Zickel nail.

POSTOPERATIVE MANAGEMENT

In our series no patient was treated postoperatively in traction, but all were mobilized as soon as they were comfortably able and were advanced to ambulation with crutches or walker. The protocol was very similar to that used for other hip fractures (intertrochanteric or intracapsular) that have been treated by nailing. Full weight-bearing has been discouraged until there is roentgenographic evidence of fracture healing. This usually occurs at an average of 4 months, but many patients

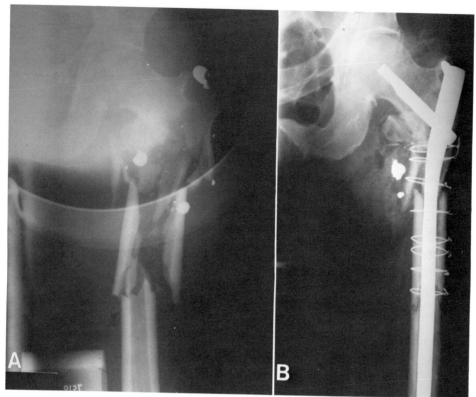

Fig 20–33—**A,** *severely comminuted proximal shaft fracture from gunshot wound.* **B,** *same patient postoperatively. Cerclage wires are used for accessory fixation.*

showed significant healing and stability as early as 2 months and were permitted full weight-bearing.

REFERENCES

1. Zickel R.E.: A new fixation device for subtrochanteric fractures of the femur: A preliminary report. *Clin. Orthop.* 54:115, 1967.
2. Zickel R.E., Mouradian W.H.: Intramedullary fixation of pathological fractures and lesions of the subtrochanteric region of the femur. *J. Bone Joint Surg.* 58A:1061, 1976.
3. Distefano V.J., Nixon J.E., Klein K.S.: Stable fixation of difficult subtrochanteric fracture. *J. Trauma* 12:1066, 1972.
4. Zickel R.E.: Subtrochanteric femoral fractures. *Orthop. Clin. North Am.* 11:555, 1980.

Chapter 21

Use of the Moore Prosthesis in the Management of Acute Fracture of the Femoral Neck

E. M. Lunceford, Jr., M.D.

Since the late 1940s and early 1950s when Austin Moore introduced the intramedullary endoprosthesis for management of "unsolved fractures" of the femoral neck, a number of design changes and technique modifications have come and gone. As many as 150 different prostheses have been available at one time or another for use by the orthopedic surgeon in treating this entity. The Moore prosthesis or a variation of it has withstood the test of time and continues to be used for femoral neck fractures. Despite some modifications in design from the original prosthetic appliance and changes in surgical indications, the long-term results of the Moore prosthesis point to an extended lifetime for this device.

Preservation of the patient's own femoral head is a desired goal, and in the younger, active patient, it is frequently achievable. Use of a vascular pedicle bone graft, as advocated by Meyers, can markedly reduce the incidence of avascular necrosis and/or nonunion. In addition, early, prompt reduction and fixation of the fractured femoral neck can often provide satisfactory functional results.[1] The incidence of nonunion has been reported by Fielding et al.,[2] Kimbrough et al.,[3] Lunceford and Emmett,[4] and Meyers et al.[1] to be less than 5%, and the incidence of avascular necrosis has been reported to be only 6%–7%. If these figures are accurate, why the necessity of replacing the femoral head with a prosthesis? Unfortunately, the results reported are not universally obtainable, and therefore it behooves us to examine the efficacy of prosthetic replacement. Does endoprosthetic replacement in fracture of the femoral neck work as effectively as total hip arthroplasty? In an effort to answer this perplexing question, my colleagues and I undertook a literature search, and review of patient records at the Moore Clinic in Columbia, South Carolina. Our study, which focused on long-term evaluation of Moore prosthesis replacement for fractures of the femoral neck in the elderly and for treatment of avascular necrosis with a relatively intact acetabulum, found that the Moore prosthesis yielded results similar to those obtained by the internal fixation and fracture fixation techniques described above.[5] Because of the similarity, it is imperative to review the current management of patients with fractures of the femoral neck and/or avascular necrosis of the femoral head.

INDICATIONS FOR ENDOPROSTHETIC REPLACEMENT OF THE FEMORAL HEAD

Indications for endoprosthetic replacement have remained essentially unchanged since the early 1960s. It is still important to preserve the femoral head in the younger, more active patient, but in my opinion prosthetic replacement for acute fractures is the procedure of choice in the elderly patient.[4] Following is a list of indications for which endoprosthetic replacement is preferred.

1. Old age. Persons of a physiologic age of 70 years or more who have a displaced vertical neck fracture frequently can withstand only one operation and do not tolerate the prolonged protected weight-bearing following reduction and internal fixation.

2. Mental illness. We found that prosthetic replacement has been followed by fewer complications and better long-term results in patients confined because of mental illness. These patients frequently walk the day of operation with little or no assistance. They seem to have little or no awareness of pain, and once the hip is stable, they become ambulatory.

3. Shock therapy. In patients receiving shock therapy, a reduction allows continuation of therapy.

4. Parkinson's disease. The tremor and inability to use crutches for protected weight-bearing caused by this disease led to a high percentage of fractures and complications after reduction and fixation. These patients have done better with primary prosthetic replacement.

5. Conditions requiring confinement to a wheelchair or bed. Patients with such conditions can be made more comfortable with primary prosthetic replacement, and the need for nursing care is lessened.

6. Pathologic fractures secondary to metastatic or primary malignant tumors. When a prosthesis is inserted, these patients can be made more comfortable and can be rehabilitated more quickly during the terminal stages of their disease.

7. Rheumatoid arthritis. The patient with an acute fracture responds favorably to prosthetic replacement. Prosthetic replacement permits early mobilization, thereby preserving mobility and reducing the tendency to contracture.

8. Irradiation osteitis following treatment for carcinoma of the cervix.

9. Avascular necrosis of the femoral head with intact acetabulum. This may be due to a variety of causes, including Caisson's disease.

10. Traumatic dislocation of the hip with fracture of the femoral head. An incongruous joint is inevitable and avascular necrosis is likely.

Patient evaluation is essentially the same now as it was when Moore first developed the endoprosthesis. Radioisotope scanning is interesting, and sulfur colloid evaluation of the fractured femoral neck has been reported to be helpful in determining the viability of the femoral head but has not yet proved to be the single best diagnostic study. The femoral head can be replaced using the straight-stem prosthesis, which increases the surface area over that of the shorter curved-stem prosthesis and provides greater stability of the endoprosthesis in the proximal femur (Fig 21–1). The Moore prosthesis in use today is the same prosthesis that evolved in the early and mid-1960s, with slight modifications. An attempt is made to increase the

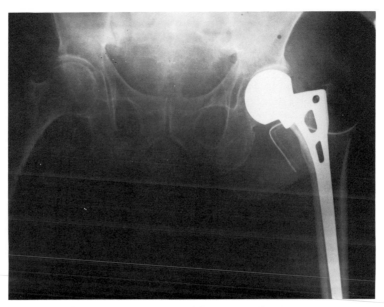

Fig 21–1—Straight stem Austin-Moore prosthesis, post operative.

stability by having various stem sizes as well as different stem lengths. A straight-stem prosthesis is used which can be applied to either the right or the left hip. The head is supplied in a spherical configuration and in sizes of 1-mm increments to achieve a better fit of the acetabulum. The anteversion can be achieved by surgical technique.

OPERATIVE TECHNIQUE

The prosthesis is best inserted via the southern exposure,[6] through an oblique skin incision over the posterior lateral thigh. The patient lies on the unaffected side, the affected hip uppermost. The patient should be stabilized on the operating table in the lateral recumbent position. The hip is prepared and draped in the usual fashion. The skin incision extends in an oblique line from the posteroinferior iliac spine to the junction of the proximal and middle thirds of the proximal femur (Fig 21–2). After the skin is incised, the scalpel is directed obliquely anteriorly in the subcutaneous tissue in the midportion of the incision toward the greater trochanter. As the hip is flexed with the skin incision made in this plane, the greater trochanter is placed in the midportion of the incisional site. The tensor fascia femoris and the fascia are incised and a hip retractor is placed over the anterior aspect of the greater trochanter to facilitate this section of the exposure. The sciatic nerve is visualized and protected. The short external rotators (the pyriformis, the gemelli, the obturator internus, and the quadratus femoris) are identified and divided near their insertion on the posterior intertrochanteric ridge. If additional exposure is needed for mobilization of the proximal femur and visualization of the acetabulum, the gluteus maximus can be detached along the linea aspera for a distance of 2–4 cm (Fig 21–3). It is helpful if this portion of the dissection is made adjacent to the bone to avoid damage to the ascending branch of the posterior femoral circumflex artery. As the dissection is carried out, digital pressure is applied to the circumflex vessels and the femur is internally rotated 30°–40°; this maneuver assists materially in reducing the amount of bleeding that occurs.

A T incision is made in the capsule paralleling the obturator internus, and the superior and inferior flaps of the capsule may be grasped with clamps to facilitate the exposure. These flaps are then retracted and the incision in the capsule is carried to the labrum of the acetabulum. The fracture site and femoral head can now be seen. The femoral neck may be transected at the appropriate level by using the prosthesis as a template, placed alongside the proximal femur to determine the location for transection of the femoral neck. Preoperative planning is essential for

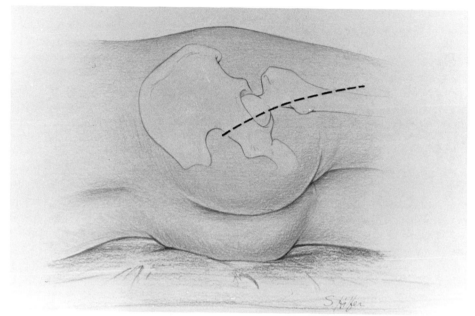

Fig 21–2—Diagram of skin incision.

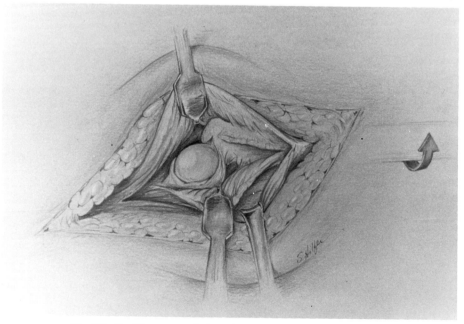

Fig 21–3—Diagram of detachment of gluteus maximus.

preservation of leg length and a comparison with the opposite hip is the ideal method for determining the appropriate level for transection of the femoral neck. The prosthetic femoral head should be placed at the same level as the normal femoral head on the opposite hip. Usually, this means that the femoral neck is transected at a level of 1–1.5 cm above the lesser trochanter. If the femoral neck is transected in this manner, it is easier to remove the femoral head from the acetabulum. The femur is then retracted anteriorly by placing a small Homan retractor over the rim of the acetabulum and retracting the proximal femur anteriorly. The fracture surface of the proximal fragment (the femoral head) is identified. The short T screw and subsequently the long T screw are placed in the femoral head and the head is then rotated sufficiently to free it from the ligamentum teres and any capsular attachment that may be present. Sharp dissection is occasionally needed to complete this portion of the procedure.

The femoral head is removed and measured to ascertain its exact size. The acetabulum is inspected and any redundant soft tissue removed and the quality of the cartilaginous surface of the acetabulum assessed. The femoral prosthetic head that has been selected by measuring the removed femoral head can be tried in the acetabulum. It is desirable to insert a prosthetic head that is 1–2 mm larger than the removed femoral head to obtain an accurate fit of the femoral prosthesis in the acetabulum. Once the trial reduction has been accomplished and the appropriate prosthesis selected, the femur is approached for insertion of the prosthesis. The proximal femur is flexed 90° and the knee is flexed 90°. The femur is internally rotated 90°. This places the leg vertically in relation to the long axis of the patient. The leg will be pointing toward the ceiling and will be perpendicular to the operating table (Fig 21–4). A rectangular slot is made by opening the pyriformis recess with a drill and placing the rectangular chisel in the pyriformis recess, then rotating it to form

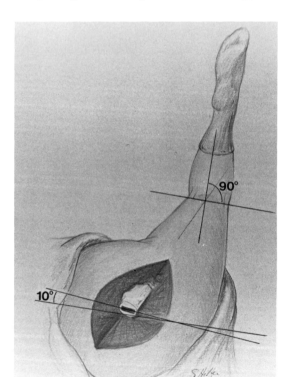

Fig 21–4—Diagram of position of leg for insertion of prosthesis.

an obtuse angle of 100° with the leg to provide 10°–15° of anteversion of the prosthetic head. The prosthesis is rotated according to this slot to reproduce the normal anatomy of the proximal femur. The bone obtained from creating the slot with the rectangular chisel may be placed in the fenestrations of the prosthesis.

A drill is used to open the medullary canal to 9, 10, or 11 mm, as necessary, for insertion of the straight-stem Moore prosthesis. The femoral broach is inserted to facilitate a press fit of the endoprosthesis in the femoral canal. Once this has been obtained and accurate positioning of the femoral neck to the prosthetic collar is ensured by using a neck facer, the prosthesis is inserted. The neck facer is used after the canal has been broached and the handle of the broach removed. The template is left in the canal, and a neck facer, either manually operated or electrically powered, is used to trim the femoral neck so that it accurately fits the collar of the prosthesis. The prosthesis is inserted after bone graft is placed in the fenestrations and the hip reduced. The hip with the prosthesis in place should be checked for stability, length, and full range of motion. Routine closure is then carried out with the capsule closed. The short external rotators can be reattached, or if they are not reattached, they will heal because of the close proximity of the proximal femur to them when the patient is lying in bed in the externally rotated position. A Hemovac drain is inserted prior to closure and removed in 24–48 hours. Blood loss during this procedure is usually 300–500 cc and rarely requires a transfusion.

In the elderly patient with severe osteoporosis, bone grafting of the medullary canal may be useful in obtaining a better press fit of the prosthesis to the femur. The bone graft can be taken from the femoral head, using the grater type of acetabular reamers which collect bone in the reamer. This graft is then inserted as a paste into the medullary canal. An alternative is to use polymethylmethacrylate. A secure press fit of the prosthesis in the femur is desirable. It is rarely necessary to use methylmethacrylate to achieve this type of fit, and I much prefer to use bone graft.

POSTOPERATIVE MANAGEMENT

Postoperatively, the patient is restricted to bed and the hip is kept in an externally rotated, slightly abducted position. A knee immobilizer is used to prevent flexion of the hip and knee. If flexion, adduction, and internal rotation can be avoided, the likelihood of a dislocation using the posterior approach is reduced. On the day following surgery patients are helped to stand with a walker, with partial weight-bearing on the affected extremity. They are encouraged and allowed to begin ambulation with partial weight-bearing that day and to progress as tolerated. Since this fracture occurs most frequently in the elderly, rehabilitation must be carried out gradually, as their physical condition permits. Frequently rehabilitation requires 1–3 weeks and may require transfer to an extended care facility for continuation of care.

The postoperative evaluation of patients having endoprosthetic replacements for the management of acute femoral neck fractures or avascular necrosis has shown results comparable to those achieved with hip nailing, but the postoperative management is easier because the individual can begin to bear weight more quickly and effectively without having to wait for bone to heal. The use of bone cement to stabilize the endoprosthesis has not proved necessary or desirable. Stabilization with bone cement or a porous surface has provided a very rigid stable fixation of the prosthesis in the femur, but it tends to produce a problem with protrusio acetabulae. For that reason, cementation or the use of porous surfaces on the endoprosthetic device is not recommended.

Owing to early ambulation, the problem of phlebothrombosis has been greatly reduced. When persons remain in bed for more than 24 hours, the likelihood of phlebothrombosis is increased, and if they are in bed for 72 hours or longer, plebothrombosis is almost certain to develop in either the popliteal, femoral, or iliac vessels. Intravascular venography has been used to document these developments, and when patients are ambulatory within 24 hours, the incidence of phlebothrombosis is markedly reduced.

REFERENCES

1. Meyers M.H., Harvey J.P. Jr., Moore T.M.: Treatment of displaced fractures of the femoral neck with the muscle pedicle transplant technique: A prospective study and analysis of 150 cases. *J. Bone Joint Surg.* 54A:1351, 1972.
2. Fielding J.W., Wilson S.A., Ratzan S.A.: A continuing end-result study of displaced intracapsular fractures of the neck of the femur treated with Pugh nail. *J. Bone Joint Surg.* 56A:1464-1472, 1974.
3. Kimbrough E.E. III, Kolibac A.L., Lunceford E.M. Jr.: Twenty-eight years' experience with multiple adjustable Moore nail fixation of fractures of the neck of the femur. *J. Bone Joint Surg.* 49A:1282, 1965.
4. Lunceford E.M. Jr.: The use of the Moore self-locking vitallium prosthesis in acute fractures of the femoral neck. *J. Bone Joint Surg.* 47A:832-841, 1965.
5. Salvati E.A., Wilson P.D. Jr.: Long term results of femoral head replacements. *J. Bone Joint Surg.* 54A:1355, 1972.
6. Moore A.T.: The self-locking metal hip prosthesis. *J. Bone Joint Surg.* 39A:811-827, 1957.

Chapter 22

Total Hip Arthroplasty for Femoral Neck Fractures

Franklin H. Sim, M.D.
Eric R. Sigmond, M.D.

The goal in the management of the patient with a displaced intracapsular hip fracture is successful union of the fracture without avascular necrosis. Ideally, reduction and internal fixation is best. However, despite significant advances in techniques of internal fixation, the incidence of nonunion and avascular necrosis remains high.[1, 2] Many surgeons wonder whether it is worth subjecting elderly people to a procedure that has a 50% chance of ultimate failure.[3, 4] Moreover, a lengthy convalescence and the inability of many elderly patients to cooperate with the prolonged non-weight-bearing that is necessary after reduction and internal fixation are factors also to be considered. For these reasons, prosthetic replacement has been advocated as a treatment method in some elderly patients with femoral neck fractures.[3, 5-16]

The indications for replacement arthroplasty are becoming more precisely defined.[4, 14, 17-28] Replacement arthroplasty is a good example of treating the patient rather than the fracture.[29] Patient age is only a relative indication because it has no correlation with the incidence of either nonunion or avascular necrosis. However, the older the patient, the less cooperative he or she may be because of senility or neuromuscular disease. Prosthetic replacement is also useful in patients with associated medical conditions that preclude a second definitive procedure. In such a patient with a high-risk fracture, prosthetic replacement would be advantageous. One type of fracture in which the risk for failure with internal fixation is high is fracture at the higher subcapital level.[30, 31] Moreover, the greater the displacement, the higher the potential for an unsuccessful outcome.[32] Also, comminution is a significant factor because of its effect on the retinacular vessels and the stability of the reduction. Inadequate or incomplete reduction in the elderly patient is a relative indication for prosthetic replacement.[26, 33]

After determining the type of patient and the type of fracture that are best treated by prosthetic replacement, the surgeon must consider the type of replacement surgery. Should the procedure involve an endoprosthesis of the Moore or Thompson variety or an articulated endoprosthesis of the Bateman type? Or should total hip arthroplasty be done? The Moore and Thompson prostheses have served well in most of these elderly patients.[5, 11, 16, 34] However, in the more active patient, acetabular wear and prosthetic loosening have caused symptoms after these procedures. While a cemented hemiarthroplasty provides secure fixation with an interference fit in the elderly patient who has a wide osteoporotic proximal femur, the rigid femoral component does increase acetabular stress and subsequent wear on the articular cartilage. In our experience, the cemented hemiarthroplasty procedure has been expedient and successful in providing limited ambulation and relief of pain after hip fracture, but the outcome has been unpredictable in previously active patients. In these patients, erosion through the acetabular cartilage developed quickly, causing pain that required conversion to a total hip arthroplasty.[35]

With the introduction of the Bateman articulated endoprosthesis, another dimension was added to replacement arthroplasty for the treatment of acute femoral neck fractures. The Mayo Clinic experience with this prosthesis has been favorable, and the results are better than those after a cemented endoprosthesis[36]; however, the functional result has not been as satisfactory as that after total hip replacement. We believe that the articulated endoprosthesis has a definite advantage over the conventional endoprosthesis in a younger and more active patient with a displaced subcapital fracture and a normal acetabulum who does not meet the criteria for internal fixation.

A more recent concern in the management of these fractures is the role of total hip arthroplasty. Previously, the functional capacity after endoprosthesis placement was widely regarded as inferior to that after successful union without avascular necrosis. However, the improved functional results and the greater predictability of total joint replacement have broadened the indications for replacement surgery in patients with displaced femoral neck fractures.

INDICATIONS

There is agreement about the use of total hip arthroplasty for patients with complications from femoral neck fractures treated by internal fixation, particularly if articular cartilage in the acetabulum is lost.[37, 38] Total hip replacement also may be indicated after endoprostheses have failed in acute fractures. Moreover, fractures of the femoral neck after performance of a resurfacing arthroplasty require total hip replacement for salvage. On the other hand, considerable controversy remains regarding the use of total hip arthroplasty as a primary treatment of acute hip fractures. The trend in the selection of type of replacement arthroplasty for femoral neck fractures from 1969 to 1981 is shown in Figure 22–1.

In the group of 721 patients treated at the Mayo Clinic with replacement arthroplasty during 1969–1981, the number of patients with cemented endoprostheses remained fairly constant. In 1970, the number of total hip arthroplasties done for these fractures increased, reaching a peak in 1973 and gradually decreasing to the present level. The number of Bateman arthroplasties done has increased gradually since 1974, and at the present time, this procedure is the most frequent arthroplasty performed in these patients. However, the long-term results of the articulated endoprosthesis are unknown.

Patient selection is the key to defining the indications for the use of total hip arthroplasty in femoral neck fractures. Patient age, associated medical problems, associated hip disease, activity status, and fracture characteristics all influence the choice of operation.

In an effort to better define the criteria and indications for management of these fractures by total hip arthroplasty, Sim and Stauffer[39] reviewed their experience with 112 patients who underwent total hip arthroplasty for acute femoral neck frac-

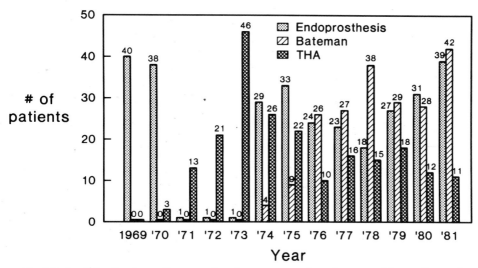

Fig 22–1—Distribution of types of replacement arthroplasty, at Mayo Clinic, for femoral neck fractures, according to year (1969–1981). THA, total hip arthroplasty.

tures at the Mayo Clinic between 1970 and 1978. It was during this time that the present criteria gradually evolved. In that series, females predominated (93 patients), and the median age of the group was 74 years (range, 40–89). The median follow-up was 1½ years. Sixty-three percent of the fractures were subcapital, 28% were midcervical, and 9% were basilar. Eighty-eight percent of the patients had Garden stage 3 or 4 displaced fractures.

Patient Characteristics

Age, activity status, and patient expectations are important considerations. The patient most likely to benefit from total hip replacement is the elderly patient who has previously been fully active and who has a high-risk femoral neck fracture that meets the criteria for prosthetic replacement. In the series reported by Sim and Stauffer,[39] 79 patients were unrestricted or mildly restricted in their activities before the injury, 25 were moderately restricted, and 6 were severely restricted. Thirty-three patients used assistive devices for ambulation before operation; 26 of these used a cane, 4 used crutches, and 3 used a walker. Two patients were unable to walk.

Associated medical conditions may encourage the use of an endoprosthesis or total hip replacement. Any medical condition that increases the risk of complications from a second operation—that is, a procedure for the revision of failed internal fixation—makes definitive treatment of the femoral neck fracture more desirable. In the Mayo Clinic series,[39] of 112 patients whose femoral neck fractures were treated with a primary total hip replacement, 67% of patients had associated cardiovascular, renal, or pulmonary problems before surgery. An average delay of 2.5 days between the time of the injury and the time of operation reflects the time required to evaluate the many medical problems in these elderly patients. Moreover, 5 patients (4.5%) had preexisting neoplastic conditions that did not involve the hip, but, because of the patients' previous high level of activity and their predicted short life expectancy, it was judged that they would benefit from the early functional restoration afforded by total hip replacement.

Associated Hip Disease

Preexisting hip disease is one of the most valid indications for primary total hip replacement.[40, 41] In Sim and Stauffer's report, the acetabulum was abnormal in more than half of the patients. Symptomatic hip disease was present in 16 patients, of whom 6 had degenerative joint disease and 5 had symptomatic rheumatoid involvement of the hip (Fig 22–2). Moreover, 3 patients had fracture of the femoral neck associated with Paget's disease of the hip. That combination has been considered to be associated with a poor prognosis after either internal fixation or endoprosthetic replacement. Our overall experience to date with total hip arthroplasty in patients with Paget's disease seems to offer a solution to this problem (Fig 22–3).[40]

Associated disease in the contralateral hip also may be a determining factor in the selection of total hip arthroplasty (Fig 22–4). Nine patients in the series reported by Sim and Stauffer had associated significant contralateral hip disease that was a factor in the selection of total hip arthroplasty. Significant osteoporosis is only a relative indication for replacement arthroplasty. The weakened bone is less likely to provide secure fixation and may result in loss of reduction and failure of the procedure. Moreover, acetabular osteoporosis is associated with medial migration of an endoprosthesis. In Sim and Stauffer's report, 79% of patients had significant osteoporosis. Moreover, in patients with metastatic tumor involvement of the hip who had actual or imminent pathologic fracture, resection with replacement arthroplasty pro-

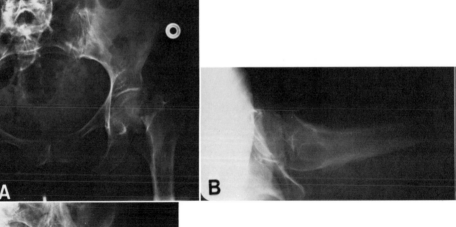

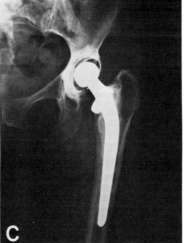

Fig 22–2—AP (A) and lateral (B) views of left hip. Patient had a Garden stage 4 displaced fracture. Patient also had rheumatoid arthritis involving multiple joints, and early narrowing of joint space is evident. C, AP view 28 months after total hip arthroplasty.

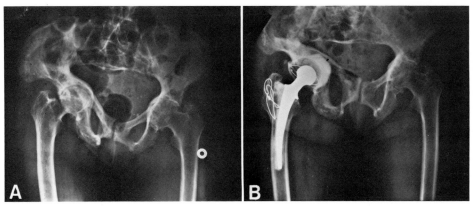

*Fig 22–3—**A,** AP view of pelvis showing extensive Paget's disease involving the right pelvis and hip and left hemipelvis. Fracture of femoral neck is evident. **B,** appearance after total hip replacement.*

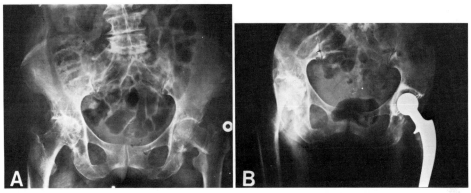

*Fig 22–4—**A,** AP view of pelvis showing severe degenerative disease of the right hip and moderate disease in the left hip. Patient had a displaced basilar neck fracture of the left hip. **B,** appearance 18 months after left total hip arthroplasty. Patient now has a fracture of the femoral neck of the right degenerative hip.*

vides relief of pain and allows early mobilization.[42] This is the treatment of choice for lesions involving the head and neck of the femur (Fig 22–5). In these patients, either hemiarthroplasty or total joint replacement may be selected. We prefer total hip arthroplasty in patients who were active before the fracture occurred and in those whose conditions are well managed medically. We believe these patients benefit more from the early restoration of function afforded by total joint replacement. When pathologic fractures involve the peritrochanteric region, various internal fixation devices are preferred. However, at times the osseous destruction is so extensive that resection with segmental prosthetic replacement is an effective way of dealing with these difficult problems. In addition, when the integrity of the acetabular bone stock is impaired by metastatic disease, collapse of the acetabulum can be avoided by hip joint replacement with acetabular reinforcement.

Many disparate factors are involved in the decision for total hip replacement in a patient with a fractured hip, and all challenge the judgment of the surgeon as to the appropriateness of this surgical procedure.

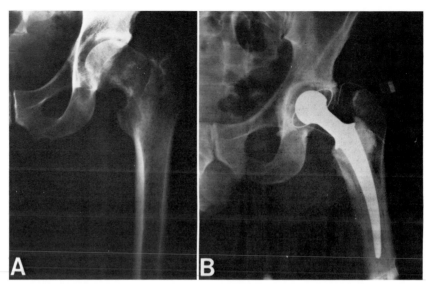

*Fig 22–5—AP views of left hip. **A,** pathologic fracture of femoral neck secondary to metastatic breast carcinoma. **B,** after Charnley total hip replacement.*

CONTRAINDICATIONS

The fewer criteria that the patient meets, the less the indication for primary treatment of the hip fracture by total hip replacement. For instance, our experience suggests that, for the minimally active or nonambulatory elderly osteoporotic patient with a fresh femoral neck fracture, a cemented endoprosthesis is an effective surgical procedure. (The general medical status of many of these patients is inadequate to withstand the extra burden of the additional surgical procedure.) Moreover, in a younger, more active patient with a fracture of the femoral neck who expects to remain active in strenuous work and recreational activities, and in whom reduction and internal fixation has been excluded as viable treatment, an articulated endoprosthesis of the Bateman type is preferred. Probably the strongest contraindication to total hip arthroplasty in the management of these fractures is a history of previous hip sepsis.

ADVANTAGES

The main advantage of total hip arthroplasty in the management of these patients is the predictability of the functional restoration afforded by the procedure. In a Mayo Clinic series, 81% of patients had no pain and 18% had mild discomfort (Fig 22–6).[39] After the operation, 61% had no restriction or were mildly restricted in their activity levels, 30% were moderately restricted, and 9% were severely restricted (Fig 22–7). Most of the patients maintained their previous levels of activity, but 13 improved and 33 were worse. The decrease in activity was generally due to deterioration of associated medical conditions. In retrospect, an endoprosthesis or Bateman arthroplasty probably would have been better in these patients. After total hip replacement, 45% of the patients used no support and 55% used some assistive device: 40% a cane for distance walking only, 3% a cane full-time, 4% crutches, and 8% a walker (Fig 22–8). The range of motion in 100 patients was recorded postoperatively: 47% had 100° or more, 45% had 90°–100°, and 8% had less than 90°.

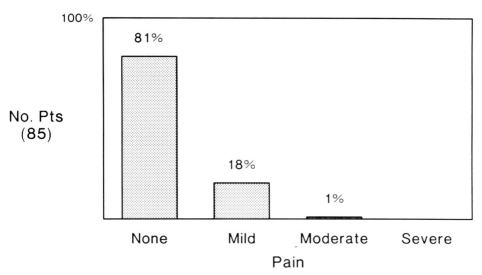

Fig 22–6—Distribution of pain in 85 patients after total hip arthroplasty for femoral neck fractures.

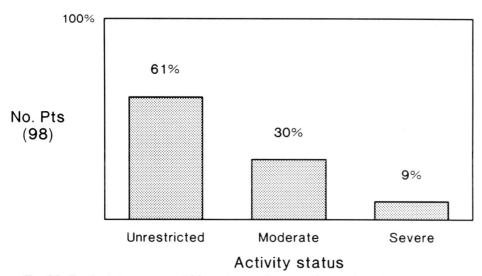

Fig 22–7—Activity status of 98 patients after total hip arthroplasty for femoral neck fractures.

Probably the most significant advantage of this procedure is that it involves one operation to treat two conditions and therefore is ideal in patients with preexisting hip disease such as rheumatoid arthritis (Fig 22–9), osteoarthritis (Fig 22–10), or Paget's disease and neoplastic involvement of the hips.

DISADVANTAGES

One of the main disadvantages of using total hip arthroplasty for primary treatment of femoral neck fractures is the greater surgical trauma associated with the procedure; moreover, if a serious complication occurs, the results may be catastrophic. Therefore, the morbidity of replacement arthroplasty for acute femoral

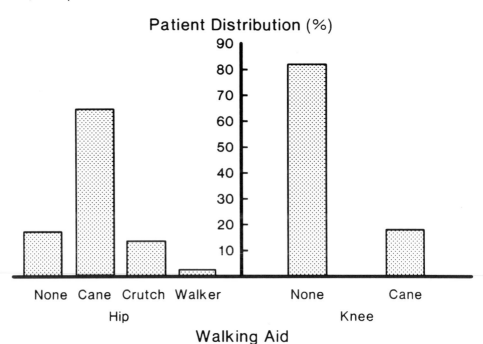

Fig 22–8—*Use of walking aids by 85 patients after total hip arthroplasty.*

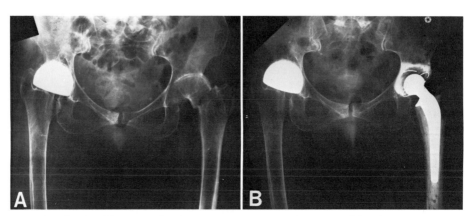

Fig 22–9—**A,** *AP view of pelvis showing acute fracture of the femoral neck in a patient with rheumatoid arthritis of the hips. There is a painful cup arthroplasty of right hip.* **B,** *view after left total hip replacement.*

neck fractures in the elderly population must be considered. While the incidences of medical and surgical complications are high regardless of the type of implant, the surgical complication rate is greater in patients undergoing total hip arthroplasty than in patients undergoing Bateman arthroplasty (22% vs. 11% at the Mayo Clinic). Moreover, the operative time is prolonged another 20 minutes (96 vs. 116 minutes), with about twice the loss of blood (551 vs. 1,250 ml), in total hip replacement. These differences are also evident when one compares the minimal surgical exposure and operative time to internally fix a hip fracture. In addition, the well-documented systemic effects of methylmethacrylate may be an added burden to the elderly patient.[43, 44]

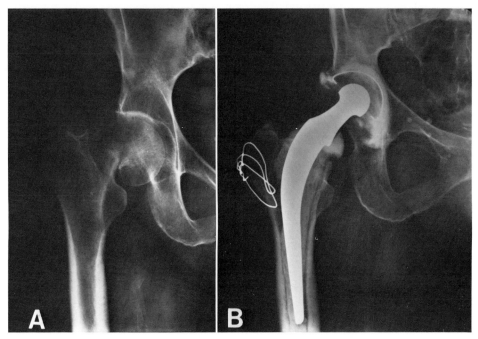

Fig 22–10—AP views of right hip. **A,** *displaced intracapsular fracture with associated symptomatic degenerative joint disease and evidence of loosening of the femoral component.* **B,** *view 16 months after total hip replacement. (**B** from Sim F.H., Stauffer R.N.: Management of hip fractures by total hip arthroplasty. Clin. Orthop. 152:191-197, 1980. Reproduced by permission of J.B. Lippincott Co.)*

SURGICAL TECHNIQUE

The surgical technique for total hip arthroplasty is well standardized; the anterolateral, posterolateral, and transtrochanteric approaches have been thoroughly described.[45, 46] Currently, we prefer the anterolateral approach.

Either general or spinal anesthesia is used. The patient is placed in the lateral decubitus position with the pelvis fixed as securely as possible at right angles to the plane of the floor and table. The perineal region is draped out of the surgical field by using nonpermeable "U" drapes. In thin patients, the head of the fibula should be padded to avoid inadvertent pressure on the peroneal nerve. During draping, a pocket made from a half sheet is placed at the side of the table to accept the leg during dislocation.

After satisfactory preparation and draping, a straight lateral incision is made and extended 10 cm proximal and distal to the greater trochanter. The incision is deepened to expose the fascia lata and the combined muscle mass of the gluteus maximus and the tensor fascia lata. The fascia lata is split and the avascular plane between the gluteus maximus and the tensor fascia lata is located. The incision is extended through this plane. The greater trochanter bursa is then excised, revealing the insertion of the gluteus medius and minimus on the greater trochanter. The anterior half of the insertion of the medius is released, as is the entire insertion of the minimus. The loose connective tissue that covers the anterior part of the hip capsule is then cleaned from its surface, and the reflected head of the rectus femoris is identified on the superior margin of the acetabulum. The reflected head is released, and a periosteal elevation is used to strip the gluteus minimus and medius from the iliac crest. A self-retaining retractor is then inserted into the bone of the iliac crest to retract these muscles. The anterior hip capsule is excised as is necessary to dislocate the hip and remove the fractured head. The hip is then dislocated, and the neck cut is made.

The trial prosthesis is held in the correct position anterior to the femur, and the collar is used to direct the cut along the neck. The femur is then pulled posteriorly with a bone hook to expose the acetabulum. The acetabulum is reamed out progressively to the appropriate depth and diameter. Modern cement techniques are utilized. Irrigating the joint with water is especially helpful to rid the wound of bony and hematogenous debris. After the acetabulum is cemented in approximately 10° of anteversion, the femoral shaft is prepared to receive its component. Proper seating of the component collar on the calcar is sought, and about 10°–15° of anteversion is achieved with neutral or slight valgus positioning of the component. Use of a bone plug and water irrigation assists the penetration of the cement into the canal. Trial reductions before cementing help to obtain the proper tightness of fit. The neck length of the femoral component varies with the level of the fracture.

The femoral component is then cemented in place by using a low-viscosity cement with pressurized injection from a cement gun, and a rubber dam (a wet surgical glove) is used to cover the opening of the femoral canal to ensure adequate filling of the proximal canal. The wound is closed in the standard fashion using absorbable sutures to reattach the gluteus medius and minimus muscles to the greater trochanter. Drains are routinely used. The patient is placed on an abduction splint or a cradle to avoid adduction of the extremity.

PITFALLS: PREVENTION AND TREATMENT

Complications in total hip surgery, although relatively rare, are far more significant than those in internal fixation. Moreover, the patients that undergo total hip arthroplasty as primary treatment for a fracture tend to be more frail than the general population undergoing elective total hip arthroplasty. Replacement arthroplasty of any variety exposes the patient to a wider range of complications than are seen after internal fixation, such as dislocation and nerve injuries.

Complications of total hip surgery for femoral neck fractures, however, are no different from those following standard elective total hip arthroplasties. These may be categorized as intraoperative, postoperative, and late.[47] Of the 112 patients in the Mayo Clinic series reported on by Sim and Stauffer, 42% had postoperative complications: 20% medical and 22% surgical. Complications specific to the total hip arthroplasty include nerve injury, bleeding and hematoma, phlebitis, embolism, dislocation, and subluxation. The incidence of clinical phlebitis and pulmonary embolism has ranged from 4% to 30%.[48] In the series of 112 patients undergoing total hip replacement for acute fracture at the Mayo Clinic, one had clinical phlebitis and five had pulmonary embolism.[39] We advocate prophylactic anticoagulation to prevent these complications.[49] Our choice is aspirin for men and sodium warfarin for women. One of the risks in anticoagulation is wound hematoma, but the benefits outweigh this risk. In the series reported by Sim and Stauffer,[39] five patients had wound hematomas, one of whom required drainage. Careful hemostasis at surgery and the use of suction drainage after the operation, as well as use of an elastic spica bandage, provide effective prevention.

Postoperative dislocation and subluxation occur in approximately 2% of patients undergoing total hip arthroplasty, but the rate is higher when the patient has had previous failed surgery.[50] A similar dislocation rate after performance of the Bateman articulated endoprosthesis procedure has been reported.[51] Patients in the series reported by Sim and Stauffer[39] who underwent total hip arthroplasty for fracture had a very high dislocation rate (12 of 112). Ten of the 12 patients were treated successfully by closed reduction, but one inactive patient had recurrent dislocation that remains unreduced. Another patient required open reduction 4 months after the initial operation. The high incidence of dislocation may be related to the normal status of the soft tissues about the fractured hip and the excellent range of motion achieved, compared with the contracted tissues usually seen in patients undergoing hip replacement electively.

Proper positioning of the acetabular and femoral components is essential for the stability of the hip. When an anterior approach is used, care must be taken to avoid excessive anteversion of the cup and femoral prosthesis. To avoid this problem, careful attention to technical details is essential. Most of the hip capsule should be preserved, and only enough of the anterior part removed to allow dislocation. Intraoperative and postoperative factors are important in the prevention of dislocation. Conversely, when the posterior approach is used, retroversion of either the femoral or the acetabular component predisposes to dislocation. Moreover, it is essential to control the positioning of the leg after the operation. Adduction and external rotation may result in dislocation after an anterior approach, and adduction and internal rotation are detrimental after the posterior approach. In either case, an abduction pillow or a lower extremity cradle is utilized to position the limb properly.

Most patients have high expectations after total hip arthroplasty, and inequality of leg length can cause a patient to be dissatisfied. While it is essential to obtain adequate tension between the components to prevent dislocation, precise measurement of length by distracting the hip before excising the capsule allows measurement from fixed points on the pelvis and trochanter. In one series,[52] 83% of patients had equal leg lengths, and only four patients had differences greater than one-half inch.

Peripheral nerve injury after total hip arthroplasty occurred in 0.7% of the 2,012 arthroplasties done at the Mayo Clinic.[53] In the series of total hip replacements for fractures reported by Sim and Stauffer,[39] two patients had nerve injuries: one had a peroneal nerve injury and the other had sciatic palsy. Significant heterotopic bone formation is uncommon—only 11 of 3,204 arthroplasties in the Mayo Clinic series required revision for this complication.[54] Of the 112 patients who underwent total hip arthroplasty for fractures, ten had mild and two had extensive heterotopic bone formation. The patient with a history of heterotopic bone formation or the patient who has a high risk for this complication, such as one with rheumatoid spondylitis or Paget's disease, may benefit from low-dose radiation therapy during the postoperative period.

Infection early or late is probably the most catastrophic complication. In a Mayo Clinic series of total hip arthroplasties,[55] the incidence of deep infection was 1.3%. Moreover, 43 patients had superficial infections that responded to treatment. In Sim and Stauffer's report on 112 patients,[39] the only postoperative infection was one superficial infection, and that responded to local debridement and the use of antibiotics. This compares favorably with the rate reported by Coventry and colleagues[49] in a series of patients who underwent total hip arthroplasty and contrasts with the 4.1% rate of infection in a series of patients who underwent cemented hemiarthroplasty at the Mayo Clinic.[17] Preventative measures include the preoperative and postoperative use of antibiotics, irrigation with antibiotic solutions, and techniques to remove bacteria from the ambient air. Most important is meticulous surgical technique. When infection is recognized, salvage of the hip arthroplasty may be difficult. With early recognition of an acute deep sepsis, thorough debridement and closure over tube irrigation, combined with high-dose specific antibiotics, is warranted. However, management of a patient who has infection generally requires removal of the prosthesis. Unfortunately, infection may be very difficult to eradicate.

Problems secondary to osteotomy of the trochanter include nonunion, avulsion, and bursitis. Trochanteric problems were responsible for 14 of 125 reoperations in a series of 3,204 arthroplasties done at the Mayo Clinic.[54] The incidence of nonunion ranges from 4% to 18%. In the series of 112 patients reported on by Sim and Stauffer who underwent total hip arthroplasty for fracture, three had nonunion of the trochanteric osteotomy, one of whom required reattachment. Six patients had evidence of broken trochanteric wires on roentgenograms. At present, we prefer to use the anterolateral approach and to avoid trochanteric osteotomy. In addition to the complications already mentioned, late complications include prosthetic loosening, stem failure, and cement fracture.[47]

Follow-up of the original 333 consecutive total hip arthroplasties done at the Mayo Clinic by the Charnley technique indicated that the roentgenographic loosening rate of the femoral component at 5–10 years after surgery was 29.9%. The rate of roentgenographic loosening of the acetabular component at 10 years was 11.3%. Fourteen hips (6.1%) required revision by 10 years because of loosening of the femoral component. Seven reoperations (3%) for loose acetabular components were needed by 10 years.[56] For most patients undergoing total hip arthroplasty for fracture of the femoral neck, the longevity of the prosthesis should be adequate, and even in a younger patient, there is less concern for late loosening. Of 112 patients in the series reported by Sim and Stauffer, only one required revision for loosening at 5 years.

COMMENT

In the past, criteria for the management of a displaced intracapsular hip fracture by internal fixation or replacement arthroplasty were not well defined. Moreover, if the patient was a candidate for prosthetic replacement, there was no consensus on the type of replacement surgery that should be done. The results in the series reported by Sim and Stauffer indicate that total hip arthroplasty has a definite place in the treatment of properly selected patients who have acute femoral neck fractures. In the series of 721 patients treated at the Mayo Clinic since 1979 by replacement arthroplasty, the number of cemented endoprosthesis procedures has remained fairly constant. The enthusiasm for total hip arthroplasty in the early 1970s led to the increased use of total hip replacement for these fractures, the number reaching a peak in 1973 and gradually decreasing to the present level as specific criteria and indications evolved. However, the Bateman articulated endoprosthesis procedure has seen gradually increased usage since 1974 and, at the present time, is the operation most frequently performed at the Mayo Clinic for a femoral neck fracture. Although the results are satisfactory, the long-term outcomes of the articulated endoprosthesis procedures are yet to be determined.

Patient selection is the key to defining the indications for treatment of femoral neck fractures with total hip arthroplasties, and this selection remains a challenge to the surgeon. Our experience indicates that total hip arthroplasty has a definite place in the management of these patients; however, it is probably best reserved for the active elderly patient who has a fracture in which standard internal fixation is likely to fail, or for the patient with significant preexisting hip disease. One must weigh the predictable excellent functional restoration afforded by total hip replacement against the morbidity and possible complications in this elderly population. With widespread use of total hip arthroplasty as the primary treatment for femoral neck fractures, one might expect the morbidity to increase to unacceptable levels.

REFERENCES

1. Albright J.P.: Treatment for fixation complications: Femoral neck fractures. *Arch. Surg.* 110:30-36, 1975.
2. Meyers M.H., Harvey J.P., Jr., Moore T.M.: Treatment of displaced subcapital and transcervical fractures of the femoral neck by muscle-pedicle-bone graft and internal fixation: A preliminary report on one hundred and fifty cases. *J. Bone Joint Surg. [Am.]* 55:257-274, 1973.
3. Hargadon E.J., Pearson J.R.: Treatment of intracapsular fractures of the femoral neck with the Charnley compression screw. *J. Bone Joint Surg. [Br.]* 45:305-311, 1963.
4. McNeur J.C.: The treatment of subcapital fractures of the neck of the femur with a nail-plate and wedge osteotomy. *J. Bone Joint Surg. [Br.]* 35:188-191, 1953.
5. Anderson L.D., Hamsa W.R. Jr., Waring T.L.: Femoral-head prostheses: A review of three hundred and fifty-six operations and their results. *J. Bone Joint Surg. [Am.]* 46:1049-1065, 1964.
6. Barr J.S., Compere E.L., Ghormley R.K., et al.: A symposium on hip joint prostheses. *Instr. Course Lect.* 15:1, 1958.
7. Barr J.S., Donovan J.F., Florence D.W.: Arthroplasty of the hip: Theoretical and practical considerations with a follow-up study of prosthetic replacement of the femoral head at the Massachusetts General Hospital. *J. Bone Joint Surg. [Am.]* 46:249-266, 1964.
8. Carnesale P.G., Anderson L.D.: Primary prosthetic replacement for femoral neck fractures. *Arch. Surg.* 110:27-29, 1975.
9. Ford L.T., Key J.A.: Replacement prosthesis for fractures of the neck of the femur. *J. Iowa State Med. Soc.* 45:597-600, 1955.
10. Hinchey J.J.: An evaluation of prosthetic replacement in management of fresh fractures of the neck of the femur. *Instr. Course Lect.* 17:121-127, 1960.
11. Hinchey J.J., Day P.L.: Primary prosthetic replacement in fresh femoral-neck fractures: A review of 294 consecutive cases. *J. Bone Joint Surg. [Am.]* 46:223-240, 1964.
12. Mahoney J.W., Mulholland J.H., Jahr J., et al.: Immediate Moore prosthetic replacement in acute intracapsular fractures. *Am. J. Surg.* 95:577-580, 1958.
13. McElvenny R.T.: Concepts and principles in the treatment of intracapsular fractures of the hip. *Am. J. Orthop.* 2:161-164; 172, 1960.
14. Nicoll E.A.: The unsolved fracture, editorial. *J. Bone Joint Surg. [Br.]* 45:239-241, 1963.
15. Salvati E.A., Wilson P.D. Jr.: Long-term results of femoral-head replacement. *J. Bone Joint Surg. [Am.]* 55:516-524, 1973.
16. Thompson F.R.: Two and a half years' experience with a Vitallium intramedullary hip prosthesis. *J. Bone Joint Surg. [Am.]* 36:489-502, 1954.
17. Bradford C.H., Kelleher J.J., O'Brien P.I., et al.: Primary prosthesis for subcapital fractures of the neck of the femur: Preliminary report. *N. Engl. J. Med.* 251:804-807, 1954.
18. Coventry M.B.: Fresh fracture of the hip treated with prosthesis. *Instr. Course Lect.* 16:292-298, 1959.
19. D'Arcy J., Devas M.: Treatment of fractures of the femoral neck by replacement with the Thompson prosthesis. *J. Bone Joint Surg. [Br.]* 58:279-286, 1976.
20. Deyerle W.M.: Multiple-pin peripheral fixation in fractures of the neck of the femur: Immediate weight-bearing. *Clin. Orthop.* 39:135-156, 1965.
21. Jensen J.S., Holstein P.: A longterm follow-up of Moore arthroplasty in femoral neck fractures. *Acta Orthop. Scand.* 46:764-774, 1975.
22. Johnson J.T.H., Crothers O.: Nailing versus prosthesis for femoral-neck fractures: A critical

review of long-term results in two hundred and thirty-nine consecutive private patients. *J. Bone Joint Surg. [Am.]* 57:686-692, 1975.

23. Lindholm R.V., Puranen J., Kinnunen P.: The Moore Vitallium femoral-head prosthesis in fractures of the femoral neck. *Acta Orthop. Scand.* 47:70-78, 1976.

24. Lunt H.R.W.: The role of prosthetic replacement of the head of the femur as primary treatment for subcapital fractures. *Injury* 3:107-113, 1971.

25. Raine G.E.: A comparison of internal fixation and prosthetic replacement for recent displaced subcapital fractures of the neck of the femur. *Injury* 5:25-30, 1973.

26. Scheck M.: Intracapsular fractures of the femoral neck: Comminution of the posterior neck cortex as a cause of unstable fixation. *J. Bone Joint Surg. [Am.]* 41:1187-1200, 1959.

27. Søreide O., Lerner A.P., Thunold J.: Primary prosthetic replacement in acute femoral neck fractures. *Injury* 6:286-293, 1975.

28. Tillberg B.: Treatment of fractures of the femoral neck by primary arthroplasty. *Acta Orthop. Scand.* 47:209-213, 1976.

29. Lunceford E.M. Jr.: Use of the Moore self-locking Vitallium prosthesis in acute fractures of the femoral neck. *J. Bone Joint Surg. [Am.]* 47:832-841, 1965.

30. Fielding J.: Displaced femoral neck fractures. *Orthop. Rev.* 2:11, 1973.

31. Fielding J.W., Wilson S.A., Ratzan S.: A continuing end-result study of displaced intracapsular fractures of the neck of the femur treated with the Pugh nail. *J. Bone Joint Surg. [Am.]* 56:1464-1472, 1974.

32. Barnes R., Brown J.T., Garden R.S., et al.: Subcapital fractures of the femur: A prospective review. *J. Bone Joint Surg. [Br.]* 58:2-24, 1976.

33. Scheck M.: Management of fractures of the femoral neck. *J. Bone Joint Surg. [Am.]* 47:819-829, 1965.

34. Whittaker R.P., Abeshaus M.M., Scholl H.W., et al.: Fifteen years' experience with metallic endoprosthetic replacement of the femoral head for femoral neck fractures. *J. Trauma* 12:799-806, 1972.

35. Beckenbaugh R.D., Tressler H.A., Johnson E.W. Jr.: Results after hemiarthroplasty of the hip using a cemented femoral prosthesis: A review of 109 cases with an average follow-up of 36 months. *Mayo Clin. Proc.* 52:349-353, 1977.

36. Cabanela M.E., VanDemark R.E. Jr.: Unpublished data.

37. Hunter G.: Treatment of fractures of the neck of the femur. *Can. Med. Assoc. J.* 117:60-61, 1977.

38. Hunter G.A.: A further comparison of the use of internal fixation and prosthetic replacement for fresh fractures of the neck of the femur. *Br. J. Surg.* 61:382-384, 1974.

39. Sim F.H., Stauffer R.N.: Management of hip fractures by total hip arthroplasty. *Clin. Orthop.* 152:191-197, 1980.

40. Stauffer R.N., Sim F.H.: Total hip arthroplasty in Paget's disease of the hip. *J. Bone Joint Surg. [Am.]* 58:476-478, 1976.

41. Vahvanen V.: Femoral neck fracture of the rheumatoid hip joint: A study of 20 operatively treated cases. *Acta Rheum. Scand.* 17:125-136, 1971.

42. Sim F.H., Hartz C.R., Chao E.Y.S.: Total hip arthroplasty for tumors of the hip. *Hip* 4:246-259, 1976.

43. Pazzaglia U., Ceciliani L., Mora R.: Reaction to methylmethacrylate in bone metastases treated by surgical curetting and filling with acrylic cement: Histological study of a case. *Arch. Orthop. Trauma Surg.* 101:145-149, 1983.

44. Sherman R.M., Byrick R.J., Kay J.C., et al.: The role of lavage in preventing hemodynamic and blood-gas changes during cemented arthroplasty. *J. Bone Joint Surg. [Am.]* 65:500-506, 1983.

45. Edmonson A.S., Crenshaw A.H.: *Campbell's Operative Orthopaedics,* ed 6. St. Louis, C.V. Mosby Co., 1980, vol. 1, pp. 69-74.

46. Eftekhar N.S.: *Principles of Total Hip Arthroplasty.* St. Louis, C.V. Mosby Co., 1978, pp. 35-55.

47. Lowell J.D.: Complications of total hip replacement. *Hip* 4:224-245, 1976.

48. Evarts C.M., Feil E.I.: Thromboembolism after elective surgery of the hip: Detection, natural history, prophylaxis, and results with low molecular weight dextran. *Orthop. Clin. North Am.* 2:167-174, March, 1971.

49. Coventry M.B., Beckenbaugh R.D., Nolan D.R., et al.: 2,012 total hip arthroplasties: A study of postoperative course and early complications. *J. Bone Joint Surg.* [*Am.*] 56:273-284, 1974.

50. Evanski P.M., Waugh T.R., Orofino C.F.: Total hip replacement with the Charnley prosthesis. *Clin. Orthop.* 95:69-72, 1973.

51. Long J.W., Knight W.: Bateman UPF prosthesis in fractures of the femoral neck. *Clin. Orthop.* 152:198-201, 1980.

52. Knight W.E.: Accurate determination of leg lengths during total hip replacement. *Clin. Orthop.* 123:27-28, 1977.

53. Weber E.R., Daube J.R., Coventry M.B.: Peripheral neuropathies associated with total hip arthroplasty. *J. Bone Joint Surg.* [*Am.*] 58:66-69, 1976.

54. Nolan D.R., Fitzgerald R.H., Jr., Beckenbaugh R.D., et al.: Complications of total hip arthroplasty treated by reoperation. *J. Bone Joint Surg.* [*Am.*] 57:977-981, 1975.

55. Coventry M.B.: The treatment of fracture-dislocation of the hip by total hip arthroplasty. *J. Bone Joint Surg.* [*Am.*] 56:1128-1134, 1974.

56. Coventry M.B., Stauffer R.N.: Long-term results of total hip arthroplasty. *Hip* 10:34-41, 1982.

Chapter 23

Medial Displacement Fixation for Unstable Intertrochanteric Fractures of the Hip

Joseph H. Dimon, III, M.D.

On Armistice Day, 1959, while performing an open reduction of an unstable intertrochanteric fracture, I became aware of the nature of this fracture. The femoral shaft shifted medially during my attempts at reduction and fixation, and it was only after much time and effort that I was able to pull the shaft laterally and secure it to the Jewett nail. In discussing this case with Dr. Otto Aufranc, Chief of the Massachusetts General Hospital Fracture Service, he pointed out that based on the fracture's behavior in the operating room, we could anticipate the shaft shifting medially postoperatively. (The Jewett nail subsequently was driven through the femoral head into the acetabulum as the shaft shifted medially.) Dr. Aufranc suggested that in situations like this, the shaft should be allowed to shift medially at the time of surgery.

I applied the technique of medial displacement and impaction of the shaft in unstable intertrochanteric fractures after I joined Drs. James Funk and Robert Wells in practice at the Peachtree Orthopaedic Clinic in Atlanta, Georgia in 1960.

Several years later, as I was discussing this method of fixation of difficult intertrochanteric fractures with Dr. Jack Hughston of Columbus, Georgia, he remarked that he did indeed think it was a good procedure and had suggested it in a letter to the Duke Piedmont Orthopaedic Society letter and in a Correspondence Club letter several years earlier. Dr. Hughston and I then collaborated on a detailed study of more than 300 consecutive intertrochanteric fractures operated on at the Peachtree Orthopaedic Clinic and the Hughston Clinic. This study was published in the April 1967 issue of the *Journal of Bone and Joint Surgery*. Our conclusions are described in the following paragraphs.

1. Essential to the identification of most unstable intertrochanteric fractures is the recognition of four basic components: the femoral head and neck, a medial calcar-lesser trochanteric fragment, a posterior greater trochanteric fragment, and the femoral shaft (Fig 23–1).

2. In many cases of intertrochanteric fracture instability, the shaft of the femur migrates medially and proximally, and/or the fracture deforms into varus in

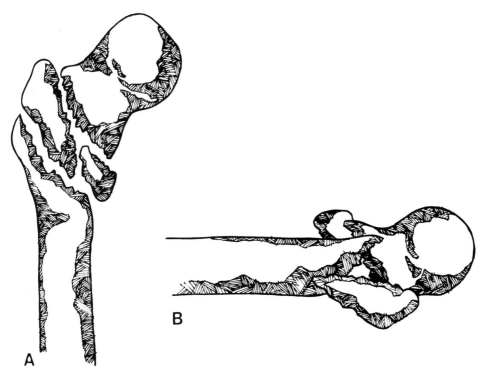

Fig 23–1—The characteristic four parts of the unstable intertrochanteric fracture.
A, *AP view of right hip showing the four-part fracture (head-neck segment, calcar and lesser trochanter fragment, greater trochanteric segment, and shaft).* **B,** *lateral view. Medial calcar and lesser trochanteric fragment is pulled anteriorly by the iliopsoas and the posterior greater trochanteric fragment is pulled back by the external rotators.*

order to close the medial and posterior gaps that create instability of intertrochanteric fractures.

3. Unstable intertrochanteric fractures that have been reduced anatomically and fixed with a solid nail plate device such as a Jewett nail are associated with a high incidence of fixation complications because of migration of the shaft medially and proximally or varus deformity of the fracture thereby closing the medial and posterior gaps which create instability of intertrochanteric fractures (Fig 23–2).

4. Fixation of stable intertrochanteric fractures results in few complications, regardless of the fixation device.

5. Fixation of unstable intertrochanteric fractures by medial displacement with impaction markedly lowers the fixation complication rate when a Jewett nail (solid nail plate device) is used (Fig 23–3).

In the last few years, the use of sliding nail and sliding compression screw devices has reduced the fixation complication rate. These devices compensate as the fracture fragments collapse into a more stable position (Fig 23–4). In addition, penetration of the head and acetabulum is markedly reduced. The use of the telescoping type of devices has decreased the indications for a primary medial displacement osteotomy. Therefore, the surgeon may elect to perform the technically less difficult and less traumatic conventional anatomical reduction and fixation procedure using these devices. If reduction and fixation is selected, the additional use of a slotted side plate with yoking of the lateral cortex further accommodates fracture impaction.

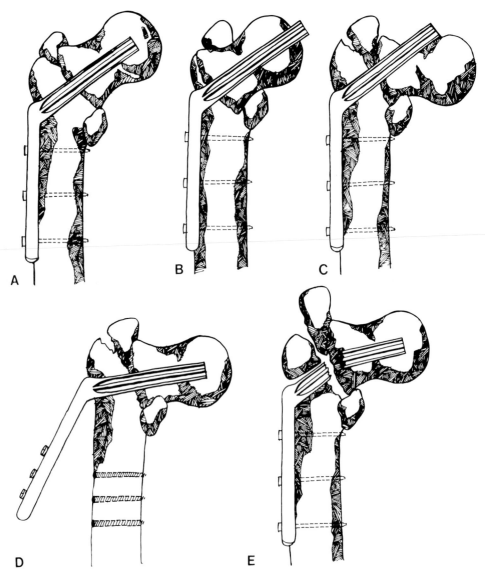

Fig 23–2—Conventional reduction with Jewett fixation for unstable intertrochanteric fractures, and complications that may occur. **A,** *Jewett nailing after anatomical reduction.* **B,** *medial migration of shaft to close gaps results in penetration of the Jewett nail through femoral head and into acetabulum.* **C,** *varus collapse of unstable fracture results in nail cutting out of head and neck.* **D,** *varus collapse of fracture results in screw heads pulling off.* **E,** *breakage of Jewett nail as fracture collapses into varus.*

Achieving stability initially by displacement fixation depends on the surgeon's evaluation of the situation. He or she must determine whether or not the procedure is necessary and must weigh the difficulties involved.

INDICATIONS

When instability of the intertrochanteric fracture is recognized on roentgenographic examination, digital palpation at surgery, or medial shift of the shaft during

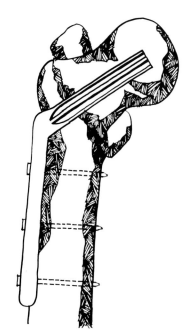

Fig 23–3—Jewett nail fixation of unstable fracture after impaction fixation of the fracture, closing gaps.

the nailing procedure, medial displacement of the shaft with vertical impaction and fixation should be considered initially to improve contact between the fracture fragments and achieve stability.

The complication rate of fixation of the unstable intertrochanteric fracture *will* be decreased by initial medial displacement fixation when a fixed nail plate combination such as a Jewett nail is used. Therefore, medial displacement fixation should be carried out in this instance.

The complication rate *may* be decreased by initial medial displacement fixation of the unstable intertrochanteric fracture if a sliding nail or sliding compression screw device is used. Using a slotted side plate with yoking of the lateral cortex may further decrease the complication rate (Fig 23–5).

CONTRAINDICATIONS

Intertrochanteric fractures that are thought to be stable do not require medial displacement fixation.

Unstable intertrochanteric fractures in young patients with strong bone, where preservation of length is of major importance, should be stabilized anatomically without displacement fixation and should be protected for a prolonged period of time by supplemental traction, as necessary, and prolonged partial weight-bearing.

Unstable intertrochanteric fractures should not be displaced medially if one does not have the appropriate equipment. Short Jewett nails, 2–3 inches long, or similar compression screws and barrels allowing telescoping down to 2–2½ inches in overall length, should be available in case they are required.

Unstable intertrochanteric fractures should not be displaced medially if the operating surgeon is unfamiliar or uncomfortable with the technique.

ADVANTAGES OF THE MEDIAL DISPLACEMENT FIXATION TECHNIQUE

The advantage of initial medial displacement fixation of unstable intertrochanteric fractures is that an unstable fracture is converted to a stable fracture through

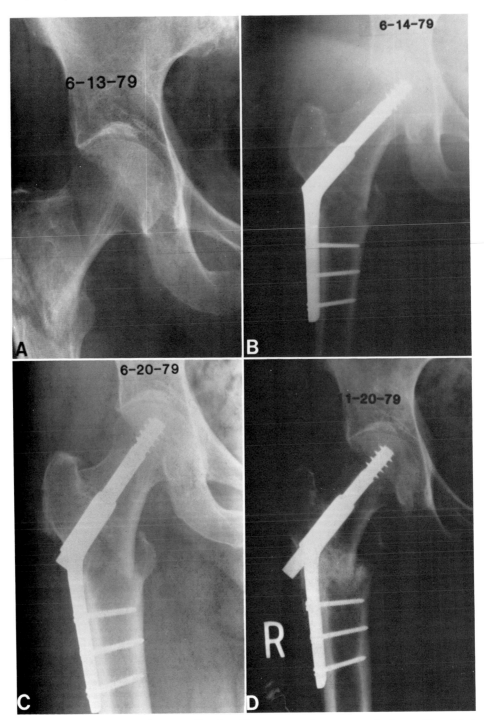

*Fig 23–4—Unstable fracture fixed with compression screw device without initial displacement and impaction. **A,** AP view of fracture prior to reduction. **B,** AP view after anatomical reduction and compression screw fixation. **C,** AP view showing spontaneous medial displacement of shaft and telescoping of compression screw device. **D,** AP view showing further spontaneous medial displacement of shaft and telescoping of compression screw device with fracture healing.*

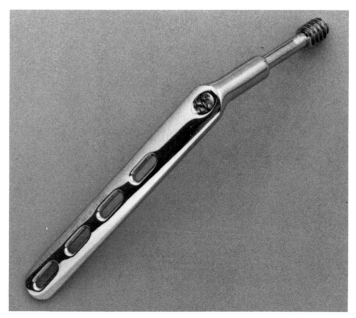

Fig 23–5—Compression screw device with slotted side plate.

better bony contact. More rapid healing is promoted, less stress is borne by the internal fixation device during the fracture healing period (which decreases device failure), and there is less shifting of the fracture after fixation. These factors result in a decreased incidence of fixation complications.

DISADVANTAGES OF THE MEDIAL DISPLACEMENT FIXATION TECHNIQUE

Technically, the procedure is more difficult than anatomical fixation until the surgeon becomes familiar with the procedure.

There may be some associated shortening of the extremity. (Shortening of up to 1 inch may occur, but this has not significantly interfered with the elderly patient's function after healing of the intertrochanteric fracture.) However, if a valgus neck shaft angle is achieved, then the shortening from telescoping at the fracture site is usually reduced.

A valgus configuration of the knee may be accentuated by the medial displacement of the shaft of the femur.

SURGICAL PROCEDURE

The patient is placed on the fracture table to allow use of the image intensifier or of standard anteroposterior and lateral roentgenography of the hip. The operating surgeon reduces the fracture by his or her preferred manipulative technique. During reduction, instability may be confirmed if the shaft shifts medially.

The hip is approached laterally by opening the tensor fascia. The vastus lateralis is split in its posterior third and elevated subperiosteally. The origin of the vastus lateralis below the greater trochanter may require division and elevation for exposure. The fracture site is then examined manually. Instability is confirmed by medial displacement of the shaft on pressure or by palpating comminution posteriorly and medially (to detect absence of cortical bone). The surgeon then decides whether or not to proceed with the medial displacement technique, taking into consideration the internal fixation devices available and his or her familiarity with the procedure.

If medial displacement is to be carried out, the procedure is as follows:

Step 1.*—Several drill holes are made in the lateral femoral cortex slightly above the level of the lesser trochanter. These drill holes are placed in the lateral femoral cortex so that an osteotomy may be made, to allow the greater trochanteric to be reflected superiorly and/or posteriorly. The drill holes are usually placed transversely, but if there is a spontaneous fracture into this area, their placement can be altered to facilitate the reflection of the greater trochanter.

Step 2.*—The osteotomy is completed with a wide osteotome or saw. The multiple drill holes are then connected by an osteotome or, preferably, an oscillating saw, to minimize the possibility of splitting the cortex and unnecessary loss of support bone (Fig 23–6,A).

Step 3.—The major greater trochanteric fragment is reflected proximally. The greater trochanteric fragment and cut portion of the femur are then reflected proximally or posteriorly to expose the head and neck fragment end on.

Step 4.—The surgeon visualizes the neck end-on and inserts the guide wire slightly inferiorly and posteriorly in the head and neck. If a dead-center position is obtained, it should be accepted. Because of the small cross-sectional area of the head and neck, it is difficult to pass a guide wire or fixation device in exactly the correct position. The intramedullary cancellous bone appears red and within the circle of cortical bone of the neck. Some cancellous bone may have to be removed with a curet or a rongeur to permit adequate visualization of the neck (Fig 23–6,B).

Step 5.—The capsule and other soft tissues are debrided from the spike of the proximal fragment. Debridement sometimes requires sharp dissection, as the fibers of the hip capsule may extend down the spike and there may be dense tendinous bands from the iliopsoas tendon. If the head and neck fragment is flexed, the spike may be buried in the anterior soft tissues. If so, the spike must be freed with an elevator or blunt instrument. If better control of the head and neck is necessary, a large Steinmann pin can be inserted into the head and neck junction, giving the operator a "handle" on the head and neck. However, this is usually not necessary.

Step 6.—Any bony fragments are removed from the femoral canal with a curet. The shaft fragment may have to be adducted and externally rotated to clean out the medullary canal.

Step 7.—The spike of the proximal fragment is impaled in the medullary canal of the shaft fragment. Traction may be required, and one may need to use a periosteal elevator as a lever to shift the spike of the proximal fragment into the medullary canal of the shaft. Occasionally the spike is of such length that it may impede impaction if the head and neck fragment shifts into a valgus position. In these cases, a portion of the spike should be removed with a rongeur.

Step 8.—Traction is released and the spike impacted in the shaft fragment. Traction must be released at the foot of the fracture table. This must be taken into account during initial positioning of the traction stirrup so that it can be easily performed by the assisting personnel. When the traction is released, the surgeon reaches through the drapes, grasps the knee, and manually impacts the fracture fragments.

---

*Steps 1 and 2 may not be necessary if a spontaneous fracture through the trochanter has already occurred.

Step 9.—The fixation device is inserted over the guide wire. A short screw or nail may be necessary, as determined by checking the guide wire insertion length (Fig 23–6,C).

Step 10.—Rotation is checked by noting the AP and lateral profiles of the head and neck. Leg rotation is adjusted as necessary. Fixation is to be avoided if there is excessive internal or external rotation. If on the AP fluoroscopy view one sees a long neck profile, one should assume the head and neck fracture is in neutral or some internal rotation. The kneecap should be palpated through the drapes and the rotation adjusted accordingly. (Care must be taken not to fix the fracture in internal rotation. External rotation is much better tolerated functionally than internal rotation.)

Step 11.—The yoke in the lateral cortex is cut with a rongeur. This allows vertical compression and takes advantage of the mechanics of the slotted side plate. A U-shaped hole is made in the lateral cortex of the distal shaft so that after application of the side plate, further vertical compression of the distal segment is possible; that is, the lateral cortex of the distal shaft is not blocked at the nail plate junction. This yoking of the lateral cortex can be done with a rongeur, or one can make multiple drill holes and then use a rongeur (Fig 23–6,D and E).

Step 12.—The angled slotted side plate is applied, usually at 135°–150°. A short barrel may be required. If the fracture fragments are in valgus, the surgeon may consider using a 150° angled side plate. If the fracture tends to set up in a coxa norma, then a 135° angled side plate should be used. If side plates of other angles are available, the one chosen should have an angle that yields good contact with the femoral shaft without the use of force.

Step 13.—The fracture site is again impacted, as described under step 8.

Step 14.—The plate is secured by inserting the screws. If a DCP plate is used, compression is achieved with screw insertion. If a slotted side plate is used (my preferred method), the screws should be inserted in the distal end of the slots, away from the fracture site. This placement will allow further vertical compression, as the unstable fracture may collapse a little more, even after initial impaction.

Step 15.—The final compression screw is inserted (only applicable when a compression screw device is utilized) (Figs 23–6,F and G). I recommend leaving the final compression screw in place in most cases to prevent disengagement of the hip screw and the barrel. Occasionally the final compression screw may loosen and fall in the soft tissues. This is a relatively minor complication when compared with disengagement of the hip screw and the barrel (Fig 23–7).

During a conventional hip nailing procedure, as the lateral cortex is reamed to accept the internal fixation device, or as the side plate is inserted, the femoral shaft may displace medially, confirming instability. If such displacement occurs, *the surgeon should not change this position of stability.* The fracture fragments should be nailed in situ, or the surgeon may proceed with a formal displacement impaction procedure.

PITFALLS AND THEIR PREVENTION

Compression not Obtained at Fracture Site.—Compression may not be obtained at the fracture site if a fragment of bone in the medullary canal prevents telescoping of the spike into the shaft. This complication may be prevented by clearing the medullary canal with a curet or hemostat before telescoping the fragments.

Compression may not be obtained at the fracture site because of soft tissue remaining attached to the spike of the proximal fragment. The soft tissues should be debrided from the spike with a periosteal elevator, scalpel, and rongeur.

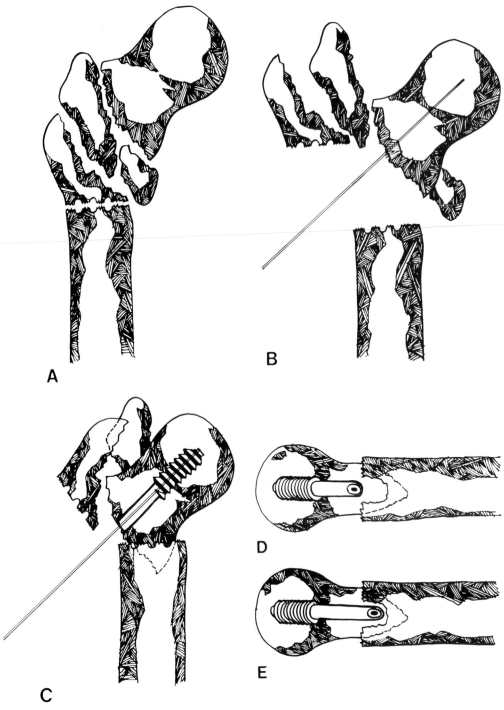

*Fig 23–6—Sequential steps in displacement osteotomy and impaction proce-
dure.* **A,** *osteotomy created through drill holes.* **B,** *placement of guide wire.* **C,**
*insertion of screw over guide wire after tapping and insertion of spike in femoral
shaft canal.* **D,** *yoking of lateral cortex below area of plate insertion over screw.*
E, *yoking allows further vertical impaction of shaft at plate-screw junction.*

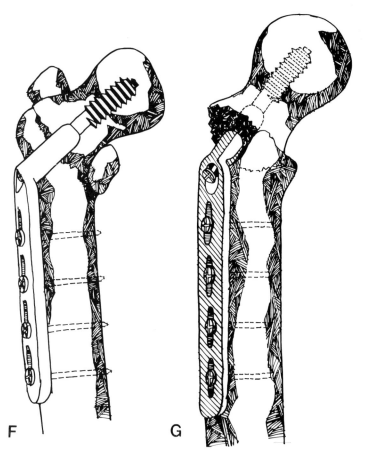

Fig 23–6—**F,** *final application of compression screw device after yoking and impaction of the fracture.* **G,** *compression screw device, lateral yoking, and slotted side plate allow further compression of fracture without fixation complications during the postoperative phase.*

INSUFFICIENT COMPRESSION AT FRACTURE SITE.—Compression at the fracture site may be insufficient due to blockage of the shaft's proximal (vertical) migration at the nail plate junction. Use of a slotted side plate with yoking of the lateral cortex may prevent this complication.

EXCESSIVE ROTATION.—The head-neck profile and the knee position must be compared before the side plate is secured to the femur. The surgeon should err on the side of external rotation when in doubt.

IMPROPER PLACEMENT OF DEVICE.—The screw or nail must be placed either dead center or slightly posteriorly and inferiorly. The tip of the nail or screw should be within 10 mm of subchondral bone. Guide wires should be reinserted until the desired position is definitely obtained.

POOR FIXATION OF THE PROXIMAL FRAGMENT.—This may be due to poor bone or multiple screw or nail insertions. The surgeon should accept only accurate positioning of the guide wires so that only one screw or nail placement is necessary. Methylmethacrylate may be used for supplemental fixation, if necessary.

GUIDE WIRE BACKS OUT AFTER REAMING.—The threaded tip of the guide wire is passed into acetabular subchondral bone. If the guide wire is nevertheless removed

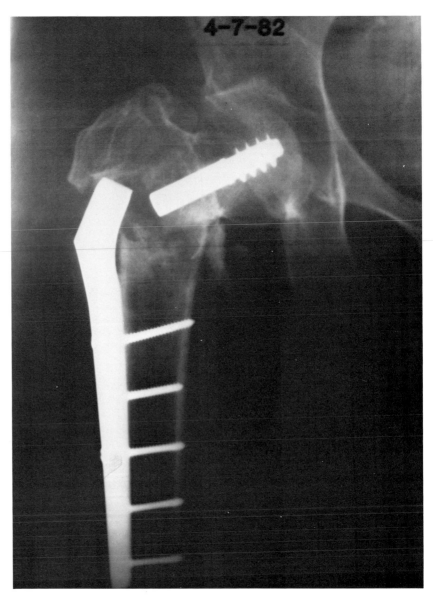

Fig 23–7—AP view showing disengagement of lag screw from barrel.

by the reamer, the barrel of the lag screw (reversed position) may be inserted into the head and neck as a guide for its exact replacement.

HEAD AND NECK SEGMENT SPINS WITH COMPRESSION SCREW INSERTION.—A Steinmann pin is inserted directly into the head at the head and neck junction to achieve temporary stability.

MANAGEMENT OF MAJOR COMPLICATIONS OCCURRING INTRAOPERATIVELY OR POSTOPERATIVELY

FRAGMENTATION OF THE HEAD AND NECK SEGMENT.—If fragmentation of the head and neck portion occurs or if osteopenic bone does not allow fixation, the head

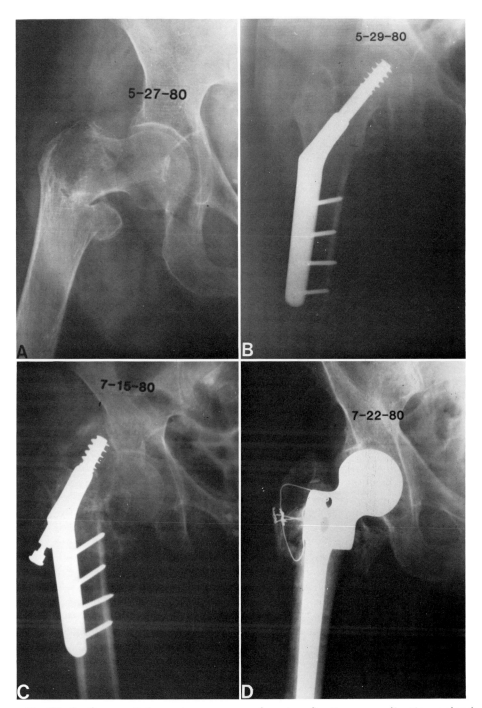

Fig 23–8—Sequential roentgenograms showing fixation complication solved by insertion of Leinbach prosthesis. **A,** AP view of unstable intertrochanteric fracture. **B,** AP view after insertion of compression screw device without initial displacement fixation. **C,** collapse of fracture into varus with screw cutting out of head and neck. **D,** Leinbach prosthesis inserted.

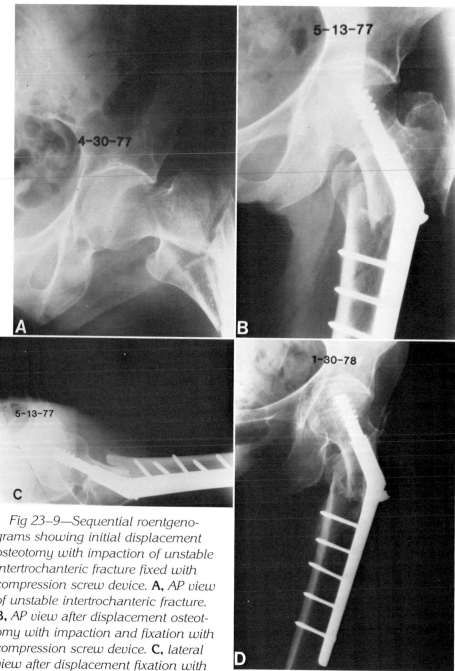

*Fig 23–9—Sequential roentgenograms showing initial displacement osteotomy with impaction of unstable intertrochanteric fracture fixed with compression screw device. **A,** AP view of unstable intertrochanteric fracture. **B,** AP view after displacement osteotomy with impaction and fixation with compression screw device. **C,** lateral view after displacement fixation with impaction and insertion of compression screw device. **D,** AP view showing healing of fracture.*

and neck portion may be replaced by a Leinbach, Averett, or other appropriate femoral prosthesis.

PENETRATION OF THE HEAD AND ACETABULUM.—If the nail or screw penetrates the head and acetabulum or cuts through the head and neck segment postoperatively, a Leinbach, Averett, or other appropriate femoral prosthesis (and matching polyethylene socket, if necessary) may be used (Fig 23–8).

NONUNION.—If nonunion develops with or without device failure, and if there remains good head and neck stock and a good hip joint, renailing with valgus fixation and bone grafting with a compression screw and slotted side plate as well as other osteotomy techniques should be considered.

COMMENT

Increasing attention has been given to the management of unstable intertrochanteric fractures over the past 20 years. It has been demonstrated that if internal fixation of this fracture is accomplished with a solid nail plate device, the complications of fixation will be markedly reduced by initial medial displacement fixation, whereas if a telescoping device such as a compression hip screw is used, fixation complications will be decreased *whether or not* initial medial displacement fixation is carried out.

When the surgeon is presented with an obviously unstable fracture, it is reasonable to seriously consider stabilizing the fracture initially by medial displacement and impaction with a sliding compression hip screw device and a slotted side plate. This approach provides the most favorable factors for fracture stability and healing, as well as maintaining the integrity of the metal fixation (Fig 23–9).

If one elects not to perform initial medial displacement fixation for unstable intertrochanteric fractures, it is my opinion that the fracture should be stabilized with a telescoping device such as a compression hip screw, to guide the fracture as it compresses medially and axially. A slotted side plate should be utilized with appropriate yoking of the lateral cortex to allow further compression and stabilization at the fracture site (Fig 23–10).

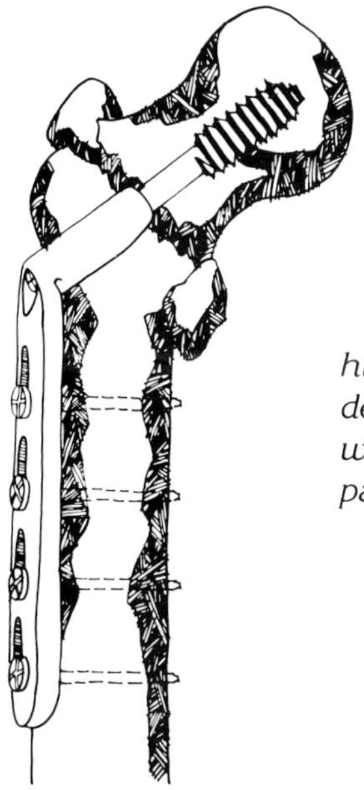

Fig 23–10—AP view of unstable hip fixed with compression screw device and slotted side plate, but without initial displacement and impaction.

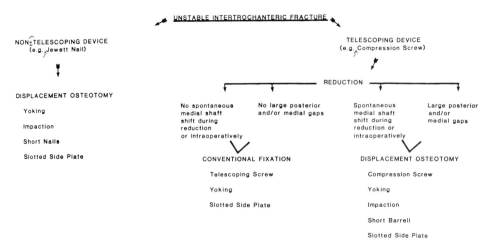

Fig 23–11—Author's current recommendations for management of the stable intertrochanteric fracture. A telescoping device is preferred.

Long-term application of thē principles described in this chapter should improve the results of operative treatment for unstable intertrochanteric fractures (Fig 23–11).

ACKNOWLEDGMENT

Drawings in this chapter are by Kathy and Achim Seifert.

BIBLIOGRAPHY

1. Aufranc O.E., Jones W.N., Turner R.H.: Severely comminuted intertrochanteric hip fracture. *JAMA* 199:140-143, 1967.
2. Bonamo J.J., Accettola A.B.: Treatment of intertrochanteric fractures with a sliding nail-plate. *J. Trauma* 22:205-215, 1982.
3. Bong S.C., Lau H.K., Leong J.C., et al.: The treatment of unstable intertrochanteric fractures of the hip: A prospective trial of 150 cases. *Injury* 13:139-146, 1981.
4. Cameron H.U., Graham J.D.: Retention of the compression screw in sliding screw plate devices. *Clin. Orthop.* 146:219-221, 1980.
5. Dimon J.H., Hughston J.C.: Unstable intertrochanteric fractures of the hip. *J. Bone Joint Surg.* 49:440-450, 1967.
6. Doherty J.H. Jr., Lyden J.D.: Intertrochanteric fractures the hip treated with the hip compression screw: Analysis of problems. *Clin. Orthop.* 141:184-187, 1979.
7. Doppelt S.H.: The sliding compression screw: Today's best answer for stabilization of intertrochanteric hip fractures. *Orthop. Clin. North Am.* 11:507-523, 1980.
8. Ecker M.L., Joyce J.J. III, Kohl E.J.: The treatment of intertrochanteric hip fractures using a compression screw. *J. Bone Joint Surg.* 57:23-27, 1975.
9. Friedenberg Z.B., Gentchos E., Rutt C.: Fixation in intertrochanteric fractures of the hip. *Surg. Gynecol. Obstet.* 132:225-228, 1972.
10. Green J.P.: Union of intertrochanteric osteotomies. *J. Bone Joint Surg.* 49:448-494, 1967.
11. Greider J.L. Jr., Horowitz M.: Clinical evaluation of the sliding compression screw in 121 hip fractures. *South. Med. J.* 73:1343-1348, 1980.
12. Hang Y.S., Lin G.D.: Sliding screw plate in the treatment of intertrochanteric fracture of the femur. *Taiwan I Hsueh Hui Tsa Chih* 79:405-415, 1979.
13. Harper M.C.: The treatment of unstable intertrochanteric fractures using a sliding screw-medial displacement technique. *J. Trauma* 22:792-796, 1982.

14. Harrington K.D.: The use of methylmethacrylate as an adjunct in the internal fixation of unstable comminuted intertrochanteric fractures in osteoporotic patients. *J. Bone Joint Surg.* 57:744-750, 1975.
15. Hessels G.J.: Unstable intertrochanteric fractures. *Acta Orthop.* 41:66-71, 1975.
16. Heyse-Moore G.H., MacEachern A.G., Evans D.C.: Treatment of intertrochanteric fractures of the femur: A comparison of the Richards screw-plate with the Jewett nail-plate. *J. Bone Joint Surg.* 65:262-267, 1983.
17. Holland W.R., Weiss A.B., Daniel W.W.: Medial displacement osteotomy for unstable intertrochanteric femoral fractures. *South. Med. J.* 70:576-578, 1977.
18. Hunter G.A., Krajbich I.J.: The results of medial displacement osteotomy for unstable intertrochanteric fractures of the femur. *Clin. Orthop.* 137:140-143, 1978.
19. Jacobs R.R., Armstrong H.J., Whitaker J.H., et al.: Treatment of intertrochanteric hip fractures using a compression hip screw and a nail plate. *J. Trauma* 16:599-603, 1976.
20. Jacobs R.R., McClain O., Armstrong H.J.: Internal fixation of intertrochanteric hip fractures: A clinical and biomechanical study. *Clin. Orthop.* 146:62-70, 1980.
21. Kyle R.F., Gustilo R.B., Premer R.F.: Analysis of six hundred and twenty-two intertrochanteric fractures. *J. Bone Joint Surg.* 61:216-221, 1979.
22. Laros G.S.: Intertrochanteric fractures: The role of complications of fixation. *Arch. Surg.* 110:37-40, 1975.
23. Laskin R.S., Gruber M.A., Zimmerman A.J.: Intertrochanteric fractures of the hip in the elderly: A retrospective analysis of 236 cases. *Clin. Orthop.* 141:188-195, 1979.
24. Morrison D., Mrstik L.L., Weingarden T.L.: Management of unstable intertrochanteric fractures of the hip. *J. Am. Osteopath. Assoc.* 10:793-802, 1977.
25. Naiman P.T., Schein A.J., Siffert R.S.: Medial displacement fixation for severely comminuted intertrochanteric fractures. *Clin. Orthop.* 62:151-155, 1969.
26. Rao J.P., Banzon M.T., Weiss A.B., et al.: Treatment of unstable intertrochanteric fractures with anatomic reduction and compression hip screw fixation. *Clin. Orthop.* 175:65-71, 1983.
27. Roberts A., Rooney T., Loupe J., et al.: A comparison of the functional results of anatomic and medial displacement valgus nailing of intertrochanteric fractures of the femur. *J. Trauma* 12:341-346, 1972.
28. Schatzker J., Ha'eri G.B., Chapman M.: Methylmethacrylate as an adjunct in the internal fixation of intertrochanteric fractures of the femur. *J. Trauma* 18:732-735, 1978.
29. Stern M.B., Goldstein T.B.: Primary treatment of comminuted intertrochanteric fractures of the hip with a Leinbach prosthesis. *Int. Orthop.* 3:67-70, 1979.
30. Stern M.B., Goldstein T.B.: The use of the Leinbach prosthesis in intertrochanteric fractures of the hip. *Clin. Orthop.* 128:325-331, 1977.
31. Wardle E.N.: The prevention of deformity in intertrochanteric fractures of the femur. *Postgrad. Med J.* 43:385-399, 1967.
32. Wilson H.S. Jr., Rubin B.D., Helbig F.E., et al.: Treatment of intertrochanteric fractures with the Jewett nail: Experience with 1,015 cases. *Clin. Orthop.* 148:186-191, 1980.
33. Wolfgang G.L., Bryant M.H., O'Neill J.P.: Treatment of intertrochanteric fracture of the femur using sliding screw plate fixation. *Clin. Orthop.* 163:148-158, 1982.

Chapter 24

Osteonecrosis of the Femoral Head Following Hip Fractures

Marvin H. Meyers, M.D.

Osteonecrosis of the femoral head is a common complication following intracapsular fracture of the femoral neck. It is the result of ischemia, presumably due to injury of the major arteries that supply the head of the femur. The incidence of osteonecrosis is highest after displaced subcapital fractures and decreases progressively at the fracture levels more distally. The lowest incidence is seen following fracture at the basal neck level. Osteonecrosis of the femoral head after intertrochanteric fractures is rare. In most reported series, there is a high incidence of nonunion, and some 30% of displaced intracapsular fractures that go on to osseous union will show late segmental collapse (Fig 24–1). This accounts for the term, "the unsolved fracture."[1] Only 10% of undisplaced intracapsular fractures progress to late segmental collapse. Frequently the femoral head in the ununited fracture is avascular but does not progress to late segmental collapse. I have not seen late segmental collapse of the femoral head in an ununited fracture.

Although the incidence of osteonecrosis appears to be high after displaced intracapsular fractures, most such fractures will unite following manipulation and firm internal fixation if anatomical reduction can be achieved. Whereas osteonecrosis is an early phenomenon, segmental collapse of the anterosuperior weight-bearing surface of the head is a late phenomenon. A prerequisite for segmental collapse is osseous union of the fracture.

The unacceptable high incidence of late segmental collapse has led many orthopedic surgeons to adopt a pessimistic attitude toward manipulation and internal fixation as the treatment of choice for subcapital and transcervical fractures. Consequently, they routinely treat these fractures in the elderly patient with replacement arthroplasty. There is disagreement concerning the cause, diagnosis, preventative treatment, and management of this troublesome complication.

PATHOPHYSIOLOGY

As illustrated in chapter 4, the major arteries supplying the femoral head are vulnerable to injury because of their location in the superoposterior aspect of the proximal portion of the femoral neck at the head and neck junction. This area is frequently incorporated in the fracture. The arteries may be torn at the time of displacement or may be crushed between the head and neck fragments as the head

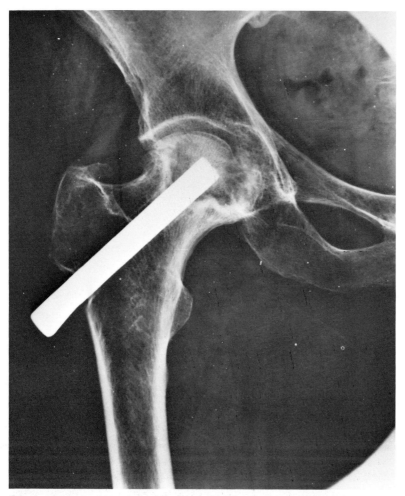

Fig 24–1—Late segmental collapse after healed subcapital fracture femoral neck 2 years following reduction and fixation with Smith-Peterson nail.

rotates posteriorly and inferiorly. The posterior aspect of the proximal neck is severely comminuted in 70% of displaced fractures, which places at risk the major vessels supplying the femoral head.[2] The lateral epiphyseal arteries are the main source of vascular supply to the femoral head and may be crushed at their entrance to the femoral head, accounting for the 10% incidence of late segmental collapse in undisplaced and impacted femoral neck fractures.

Other causes have been suggested for postfracture osteonecrosis of the femoral head. However, it is difficult to validate their contribution since there are no statistically significant studies available to support such claims. The criteria for determining osteonecrosis of the femoral head are variable and tests for verification are often difficult to perform.

Vigorous manipulation or multiple attempts to reduce displaced fractures may cause damage to the femoral head arteries that have survived the original injury.

Many orthopedic surgeons believe that early treatment of femoral neck fractures can reduce the incidence of osteonecrosis and late segmental collapse. In several reports, there was no difference between early surgery and late surgery with respect to avascular necrosis and late segmental collapse.[2,3] In my experience, delaying surgery for several days in order to evaluate the medical status of the patient and stabilize medical problems will not cause an increase in the incidence of osteonecrosis.

Hemarthrosis following fracture has been reported as a possible major cause of avascular necrosis due to tamponade of the retinacular vessels.[4] A recent report refutes the claim that significant hemarthrosis of the hip joint follows intracapsular fracture.[5] Intra-articular pressures were too low to cause tamponade of the retinacular vessels.

Garden concluded that malreduction was more important than ischemia in the production of late segmental collapse.[6] Although malreduction may increase the incidence of nonunion, it is more likely that ischemia is the underlying cause of late segmental collapse. Calandruccio and Anderson do not believe that anatomical reduction and fixation decreases the underlying incidence of avascular necrosis.[7] However, they stated that fixation of the fracture with malreduction of the head may increase the incidence of avascular necrosis.

It has been suggested that internal fixation may damage intraosseous vessels, thereby causing avascular necrosis and segmental collapse in intertrochanteric fractures (see Fig 4–4)[8] and in intracapsular fractures (Fig 24–2).[9] The evidence for this effect is circumstantial.

There is general agreement that osteonecrosis occurs in a high percentage of displaced subcapital and transcervical fractures of the femoral neck, that revascularization may be complete or incomplete, and that late segmental collapse occurs in a high percentage of cases in which the entire head has not been revascularized.

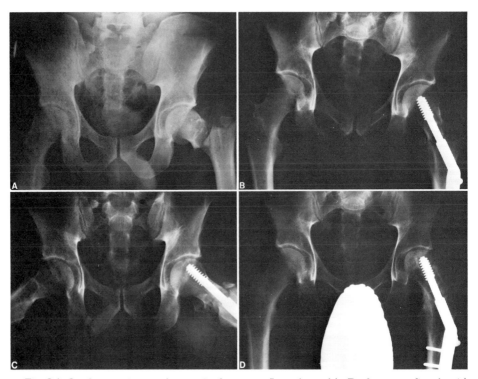

*Fig 24–2—***A,** *cervicotrochanteric fracture (basal neck).* **B,** *fracture fixed with sliding compression nail.* **C,** *lateral x-ray view after surgery.* Note *nail close to entry point of lateral epiphyseal vessels.* **D,** *x-ray film 2 years after injury showing late segmental collapse of the head.*

PATHOGENESIS

The pathology and pathogenesis of osteonecrosis of the femoral head following intracapsular fracture of the hip have been described by Coleman and Compere[10] and Catto.[11] The following is a summation of their reports.

Normally there is a patchy absence of osteocytes in trabecular bone and of chondrocytes in articular cartilage, especially in the deeper cartilaginous layers of

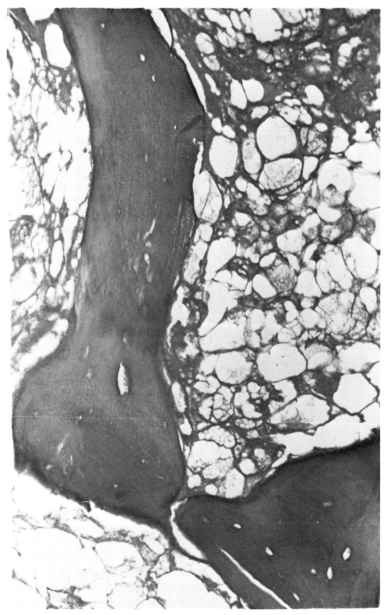

Fig 24–3—Histologic section showing osteonecrosis of the femoral head. Trabeculae are devoid of osteocytes. The marrow shows loss of hematopoietic cells and coalescence of fat. (From Meyers. M. H.: Proceedings of the Hip Society, 1983. Reproduced by permission.)

the femoral head. The fate of the head is apparently determined at the time of the fracture.

In the first 5 days, there is fibrin deposition, edema, and organizing hemorrhage at the fracture site. There are multiple fragments of viable and necrotic bone on the fracture surfaces. Ischemia is evidenced by the decreased number of lacunar osteocytes and the progressive eosinophilic appearance of the marrow.

From day 5 to day 14, devascularized bone marrow shows an increased loss of trabecular osteocytes, absence of hematopoietic elements, loss of lipocytes, necrosis of blood vessels, and coalescence of fat cells (Fig 24–3). New bone formation

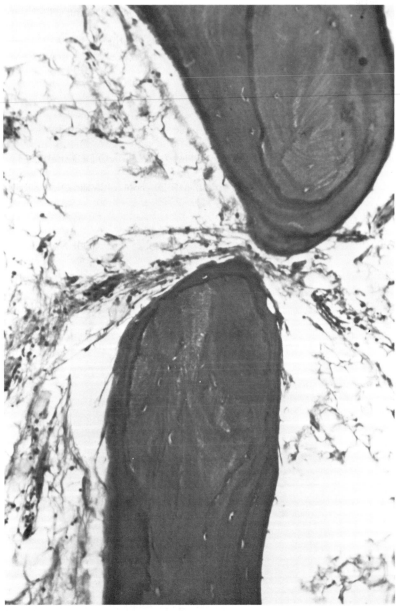

Fig 24–4—Note some trabecular areas with empty lacunae surrounded by new bone. The marrow is fatty, fibrous, and lacks hematopoietic elements. (From Meyers M. H.: Proceedings of the Hip Society, 1983. Reproduced by permission.)

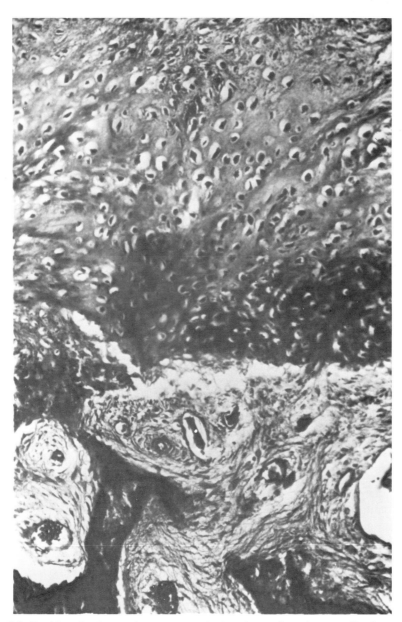

Fig 24–5—Histologic section at granulation front showing cartilaginous zone with increased number of bone vessels just below. (From Meyers M. H.: Proceedings of the Hip Society, 1983. Reproduced by permission.)

may be seen at the fracture site. The new bone is invariably on the distal fracture surface. When new bone formation is present on the proximal fracture surface, the head fragment is probably viable.

A conclusion cannot be reached concerning viability of the femoral head based on histologic evidence until approximately 14 days after the necrosis. There usually is invasion of the bone by vascular connective tissue at the fracture surface and fibrosis with new bone formation on the distal fracture site. The marrow and trabecular elements are acellular.

From 1 to 6 months, there is evidence of "creeping substitution"[12] (replacement of dead trabeculae) and creeping apposition" (Fig 24–4) (surrounding of dead trabeculae by new bone).[13] Revascularization of the necrotic femoral head segment is a slow process. Some believe it is a limited process and that as the granulation front proceeds proximally the combination of loading forces, absorption of osteonecrotic trabeculae, and fatigue fractures of weakened trabeculae stimulate a fibrocartilaginous zone which stops the progression of revascularization and reossification (Fig 24–5).[7]

Late segmental collapse of the load-bearing portion of the femoral head (anterosuperior surface) represents a complication of osteonecrosis.

Chondrocyte loss indicative of cartilage necrosis is seen a few weeks following fracture. The loss may be minimal or extensive and is dependent on the biochemical impairment caused by diminution of physical stress, as well as a decrease in diffusion of solutes from the synovial fluid. Joint motion promotes diffusion.[14] A humoral factor may play a limited role in chondrocyte degeneration since subchondral vessels are thought to supply some nourishment to articular cartilage,[15] and this source would be cut off in an avascular head.

DIAGNOSIS

Routine evaluation by roentgenograms may not be helpful in the first few months following fracture. Although the head fragment may be avascular, the x-ray films may reveal no change in x-ray density. However, if the patient is relatively inactive, there will be disuse atrophy of the viable distal femoral neck and metaphyseal bone, which will cause demineralization, resulting in a relative increase in the radiographic density of the head fragment, since the real osseous density in the avascular head in unchanged (Fig 24–6). This change in density may be visible in the first 4–6 weeks. Improvement in rehabilitation methods and early weight-bearing can minimize disuse atrophy. Consequently, the density in the distal vascularized bone may not change or the early relative increase in density may be transient. After osseous union of the fracture and revascularization of a dead head, a real (absolute) increase in the density of the femoral head due to creeping apposition (new bone surrounding dead trabeculae) can take place (see Fig 24–4). The femoral head may now be considered viable. Patchy areas of increased density or the appearance of an infarct are characteristic of incomplete revascularization (see Fig 24–1). In most cases this stage is followed within 2–3 years by segmental collapse of the anterosuperior weight-bearing segment of the femoral head.

Bone scans may provide supportive or diagnostic evidence of viability. Technetium 99m methyl diphosphonate and technetium 99m sulfur colloid are the radioisotopes used most often for demonstrating viability (Fig 24–7). The former is taken up in the mineralization process and the latter is phagocytized by the retinaculoendothelial cells of the marrow.

CAN OSTEONECROSIS AND LATE SEGMENTAL COLLAPSE BE PREVENTED?

In my opinion, osteonecrosis of the femoral head is primarily due to extensive damage to the vascular supply of the femoral head at the time of the fracture. There is no significant evidence that other factors, including early open reduction and rigid internal fixation, manipulation, or anatomical reduction, will reduce the incidence of or prevent osteonecrosis.

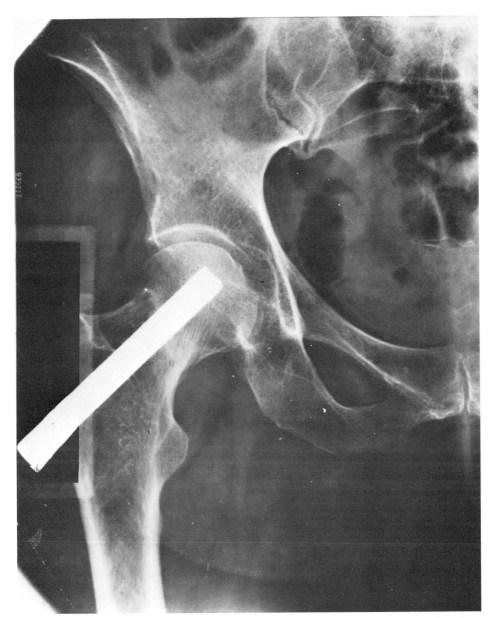

Fig 24–6—Six-week-old subcapital fracture with early evidence of union. The femoral head appears denser than the metaphysis, consistent with ischemia of the head fragment.

Sevitt reported that 85% of the femoral heads in fresh displaced intracapsular fractures studied by arteriographic and histologic techniques demonstrated total or subtotal osteonecrosis.[16]

Segmental collapse is a late phenomenon that occurs within 2 years of the fracture in most cases. Late segmental collapse is uncommon after 3 years and does require union of the fracture. If osteonecrosis is recognized early, various surgical measures have been suggested to prevent collapse. These are discussed in the following section.

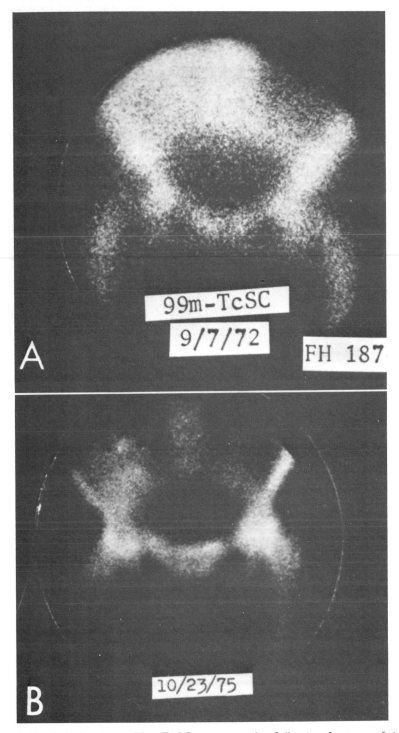

Fig 24–7—**A,** technetium 99m TcSC scan one day following fracture of right hip showing minimal activity with good uptake on the left (uninjured) side. **B,** technetium 99m MDP scan of pelvis. Bilateral avascular necrosis with marked uptake in both hips.

TREATMENT

Osteonecrosis of the femoral head in a united intracapsular fracture is not symptomatic. Some fractures will be completely revascularized and the femoral head will once again be viable, while others will not, or will become revascularized only in part.

The combination of a nonviable head and a united intracapsular fracture is not necessarily an unacceptable situation as long as late segmental collapse does not follow. Late segmental collapse is most often symptomatic. Occasionally elderly patients that develop late segmental collapse following an intracapsular fracture will function with minimal or no pain. They may require crutches or a cane to unload the hip. The more active patient, however, can be expected to become symptomatic. Pain will be the determining factor insofar as surgical correction is concerned.

The surgical options for the painful hip due to late segmental collapse are osteotomy, hemiarthroplasty, and total hip replacement. I prefer the bipolar endoprosthesis as the treatment of choice unless there are severe degenerative changes in the acetabulum. In that case, I prefer total hip replacement. Sugioka et al. in 1982 reported good results following a transtrochanteric osteotomy in 77% of cases, with a 2- to 9-year follow-up.[17] I have found this to be a satisfactory alternative operation in young patients, providing that no more than one third of the femoral head has collapsed. I have had no success with this operation when more than one third of the articular surface has collapsed.

Prior to segmental collapse, if the roentgenogram shows subtle mottled densities or a well-demarcated area of infarction in the anterosuperior stress-bearing

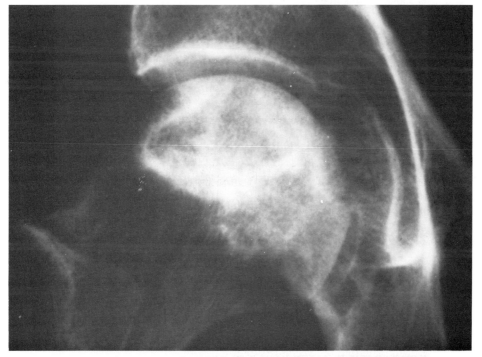

Fig 24–8—Osteonecrosis of the femoral head (stage II). (From Meyers M. H.: Instructional Courses of the American Academy of Orthopaedic Surgery. Reproduced by permission.)

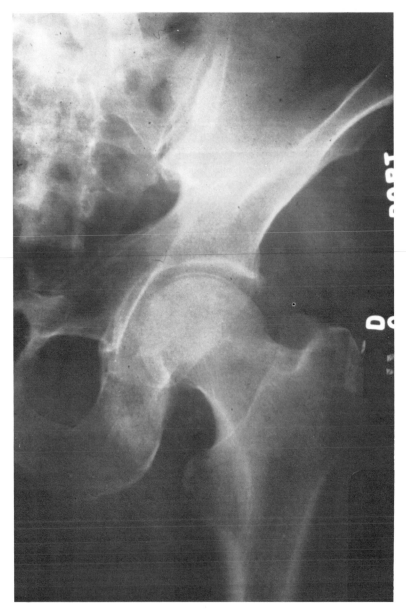

Fig 24–9—Osteonecrosis of the femoral head (stage III). Note the radiolucent crescent sign. (From Meyers M. H.: Instructional Courses of the American Academy of Orthopaedic Surgery. Reproduced by permission.)

portion of the femoral head (stage I or II of Marcus et al.[18]) the treatment options are core biopsy or multiple drilling of the head and neck of the femur (Fig 24–8).[19] There is reasonable evidence that these surgical procedures can prevent segmental collapse. However, there is little chance of success when there is a radiolucent crescent sign (stage III; Fig 24–9) or segmental collapse (stage IV). The posterior quadratus femoris pedicle graft is my preferred treatment in the vigorous patient under 50 years of age with one third or more of the femoral head involved.[20] However, the pedicle graft is usually unsuccessful in stages III and IV.

REFERENCES

1. McCarroll H.R.: Has a solution for the "unsolved fracture" been found? Problems and complications of fractures of the femoral neck. *JAMA* 153:536, 1953.
2. Meyers M.H., Harvey J.P., Moore T.M.: Treatment of displaced subcapital and transcervical fractures of the femoral neck by muscle-pedicle bone bone graft and internal fixation. *J. Bone Joint Surg.* 55A:257-274, 1973.
3. Kenzora J.E., McCarthy R.E., Lowell J.D., et al.: Hip fracture mortality: Relation to age, treatment; preoperative illness, time of surgery and complications. *Clin. Orthop.* 186:45, 1984.
4. Soto-Hall R., Johnson L.H., Johnson R.: Alterations in the intra-articular pressures in transcervical fractures of the hip. *J. Bone Joint Surg.* 46A:662, 1963.
5. Drake J.K., Meyers M.H.: Intracapsular pressure and hemarthrosis following femoral neck fractures. *Clin. Orthop.* 182:172-176, 1984.
6. Garden R.S.: Malreduction and avascular necrosis in subcapital fractures of the femur. *J. Bone Joint Surg.* 53B:183-196, 1971.
7. Calandruccio R.A., Anderson W.E.: Post-fracture avascular necrosis of the femoral head. *Clin. Orthop.* 152:49-84, 1980.
8. Rodetti B.A.: The blood supply of the femoral neck and head in relation to the damaging effects of nails and screws. *J. Bone Joint Surg.* 42:794, 1960.
9. Linton P.: On the different types of intracapsular fracture of the femoral neck. *Acta Chir. Scand. Suppl.* 86, 1900.
10. Coleman S.S., Compere C.C.: Femoral neck fractures: Pathogenesis of avascular necrosis, non-union, and late degenerative changes. *Clin. Orthop.* 20:247, 1900.
11. Catto M.: A histological study of avascular necrosis of the femoral head after transcervical fracture. *J. Bone Joint Surg.* 47B:749, 1965.
12. Phemister D.B.: Bone growth and repair. *Ann. Surg.* 102:261, 1900.
13. Bobenchko W.P., Harris W.R.: The radiographic density of avascular bone. *J. Bone Joint Surg.* 42B:626, 1960.
14. Maroudes A., Bullough P., Swanson S.A.V., et al., Permeability of articular cartilage. *J. Bone Joint Surg.* 50B:166-177, 1968.
15. McKibben B., Maroudas A.: Nutrition and metabolism, in Freeman M.A.R. (ed.): *Adult Articular Cartilage,* ed. 2. New York, Pitman Medical Publishing Co., 1979, p. 461.
16. Sevitt S.: Avascular necrosis and revascularization of the femoral head after intracapsular fractures. *J. Bone Joint Surg.* 46B:270-296, 1964.
17. Sugioka Y., Katsuki I., Hotokebuchi T.: Transtrochanteric rotational osteotomy of the femoral head for the treatment of osteonecrosis. *Clin. Orthop.* 169:115-126, 1982.
18. Marcus H.D., Enneking W.F., Massam R.A.: The silent hip in idiopathic aseptic necrosis. *J. Bone Joint Surg.* 55A:1351, 1973.
19. Ficat P.R., Arlet J.: *Ischaemia and Necrosis of Bone,* edited and adapted by David S. Hungerford. Baltimore, Williams & Wilkins Co., 1979.
20. Meyers M.H.: The treatment of osteonecrosis of the hip with fresh ostochrondral allografts and with the muscle pedicle graft technique. *Clin. Orthop.* 130:202, 1978.

Chapter 25

Pulmonary Embolism and Deep Vein Thrombosis in Patients With Hip Fractures

Lorraine Day, M.D.

It has been widely accepted that the incidence of pulmonary embolism is high after hip fracture and hip surgery. Patients with hip fracture are subjected to a period of bed rest as well as operation—both of which have been shown to increase the likelihood of thromboembolic complications. The apparent magnitude of the problem was brought to widespread attention, particularly among orthopedic surgeons, with the publication of Sevitt's and Gallagher's paper in *Lancet* in 1959.[1] These authors concluded that it was necessary to treat a wide range of patients prophylactically because pulmonary embolism (PE) was found in about 20% of autopsies at the Birmingham Accident Hospital and was "the cause of death in 40 to 50% of elderly patients who died after fracture of the femure, tibia, or pelvis." In 1966 Saltzman and Harris stated that PE "is the leading cause of death after fracture of the hip."[2] Fitts et al. in 1964 reported that 38% of patients dying after a fracture of the hip were found to have died of PE.[3] Since that time much research has been directed toward defining an effective regimen to prevent deep vein thrombosis (DVT) and PE.

Because agents used for prophylaxis and treatment of PE frequently pose substantial risks to the patient, it is important to answer the following questions: How accurate are the reported figures on the incidence of PE? What are the criteria used for the diagnosis? What is the mortality from untreated PE? What are the complications of prophylaxis or treatment?

INCIDENCE

The incidence of PE in autopsy reports shows an amazing variance from 6% to 64%.[4] When evaluating these statistics it is difficult to ascertain just how often PE was the sole cause of death or even a major contributor to death. Autopsy studies show what patients die *with*, not necessarily what they die *of*. Many patients remain in a terminal state for hours or even days before they die, and the terminal state itself is known to predispose to PE. Because PE is associated with advanced age and is a complication of many potentially fatal diseases, especially heart disease, it commonly is an incidental feature of the terminal state.

Autopsy studies have shown a much higher incidence of PE than is recognized clinically before death.[1,3,4] Therefore it has been assumed that PE is vastly underdiagnosed. A critical look at the literature, however, does not support this contention. Postmortem studies are based on a group that is disproportionately populated by the chronically ill, those with a high prevalence of heart failure, and those who are malnourished and chronically bedridden. But even in elderly debilitated patients, the incidence of PE may not be as high as previously claimed. For example, Moser et al. studied patients admitted to a respiratory intensive care unit for treatment of acute respiratory failure.[5] Such patients often have multiple risk factors for DVT and PE, including venous stasis caused by immobility, right ventricular failure, positive pressure ventilation, dehydration, and advanced age. Of 23 patients studied by radiofibrinogen leg scans, there were three (13%) who had abnormal scans in the first week. All scans performed after the first week in the other 20 patients remained normal. PE was present at autopsy in 20%, but in none of the patients was PE the principal, or even a contributory, cause of death.

Establishing an accurate incidence of death from PE is imperative in order (1) to decide the risks warranted for prophylaxis of PE and (2) to document any decrease in mortality from PE resulting from prophylaxis. One major problem in trying to determine the incidence of PE by reading reports on this subject is that the term thromboembolism is frequently used to refer to both PE and DVT. Although PE and DVT are related (just how is not totally clear), they have major differences in morbidity and mortality.

Leg vein thrombosis without PE is usually of minor consequence, although it can increase the length of hospitalization and frequently requires treatment. Its major significance, however, is as an antecedent of PE. As mentioned, most studies on this subject combine the figures for DVT and PE, incorrectly suggesting a direct relationship or a serious clinical problem in every case. DVT isolated to the calf is much more common and more benign than thrombosis that also involves the thigh. Browse showed that only 18% of patients with isotopically detected calf vein thrombosis went on to develop abnormalities on lung scan.[6] On the other hand, over 50% of patients with venous thrombosis above the knee have been found to have scintigraphic evidence compatible with PE.[7] However, not all of these are symptomatic.

One reason commonly proposed for the prevention and/or treatment of calf vein thrombosis is the likelihood that the thrombus will extend proximally from the veins of the calf to those of the thigh. But whether proximal extension occurs with any frequency has been challenged by two groups[7,8] who believe that propagation is uncommon and that only small (clinically insignificant) emboli come from distal sites. Kakkar et al. found that about 15% of thrombi initially limited to the calf ultimately extend to the thigh veins.[9]

Detection of DVT, however, is only an intermediate step, and although it has been assumed to be true, there is no proof that decreasing the incidence of DVT necessarily decreases the number of deaths from PE. In fact, studies that have used the diagnosis of DVT as the principal end point have reported a remarkably low incidence of PE.[10,11] There is really no scientific justification for continuing to highlight DVT to the extent that has been done in the recent past. Instead, a decrease in the incidence of PE, not just a decrease in the incidence of DVT, is the standard by which therapeutic regimens must be judged.

Though Fitts et al. in 1964 reported a 38% mortality from PE in patients with fracture of the hip,[3] this estimate was revised downward by Salzman and Harris,[12] who in 1976 reported that 4%–10% of patients with hip fractures who received no prophylaxis died of PE. Having studied this problem at the San Francisco General Hospital,[13] we concluded that the incidence was even lower. We analyzed the course of 565 consecutive patients with hip fracture admitted between 1971 and 1977, many of whom had multiple additional injuries. Standard treatment for hip fracture during this period was early internal fixation (usually within 1–7 days of injury) and mobilization the day after surgery. No drug or mechanical prophylaxis for thromboembolic disease was given to any patient. Patients with a prior history of PE or DVT were not treated in any special way except that a greater effort might have been made to mobilize them on the first postoperative day. No patients with hip fracture were excluded from the study.

In our study, the in-hospital mortality from all causes was 6.2% (35 of 565 patients). Of these 35 patients, 90% underwent autopsy. In five cases patients were found to have died of PE, an incidence of less than 1%. Among these five patients were three over the age of 80 (two with severe chronic brain syndrome), and one with long-standing, severe multiple sclerosis. In two additional patients, PE was initially recorded as the cause of death, but autopsies revealed that the death of both was caused by aspiration. Therefore, in three of these five patients, PE could realistically be viewed as the final event of a terminal disease.

This incidence of PE confirmed by autopsy in a typical county hospital population is substantially lower than that reported in other studies in which the diagnosis frequently was made on clinical grounds. If indeed the incidence is this low, regimens for prophylaxis not only must be effective but also must be almost risk-free in order to justify their use.

DIAGNOSIS

Is PE underdiagnosed? There is still a widespread belief that clinical assessment and routine laboratory tests are sufficient to make a correct diagnosis of PE. But there is strong evidence now that if we rely solely on such information, PE will be overdiagnosed and overtreated. For example, the Urokinase-Streptokinase Pulmonary Embolism Study reported findings in 906 patients with the presumptive diagnosis of PE who underwent pulmonary angiography.[14] Only 152 of 906 angiograms (about 20%) confirmed the presence of an embolus. Menzoian and Williams[15] reported that angiograms showed emboli in only 70 of 158 patients suspected of having PE. Therefore, on the basis of firm clinical impressions in patients with a high probability of having PE, angiography confirms the diagnosis in only 20%–50% of cases. If treatment were to be given without angiographic proof of PE, as many as 50%–80% of patients would be unnecessarily subjected to the hazards of anticoagulation.

ACCURACY OF DIAGNOSIS

If a patient is treated without adequate diagnostic evidence of PE, he will not only incur the risks of anticoagulation during the initial hospitalization, but, because of the threat of recurrent disease, he will be subjected to similar risks with every subsequent operation or hospitalization. The use of heparin in surgical practice is especially hazardous, particularly for orthopedic patients, who may have large areas of bleeding bone from fractures or operation. Thus, PE must be diagnosed with the most reliable methods available. This section reviews the accuracy of several methods of diagnosis.

Clinical Signs and Symptoms

The clinical signs and symptoms of PE are suggestive but nonspecific. The traditional symptoms of hemoptysis and pleuritic pain, which are characteristic of pulmonary infarction, are inadequate to diagnose acute PE. In many cases the clinical presentation suggests congestive heart failure, pneumonia, or, less commonly, myocardial infarction. More than half of patients with PE[16] experience chest pain (pleuritic 74%, nonpleuritic 15%), dyspnea, apprehension, and cough.[16] One study noted that chest pain often was present for 3–4 days before the diagnosis was made.[17] Hemoptysis occurred in only 28% of patients. Dyspnea, hemoptysis, or pleuritic pain occurred separately or in combination in 94% of patients, but all three symptoms were present in only 22%. Signs of DVT were present in 41%, and a pleural friction rub was present in only 18%. Many of these findings are present in a wide variety of other diseases, including congestive heart failure, pneumonia, chronic lung disease, and myocardial infarction. This nonspecificity of the clinical syndrome explains why diagnosis may be confusing. However, a history and physical examination are invaluable as the first step in the detection of this disease. In the absence of shortness of breath, chest pain, and tachypnea, PE is unlikely.

Electrocardiogram

While the ECG may be abnormal in pulmonary embolism, it is difficult to distinguish between abnormalities due to preexisting cardiac or pulmonary disease and those related to PE. In approximately 80% of patients, the ECG is of no specific value.[17] However, it is abnormal in about 85% of cases of massive PE and in 75% of cases of submassive PE, the most frequent abnormalities being elevation or depression of the ST segment or changes in the T wave. Minor changes of the ST segment or T wave have significance only if they are new findings. In some patients ECG changes may be the first evidence of PE.

Chest X-Ray

The most common abnormalities on the plain chest film are pleural effusion and pulmonary infiltrate, each of which occurs in slightly more than half of patients with acute PE. The significance of these changes may not be obvious, however, because some patients are also known or thought to have cardiac or pulmonary disease.[18] Abnormalities are seen more commonly in the lower lobes (51%) but are wedge-shaped in only a minority of cases.[17] At least two of the following—pleural effusion, infiltrate, atelectasis, or an elevated hemidiaphragm—have been found in nearly half of patients with acute PE. However, a normal chest x-ray film in a severely dyspneic patient strongly suggests PE.[16]

Arterial Oxygen Tension

A normal PO_2 (on room air) is rare in the presence of recent PE.[19] Arterial blood gases are readily determined, but it is important to remember that there are many causes for arterial hypoxemia, including pneumonia, oversedation, mucous plugs, and aspiration. Menzoian and Williams[15] showed that the mean partial pressure of oxygen in patients with a positive pulmonary angiogram was 64 mm Hg, and the mean partial pressure of carbon dioxide (PCO_2) was 30 mm Hg. In patients suspected of having PE but whose pulmonary angiograms were normal, the results were nearly

TABLE 25–1.—Arterial Oxygen Tension*		
	Po$_2$ (mm Hg)	Pco$_2$ (mm Hg)
Positive pulmonary angiogram	64	30
Negative pulmonary angiogram	63	34

*Adapted from Menzoian and Williams.[15]

identical: the mean Po$_2$ was 63 mm Hg and the mean Pco$_2$ was 34 mm Hg (Table 25–1). Even though most patients with positive angiograms had Po$_2$ values between 50 and 80 mm Hg, some had values as high as 100 mm Hg. Of the 69 patients with a Po$_2$ of 65 mm Hg or less, only 41% had positive pulmonary angiograms. Therefore, blood gas measurements are highly sensitive but nonspecific: they are useful in the management of patients who have PE but are not as helpful in the diagnosis.

Laboratory Tests

Laboratory tests are of little value in the diagnosis of PE. Early reports suggested that LDH, SGOT, and bilirubin determinations could help confirm the diagnosis,[14] but these have not proved useful. In one large series of patients with angiographically documented PE,[14] only 4% had the "diagnostic triad" of elevated LDH and serum bilirubin levels and a normal SGOT level. In addition, 50% of patients had normal LDH levels throughout their illness.

Perfusion Lung Scans

Perfusion scanning of the lung is a safe, simple, and sensitive method of defining the status of pulmonary blood flow. Blood flow is determined by imaging the movement of radioactively tagged particles (technetium 99m) as their passage is retarded in precapillary arterioles and capillaries of the lung after injection into a peripheral vein. In the diagnosis of PE, perfusion scans are highly sensitive but lack specificity, because anything that alters blood flow will give rise to an abnormal scan. Among the more common nonembolic causes of perfusion defects are cardiopulmonary disease, in particular congestive heart failure, and chronic obstructive pulmonary disease.[20] Pneumonia or atelectasis unrelated to PE also can produce perfusion abnormalities.[21] Chest x-ray films are often helpful in explaining these scan defects by revealing the intrapulmonary pathology.

On the other hand, a normal scan virtually rules out a diagnosis of PE (Fig 25–1).[22] Positive scans (suggesting PE) are correct in only 66% of patients, resulting in a false positive rate of 33%.[15]

Ventilation-Perfusion Lung Scans

Ventilation scanning involves the use of radiolabeled xenon gas to examine the ventilatory compartments of the lung and should be performed immediately after a *positive* perfusion study. Patients with a negative perfusion scan are unlikely to have PE, and a ventilation scan would not contribute useful information. During the test, the patient takes a single deep breath of a mixture of oxygen and ^{133}Xe, and the activity of the ^{99m}Tc (from the perfusion study) and the ^{133}Xe can be selectively recorded by a scintillation camera. If there is scintigraphic evidence of normal ven-

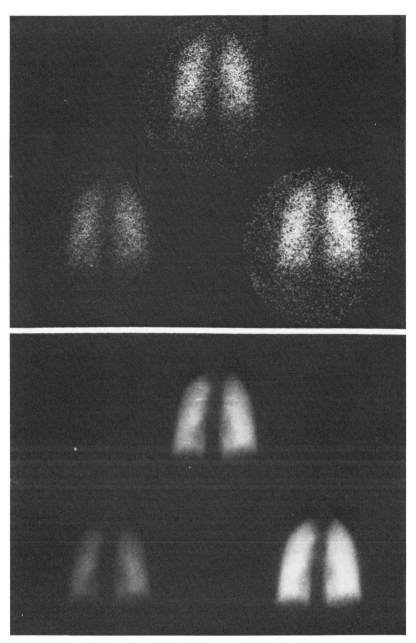

Fig 25–1—Normal ventilation-perfusion scan.

tilation in an area where a defect is demonstrable on perfusion scan, the tests are said to show a ventilation-perfusion mismatch. Diminished perfusion due to PE is associated with minimal and transient regional hypoventilation, so ventilation-perfusion mismatches are highly diagnostic of PE. Thus, in the presence of a pulmonary embolus, a defect will be visible on a perfusion scan but not on ventilation scan.

Ventilation-perfusion lung scanning has been shown to be more accurate than perfusion lung scanning alone.[23] But information is now accumulating suggesting that ventilation-perfusion lung scanning techniques are not as conclusive as was once believed.[15, 23] The highest probability estimate of PE that could be made in over 100 patients with suspected PE by perfusion scan alone was 80%. When a ventilation study was added, the probability increased to nearly 100% for patients with multiple large perfusion defects and normal ventilation. But for smaller defects with normal ventilation, the probability of PE was only 50%. If perfusion defects corresponded to known radiographic abnormalities, the probability of pulmonary embolism was only 25%.[24] Thus, scanning has been helpful in improving the accuracy of the diagnosis of PE, but it still is not as precise as pulmonary angiography. A negative scan essentially rules out PE. A major defect on a perfusion scan with a

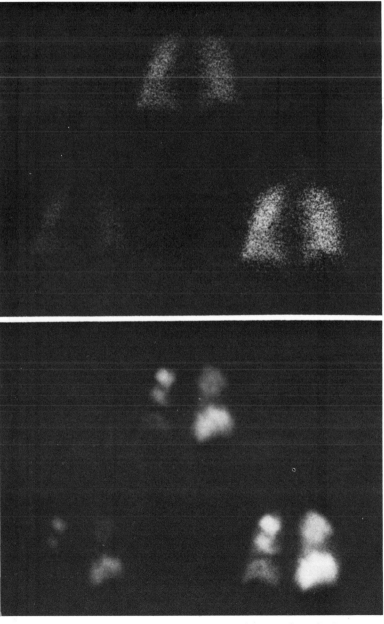

Fig 25–2—Normal ventilation scan with abnormal perfusion scan.

normal ventilation scan is virtually diagnostic of PE (Fig 25–2). But many other patients with lesser defects cannot be reliably diagnosed without angiography.

Pulmonary Angiography

Pulmonary angiography is the most precise and specific test available for the diagnosis of PE and is the standard by which all other tests must be measured (Figs 25–3 and 25–4). How accurate is this technique? As with scans, there may be observer variability and inaccuracy, but disagreement among a panel of three experts on angiograms was less than 6% in a recent study, compared with a 67% disagreement in interpretation of scan data.[17]

Since optimal selective magnification techniques allow opacification of vessels as small as 0.15 mm in diameter,[25,26] emboli of clinical importance should not be missed. This is supported by the results of postmortem examinations performed shortly after pulmonary angiography, which showed the angiographic examinations to be 100% correct.[27]

Novelline et al.[28] reported on 167 patients with normal pulmonary angiograms who were not treated and were followed for at least 6 months afterward. Not one patient died as a result of thromboembolic disease during the acute illness (20 died from unrelated causes), and none of the 147 patients that survived experienced "recurrent embolism" during follow-up. Studies comparing ventilation-perfusion

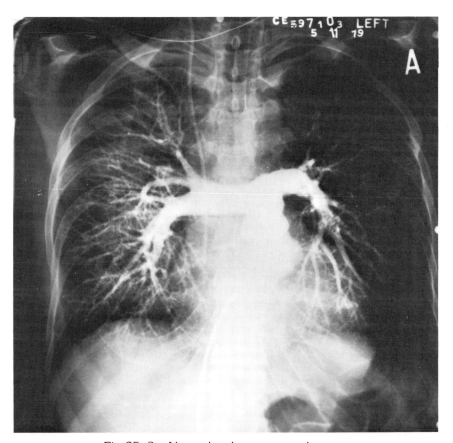

Fig 25–3—Normal pulmonary angiogram.

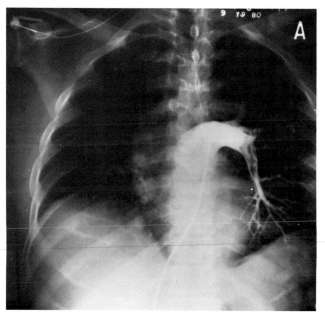

Fig 25–4—Abnormal pulmonary angiogram demonstrating absence of vascular markings. This is diagnostic of pulmonary embolism.

scanning with angiography show that between 20% and 80% of patients with lung scans suggestive of PE have normal pulmonary angiograms.[18, 23]

Ventilation-perfusion lung scanning can be used to separate many of the patients suspected of having PE and who need anticoagulant treatment from those who do not. However, a number of patients have nonspecific abnormalities on lung scan. For these patients, the risks of empirical treatment with anticoagulant drugs are probably greater than the risks of pulmonary angiography.[18] In a recent study of patients with pulmonary emboli, more than 800 pulmonary angiograms were obtained.[14, 29] The morbidity was less than 1% and the mortality was less than 0.01%, whereas mortality from anticoagulation has been reported to be as high as 2%,[30] with serious bleeding complications occurring in up to 30% of patients.

Disadvantages of the procedure include the need for professional medical and paramedical personnel as well as sophisticated equipment. Also, pulmonary angiography is invasive and a relatively expensive procedure. These disadvantages, however, will be outweighed in many cases by the procedure's accuracy, particularly when the surgeon must decide whether to anticoagulate an orthopedic patient soon after injury or surgery.

A pulmonary angiogram should be ordered when any one of the following conditions obtains:

1. A patient has pulmonary parenchymal disease.
2. A perfusion scan is negative but the clinical signs and symptoms are overwhelming.
3. Long-term or high-risk anticoagulants are contemplated.

Since the risks of angiography are less than the risks of long-term anticoagulation, patients who are not clearly categorized by lung scanning or who have abnormal chest films should undergo angiography before full anticoagulation is started.

TABLE 25–2.—Diagnosis of Pulmonary Embolism	
Means of Diagnosis	**Accuracy (%)**
Clinical signs and symptoms	20–50
Perfusion scan	50–80
Ventilation-perfusion scan	50–100
(accuracy related to defect size)	
Angiography	100

A summary of the accuracy of tests helpful in diagnosing PE is given in Table 25–2.

DIAGNOSIS OF DEEP VEIN THROMBOSIS

The clinical diagnosis of DVT is highly inaccurate. Some 50% of patients with symptoms suggestive of DVT have normal venograms.[31-33] Conversely, more than 50% of acute leg vein thrombi are not recognized clinically.[34, 35] Venography is the diagnostic standard for DVT, but because it is an invasive procedure, it does not lend itself to prospective screening or multiple examinations. In addition, the risk of inducing phlebitis by the examination itself varies between 4% and 34%.[36-38]

Iodine[125] fibrinogen scanning[39] has been reported to be accurate, sensitive, and easily repeatable, and is noninvasive (except for IV administration of the fibrinogen). Serial scans can be performed painlessly at the bedside. However, Harris et al.[40] found that only 50% of fresh thrombi seen on venograms were detected by this method in a series of patients undergoing elective hip surgery.

Impedance plethysmography (IPG), introduced in 1970 by Mullick et al.,[38] is based on blood volume changes in the leg produced by inflation and deflation of the thigh cuff. Changes in venous blood volume, measured as changes in electric resistance (impedance), are distinctly different when the deep venous system is occluded by thrombus. IPG is noninvasive, can be performed repeatedly at the patient's bedside by a technician, and has few known risks. When a thrombus is present in the popliteal or more proximal vein, the results of IPG correlate closely (95%) with venography.[41] Accuracy for detecting thrombi below the knee is much lower, however. Hull et al.[42] combined the use of leg scanning and IPG in patients with suspected venous thrombosis. One or both of these tests were positive in 81 of 86 patients with positive venograms (sensitivity, 94%) and both were negative in 104 of 114 patients with negative venograms (specificity, 91%). This study confirmed previous reports showing greater accuracy in the diagnosis of thrombi proximal to the knee than in the calf.

WHEN SHOULD PULMONARY EMBOLISM BE TREATED?

Heparin and warfarin, introduced in the 1940s, were the first drugs widely used to treat PE. The initial uncritical acceptance of these drugs, followed by enthusiastic reports of their value, made it difficult to conduct properly controlled trials of efficacy and safety. The medical community was almost universally committed to these regimens. However, many other treatments that evolved in a similar way and gained full acceptance later proved ineffective when formally assessed. There are important questions regarding the value of anticoagulation for PE that are still unanswered.

How did anticoagulation become so well accepted, and is it of benefit in the treatment of PE? One of the studies most frequently cited in support of treating PE appeared in *Lancet* in 1960.[43] The authors, Barritt and Jordan, reported the results of a controlled trial of anticoagulation (heparin and nicoumalone) versus no treatment, but abandoned it when they found that five of the first 19 untreated patients died, whereas none of the 16 treated patients died. This may be the only prospective controlled trial showing benefits from treatment, but close scrutiny of the study reveals several flaws. For example, selection was neither random nor double-blind. No information regarding the comparability of the treated and untreated patients was provided. The 40% incidence of massive pulmonary infarction among the patients who died is unusually high. Most other studies quote a 10% incidence of this complication.[44] The diagnosis of PE was based entirely on the clinical symptoms of central "chest pain, hemoptysis and faintness," yet these symptoms were present in fewer than 23% of patients with PE in a larger, more recent study using angiography to establish the diagnosis.[14] Of the five deaths reported in Barritt's and Jordan's untreated patients, one was due to cerebral infarction and two were due to sepsis.[43]

The investigators actually were criticized for conducting the trial because it was said that the benefits of anticoagulation had already been "conclusively" demonstrated by Zilliacus[45] in 1946. However, this early work failed to control important variables. For example, the patients receiving anticoagulants were mobilized after a few days, whereas the untreated patients were subjected to 40 days' enforced bed rest.

In 1977, Johnson and Charnley[46] reported results in a prospective, controlled trial of 667 patients undergoing total hip replacement, comparing anticoagulation with no treatment for PE. There were nearly four times as many recurrent emboli in the treated group (who received heparin, warfarin, or combinations of the two drugs). None of the 308 untreated patients died. This study is limited by the fact that the diagnosis of PE was made on clinical grounds without the use of scans or angiograms.

Other more recent studies have compared treated with untreated patients in the preanticoagulant era (up to 20 years ago). Dalen and Alpert[4] said that the mortality from untreated PE is 30%, but Johnson and Charnley[46] found that for patients who have recently had a hip replacement, the mortality from untreated PE is extremely low. Sabiston et al.[47] have shown that normal persons can tolerate sudden occlusion of 50% of the pulmonary vasculature without developing symptoms, so it is not surprising that PE is commonly asymptomatic. When comparing the mortality in treated and untreated patients, many authors overlook the fact that nearly 75% of deaths occur within an hour of the onset of symptoms, usually before treatment can be started.[4] If these patients are excluded from the treated groups, then the effects of "treatment" appear spectacular. One thing is certain: the real mortality from untreated PE is not known.

The risk of death does not directly correlate with the magnitude of the PE per se but is related to the presence of shock due to acute right ventricular failure after massive PE.[48] According to Alpert et al.,[48] the mortality in patients with massive PE without shock is the same as that in patients with submassive PE. In that study, patients with PE who survived long enough to have the diagnosis established and appropriate therapy begun had an excellent prognosis unless they had associated severe medical diseases. Parasakos et al.[49] believe that the best predictor of survival in PE is the presence or absence of previous heart disease. PE is often the final coup de grace in patients who are already critically ill and in whom cardiac reserve is limited. If a patient with PE who is otherwise healthy survives for at least 24 hours, his outlook is excellent.[48] Death after 24 hours occurs only in already critically ill patients, particularly those with heart disease and congestive failure.

TREATMENT OF PULMONARY EMBOLISM

It is generally agreed that the treatment of PE is medical, whether by standard anticoagulation or thrombolytic agents. Heparin, administered IV, is the agent most commonly used, with an initial anticoagulation (loading) dose of 50–100 units/kg of body weight as an IV bolus (i.e., 10,000 units for a 100-kg patient). Maintenance heparin should be given IV using an infusion pump that continuously delivers 1,000 units per hour (15–25 units/kg/hour).[50] Salzman et al.[30] have shown that intermittent doses have a higher complication rate than a continuous infusion.

The effect of heparin on whole blood coagulation is best measured by the whole blood activated clotting time (WBACT) or the activated partial thromboplastin time (APTT). Some reports suggest that maintaining the APTT greater than 1½ times the control value decreases the likelihood of recurrent thromboembolism.[50] The APPT should be checked before heparin is started, then every several hours until a maintenance dose is determined. Thereafter, the APPT should be measured daily for the duration of therapy. If the APPT exceeds 90–100 seconds the heparin dosage should be cut back promptly. The platelet count should be determined daily, and no intramuscular injections should be given to heparinized patients. Drugs that interfere with platelet function (ASA, etc.) should be avoided if at all possible.

The hematocrit should be determined before starting anticoagulation, and then every other day or more frequently as the patient's condition dictates. Orders for heparin should be written for 24 hours only and must be rewritten daily.

Prolonged anticoagulation with oral agents (warfarin, coumadin) is indicated in most patients (Table 25–3), and heparin should not be discontinued until after this is adequately regulated. The first dose of warfarin is usually given 5 days before heparin is stopped. There is no unanimity concerning the optimal duration of long-term anticoagulation, but there is a consensus that 3–6 months should be adequate.[17]

COMPLICATIONS OF ANTICOAGULATION

Heparin is responsible for the majority of drug-related deaths in reasonably healthy patients[51] and is the leading cause of adverse drug reactions in hospitalized patients (22%).[32] Many studies indicate that the incidence of dangerous bleeding from heparin, even in low-risk patients, is as high as 20%.[30] Most patients treated with heparin for PE subsequently are placed on oral anticoagulants. The latter drugs also cause complications serious enough to require hospitalization.[52]

TABLE 25–3.—Treatment of Pulmonary Embolism

Heparin:	IV bolus of 10,000 units (or 50–100 units/kg body weight). Maintenance: Continuous infusion of 20–25 units/kg/hour, IV, for 7–10 days, regulated by laboratory tests.
Coumadin:	Overlap 3–5 days with heparin. Keep prothrombin 8%–25% activity. Continue coumadin for at least 12 weeks.

Salzman et al.[30] reported that of 100 patients who received heparin in therapeutic dosages, 2% died from bleeding. Major bleeding occurred in 20% of patients, whether or not the dose of heparin was regulated with the WBACT. In a subsequent prospective trial[30] it was determined that if continuous IV heparin was given via an infusion pump the incidence of major bleeding could be reduced sevenfold, compared with administration by intermittent injection. It was also noted, coincidentally, that in 26% of patients who were given heparin for presumed PE, subsequent studies proved the diagnosis incorrect.

Elderly women are thought to be particularly susceptible to bleeding.[52] Of 42 women (average age, 59.6 years) receiving heparin in a coronary care unit, 26% experienced a major bleeding episode. Most of the bleeding was in the hip and groin, and more than half of these patients required 4 units of blood. Only 4.8% of the men experienced major bleeding.

Spontaneous retroperitoneal hemorrhage may appear clinically as an acute femoral neuropathy because the extravasated blood passes underneath the tight fascia of the iliac fossa.[53] Intracranial hemorrhage has been reported in more than 100 patients, most of whom died.[54] Spinal epidural hematoma may also occur, and sometimes can be painless. Lumbar puncture producing paraplegia has been reported, even when carried out shortly before the administration of anticoagulant drugs.[55] Arterial puncture to determine blood gas values in patients anticoagulated for pulmonary emboli can be extremely dangerous and has resulted in skin slough, infection, median and femoral neuropathies, and ischemia of the forearm muscles (Volkmann's contracture).[56] Heparin-induced thrombocytopenia is also well documented[57] and can substantially increase the risk of hemorrhagic complications.

Heparin can cause abnormal platelet aggregation in platelet-rich plasma taken from patients with heparin-induced thrombocytopenia.[57-59] The mechanics of this effect are unknown, but several investigators[57,58] have demonstrated that serum from patients with heparin-induced thrombocytopenia contains a substance or substances that, in the presence of heparin, accelerate platelet aggregation in platelet-rich plasma obtained from nonsusceptible individuals. Thrombocytopenia typically develops 2–13 days after the initiation of heparin therapy,[60] and it can lead to hemorrhagic or thrombotic complications, including major arterial occlusion, recurrent venous thromboses, and recurrent pulmonary emboli. Thromboembolic disease of the aortoiliac system with acute ischemia of the lower extremities has been reported.[60] The mortality from arterial thromboembolic complications is as high as 60%.[61] It must be treated by prompt cessation of heparin therapy.

Salzman et al.[30] reported that bleeding complications decreased when the day-to-day management of therapy was conducted by the house staff and private physicians and all patients were seen daily by a registered nurse specifically assigned to the project and who took particular note of evidence of bleeding, recurrent thromboembolism, or other untoward events. Unfortunately, this type of staffing is rarely available except in a research study.

Complications are common even when anticoagulants are administered strictly according to protocol by well-trained personnel, but deviations from protocol have been shown to be frequent. For example, an audit of anticoagulant therapy of PE and DVT reported by Meinhold et al.[62] revealed that several patients received incorrect amounts of heparin, including one patient who received 12 extra doses of heparin after an order had been written for it to be discontinued. Seventeen percent of laboratory tests ordered to monitor therapy were not reported, and the prothrombin times were properly monitored in only 50% of patients receiving warfarin. Other sources of error in heparin therapy include (1) lack of precision of the delivery pump, (2) unplanned interruption of infusion, (3) errors in making solutions, and (4) failure of infusion or charting techniques.[63]

THROMBOLYTIC AGENTS

Anticoagulation is the mainstay of therapy for acute PE but it has only a secondary role in prevention. Anticoagulants are thought to inhibit extension of the thrombus by slowing or stopping the thrombotic process and thereby decreasing the likelihood of recurrent embolic episodes. However, anticoagulation has no demonstrable immediate effect on the original embolus.

Urokinase and streptokinase are plasminogen activators that maximally activate the body's natural fibrinolytic system to dissolve fresh fibrin clots. They convert the inactive enzyme precursor plasminogen to the active enzyme plasmin, which then directly attacks the fibrin clot to dissolve it.[17, 64] The exact mechanism and molecular site of the fibrinolytic action are not known.

Thrombolytic therapy has been recommended for any patient with PE that produces a perfusion defect (single or multiple) equivalent to one lobe or more and any patient with a pulmonary embolus who is in shock or has severe pulmonary hypertension. The FDA-approved indications for streptokinase include acute massive PE, acute DTV, and arterial thrombosis and embolism.[65] Urokinase is approved only for the treatment of acute massive PE. Contraindications to the use of these agents are (1) recent major surgery (within 10 days), (2) recent trauma, including cardiopulmonary resuscitation, and (3) recent serious gastrointestinal bleeding (within 10 days).[64] Treatment is initiated with a loading dose administered through a peripheral line by a constant infusion pump. The usual loading dose for streptokinase is 250,000 units given over 20–30 minutes; for urokinase it is 4,400 IU/kg of body weight given over 10 minutes. The maintenance dose of streptokinase used in the NIH trials was 100,000 units/hour for 24 hours for PE. For urokinase, the maintenance dose was 4,400 IU/kg/hour for 12–14 hours.[66]

Laboratory monitoring is required during thrombolytic therapy only to determine the extent of systemic fibrinolysis. The best index of fibrinolysis is blood euglobulin lysis time, but the combination of the partial thromboplastin time and prothrombin time is an acceptable substitute.[67] These tests should be performed before therapy is started, 3–4 hours after it is begun, and after therapy is completed.

Bleeding is just as common a complication of thrombolytic agents as of heparin with major bleeding seen in 5%–20% of cases.[64] Many instances result from minor trauma, such as venipuncture or cutdown. Hypersensitivity reactions associated with streptokinase include urticaria, itching, flushing, nausea, headache, and anaphylaxis (1.3%–2.5%). The last of these can range in severity from minor breathing difficulty to bronchospasm, periorbital swelling, or angioneurotic edema.[64]

Urokinase does not seem to induce antibody formation, but the possibility of serious allergic reactions cannot be excluded. Fever greater than 104° F has been reported in 3.5% of patients receiving streptokinase, and febrile episodes with urokinase have occurred in 15% of patients.[64]

Thrombolytic agents have not been used extensively in orthopedic patients. Ahlberg et al.[68] reported on 34 patients with hip fracture given streptokinase for prophylaxis of thromboembolism. There were no deaths from any cause in the 34 patients, but neither was there a decrease in thrombotic episodes compared with untreated controls. No mention was made of side effects of therapy.

SURGICAL TREATMENT AND PREVENTION OF PE

Some 50% of patients with "massive" PE die within 30 minutes, 70% die within 1 hour, and more than 85% die within 6 hours.[69-71] Thus, it is essential to have a responsive medical environment with readily available diagnostic tests, including pulmonary angiography.

Mattox et al.[72] reported on 40 pulmonary embolectomies performed in 39 patients who were in extremis at the time of initiation of cardiopulmonary bypass. Despite their moribund condition, 50% of these patients lived after embolectomy. Whether or not cardiac arrest occurs secondary to pulmonary embolus is a strong indicator of survival after embolectomy. Among patients with 50% or greater obstruction of the pulmonary artery, as assessed by arteriography, the mortality following pulmonary embolectomy was 94% in patients who had had a cardiac arrest compared with 31% in those who had not arrested.[70] Use of portable cardiopulmonary bypass equipment may save some moribund patients with acute massive PE by providing support during preparation for surgery and during angiography. Angiography is strongly recommended before surgery in order to guide the surgeon to the major emboli.

Surgical Methods for the Prevention of PE

Prevention of recurrent emboli can be achieved by inferior vena cava interruption, either by ligation, plication, or by placement of an intraluminal filter. Indications for these procedures include (1) contraindications to anticoagulant therapy, (2) bleeding with anticoagulant therapy, and (3) recurrent PE on anticoagulant therapy. The Greenfield filter[73] is placed via a transvenous approach through the internal jugular vein. This is done most frequently in the radiology department under fluoroscopic control and with the patient awake. The morbidity is low, and recurrent embolization is less than 5% in most series.[74-76]

Inferior vena cava ligation, on the other hand, is accompanied by a high complication rate with an operative mortality that varies from 5% to 40%, venous stasis in 10%–50% of patients, and a recurrent embolization rate as high as 50%.[75] Ligation has largely been replaced by plication achieved by an external plastic clip that divides the lumen into multiple small channels wide enough to allow free flow of blood but too narrow for an embolus of any magnitude to pass through. Lower extremity edema is much less common with these devices than after inferior vena cava ligation.[77]

Prophylaxis of PE

There are two main methods of prophylaxis: pharmacologic and nonpharmacologic. The most commonly used pharmacologic agents are low-dose heparin, coumadin, dextran, and aspirin. When reviewing the studies on the effectiveness of each of these agents, it is important to answer the following questions:

1. Were controls used? If so, were they concurrent controls or historical controls (from some other series or some other era)?
2. Were the patients randomized and was the study double-blind?
3. Was the end point of the study a decrease in the incidence of fatal or nonfatal PE or just a decrease in the incidence of DVT?
4. Was there a decrease in the overall death rate in the group receiving prophylaxis?

5. Were the type and severity of complications accurately and completely reported?
6. Is the proposed regimen too complicated to use in the average hospital?

Surprisingly, relatively little information is available on prophylaxis of thromboembolism in patients with hip fracture. Most articles in the orthopedic literature pertain to patients with total hip replacement, an elective procedure performed in patients who are optimally prepared for surgery.

Heparin

Heparin is undoubtedly the most popular drug used for prophylaxis of PE and for therapy of established PE. Full therapeutic doses of heparin exert an anti-coagulant effect due to heparin combining with antithrombin III, a naturally occurring heparin cofactor.[17] Several steps in the clotting cascade are blocked when anti-thrombin III is unavailable. Low-dose heparin prophylaxis depends on the ability of trace amounts of heparin to augment an inhibitor of activated factor X contained in normal serum. Reports on the efficacy of heparin therapy, however, are contradictory. In a double-blind study of 52 patients with hip fracture who were randomly allocated to treatment with low-dose heparin or placebo, Moskovitz et al.[78] found that low-dose heparin afforded no protection against thromboembolism. The study also included a number of patients undergoing total hip replacement, and in these patients receiving heparin there was a reduction from 59% to 22% in "thromboembolic events." However, all of these "thromboembolic events" were DVT. There were no confirmed pulmonary emboli and no deaths in either the treated or control groups of arthroplasty patients.

Gallus et al.[79] included 46 patients with hip fracture among 350 patients treated with low-dose heparin. The end point was DVT. The authors found that low-dose heparin was less effective in patients with hip fracture than in other population groups.

Failure to prevent PE after hip fracture, total hip replacement, and above-knee amputation using low-dose heparin was also the experience of Williams et al.[80] Sharnoff[81] in 1976 reported an *increased* incidence of fatal PE in patients with hip fracture who received low-dose heparin, compared with untreated controls.

In patients undergoing total hip replacement, Harris et al.[82] and Johnson et al.[83] reported no benefit from low-dose heparin and an increased complication rate. Harris et al. discontinued the use of low-dose heparin after treating 20 patients because eight patients developed fresh thrombi while on prophylaxis, one had a pulmonary embolus, and one developed bilateral femoral arterial emboli. Johnson et al. found that the mortality from PE almost tripled after subcutaneous heparin prophylaxis, compared with no therapy.

In a multicenter trial, Kakkar et al.[84] found that low-dose heparin was more effective than no treatment in over 4,000 patients. However, less than 4% of the total were orthopedic patients. In 1,300 general surgical patients studied by Pachter and Riles,[85] no deaths were attributed to pulmonary emboli in either the patients receiving low-dose heparin or the untreated controls. Bleeding complications occurred in 10%–27% of the patients receiving heparin.

Even though low-dose heparin may be beneficial in some patients,[9] it has had no impact on the incidence of and mortality from PE in the past 25 years.[86] Furthermore, it is generally accepted that low-dose heparin is not effective as prophylaxis in patients with hip fractures.

Dextran

Another agent used for prophylaxis is dextran (either Dextran 70 or lower molecular weight dextran, Dextran 40). Although dextran has had only limited use by orthopedic surgeons in the United States, it has been the main method of prophylaxis for hip fracture in Sweden for the past 10 years. Dextran alters factor VIII, fibrin polymerization, platelet aggregability, and thrombus stabilization.[17] Few studies on the efficacy of dextran have included untreated controls, but most studies have compared dextran with other agents, such as dicumarol or low-dose heparin. The evidence regarding its effectiveness is contradictory, and DVT rather than PE has been the end point of therapy in most cases. One study comparing dextran with dicumarol[87] reported a death rate from thromboembolism of 4% even for patients who received adequate doses of dextran. All patients who died from any cause while on dextran had pulmonary edema when examined at autopsy. Fredin et al.[88] in 1982 reported a 30-day mortality of nearly 10% in patients on dextran. Potential complications of dextran therapy include renal failure, anaphylaxis, congestive heart failure, and a 10%–20% risk of wound bleeding.[12]

Coumadin

Oral anticoagulants such as coumadin gained increased acceptance after Salzman and Harris strongly recommended their use in 1966.[2] Although they reported a decrease in the incidence of PE (from 4/83 in the control group to 1/83 in the treated group), there was no statistically significant decrease in the number of total deaths in the treated group. The overall mortality was 25%, and the incidence of bleeding complications was 35%. Of note in their study was the long period of bed rest for patients postoperatively. Only 15 of the 184 patients were walking before day 20 postoperatively. This prolonged period of immobilization may have contributed to the 25% mortality and the relatively high incidence of PE in the control group.

Bergqvist et al.[87] reported on 63 patients treated prophylactically with dicumarol. Three of 63 patients on dicumarol died of PE and two patients died of hemorrhage.

Morris and Mitchell[89] confirmed the reduction of DVT and PE clinically and on postmortem examination in a trial of warfarin in elderly patients with hip fracture. No difference in total mortality rates could be shown.

Despite some evidence that coumadin is effective in preventing PE, orthopedic surgeons have been sufficiently skeptical about the risk-benefit ratio that its use has been limited.

Aspirin

In the past few years, aspirin has gained popularity as a prophylactic agent for several reasons: (1) it has been reported to be effective in some situations, (2) it is familiar to the physician and patient, and (3) it has few side effects. Aspirin is thought to act by suppressing platelet aggregation. But does it prevent PE? Zekert et al.,[90] in a double-blind trial, compared 1,500 mg of aspirin daily with placebo in 240 patients with hip fracture. Both groups were comparable with regard to age, sex, weight, and length of time from trauma to operation. The authors reported a decrease in thromboembolism in the treated group, with a profound decrease in the incidence of fatal embolism: 7% (8/120) of the patients given placebo compared with 0.8%

(1/120) of those given aspirin. However, the incidence of PE in the group receiving prophylaxis is essentially the same as in other reports of patients receiving no prophylaxis.[13, 46] DVT occurred in 14% of patients in the placebo group and 6% in the aspirin group.

Zekert's[90] results, however, were not reproduced by Snook et al.,[91] who reported on 49 patients with hip fractures, 25 of whom received placebo and 24 of whom received 600 mg of aspirin b.i.d. In the control group, 60% of patients developed DVT and 2 of 25 patients had nonfatal PE. With aspirin, 25% of patients developed DVT and one of 24 experienced a (fatal) pulmonary embolus. Thus, aspirin decreased the incidence of DVT but did not decrease the incidence of PE.

Harris et al.[82] reported on 51 patients undergoing total hip arthroplasty who received 600 mg of aspirin the day before surgery and twice daily thereafter until they were fully ambulatory. DVT developed in 38 patients receiving aspirin, many more than in the groups receiving dextran or warfarin. Later, Harris et al.[92] reported that aspirin was protective in men over age 40 undergoing total hip replacement. Still, 4 of 23 men developed DVT, which was located in the thigh in each case. No patient had a major bleeding complication while on aspirin, but there was no significant difference in the mortality from PE in the patients receiving aspirin compared with those receiving placebo.

Newer Agents

A new class of drugs potentially useful in preventing thromboembolism are the heparinoids (glucosaminoglycans), typified by sodium pentosan polysulfate (PZ68), a semisynthetic sulfated xylan from the vegetable kingdom. Preliminary results have demonstrated that administration of PZ68 increases inhibitory activity of factor Xa.[93] It is theoretically possible that the increased activity of factor Xa that develops after trauma could be counteracted with this agent.

Fredin et al.,[88] in a prospective randomized study of 100 patients with femoral neck fracture, found that the number of venous thromboses and pulmonary emboli did not differ significantly between patients on PZ68 and those on dextran, and the former experienced problems with hemorrhage. In fact, six patients had to be withdrawn from the PZ68 therapy group because of major hemorrhages. One of 27 patients on PZ68 died of PE.

Nonpharmacologic Methods for Prevention of Thromboembolism
External Pneumatic Compression Devices

Cotton and Roberts[94] pioneered the development of techniques for external pneumatic compression of the lower limbs to prevent venous thrombosis and reported significant success with this method. Many intermittent pneumatic compression devices have since been described that use varying pressures, time cycles, and power sources. Pneumatic compression while the patient is on the operating table was shown to be effective in two studies,[95, 96] but the findings were not confirmed in a multicenter study,[97] either when compression was given alone or in combination with dextran.

Effective prophylaxis in patients undergoing elective general surgical procedures has been reported with external pneumatic compression by Hills et al.[98] However, in most studies using this technique, patients having leg operations were excluded. Again, the end point of each study was the incidence of DVT, with no mention of the frequency of PE.

Compression Stockings

Compression stockings and elevation of the legs have been shown to be of no value in preventing postoperative DVT.[99] This concept has been challenged by Allan et al.,[100] who reported that when graduated compression stockings were used, there was a decrease from 40% to 15.5% in DVT in patients undergoing abdominal surgery. No fatal or nonfatal pulmonary emboli were reported, however, in both the control and treated groups.

SUMMARY

PE continues to be a challenge to the orthopedic surgeon. Its incidence in orthopedic patients in general and in patients with hip fractures in particular may not be as high as has been claimed in several well-publicized reports.[1-3] Studies that combine PE and DVT under the general heading of thromboembolism give misleading impressions of morbidity and mortality. Diagnosis of DVT is an intermediate step of intermediate importance, and it is inappropriate to use figures on the incidence of DVT to draw conclusions on the incidence of PE.

It is essential to make an accurate diagnosis of PE before subjecting the patient to the risks of anticoagulation. Even if PE has been unequivocally demonstrated, it is not clear as to just how much treatment decreases the mortality.

Information regarding prophylaxis and treatment of DVT and PE in patients undergoing general surgical procedures should not be extrapolated directly to orthopedic patients. Orthopedic patients have been shown in numerous studies to respond differently from general surgical patients to many of the regimens in common use. Because rapid changes are taking place in this field, recommendations regarding prophylaxis are hazardous. In selecting the method of therapy, it is most important to consider the risk-benefit ratio. Oral anticoagulants are difficult to control, dextran has significant side effects, and low-dose heparin is not only ineffective but can cause an increase in thromboembolic and other complications in patients with hip fractures. Zekert's study[90] of patients with hip fractures showed a reduction in fatal PE in those receiving aspirin compared with those in a control group, but this has not been supported by the findings of others.[91]

We have found that early operation and mobilization, with no other specific prophylaxis, results in a mortality from PE of less than 1% in patients with hip fractures.[13] This is as low as any figure reported by those who advocate treatment by various pharmacologic or nonpharmacologic methods.

Prophylaxis would be desirable if it really could decrease substantially this low rate of PE. But the regimen must be safe and relatively easy to administer and control, and its effectiveness must be confirmed by properly controlled trials demonstrating a decrease in the incidence of proved PE. So far, there is no persuasive evidence that this can be accomplished.

REFERENCES

1. Sevitt S., Gallagher N.G.: Prevention of venous thrombosis and pulmonary embolism in injured patients. *Lancet* 2:981-989, 1959.
2. Salzman E.W., Harris W.H., DeSanctis R.W.: Anticoagulation for prevention of thromboembolism following fractures of the hip. *N. Engl. J. Med.* 275:122-130, 1966.
3. Fitts W.T., Lehr H.B., Bitner R.L., et al.: An analysis of 950 fatal injuries. *Surgery* 56:663-668, 1964.
4. Dalen J.E., Alpert J.S.: Natural history of pulmonary embolism. *Prog. Cardiovasc. Dis.* 17:259-269, 1975.

5. Moser K.M., LeMoine J.R., Nachtwey F.J., et al.: Deep venous thrombosis and pulmonary embolism. *JAMA* 246:1422-1424, 1981.

6. Browse N.: Diagnosis of deep vein thrombosis. *Br. Med. Bull.* 342:163-167, 1978.

7. Moser K.M., LeMoine J.R.: Is embolic risk conditioned by location of deep venous thrombosis? *Ann. Intern. Med.* 94:439-444, 1981.

8. Le Quesne L.P.: Relation between deep vein thrombosis and pulmonary embolism in surgical patients. *N. Engl. J. Med.* 291:1292, 1974.

9. Kakkar V.V., Spindler, J., Flute P.T., et al.: Efficacy of low doses of heparin in prevention of deep-vein thrombosis after major surgery. *Lancet* 2:101-106, 1972.

10. Hampson W.G.J., Lucas H.K., Harris F.C.: Failure of low-dose heparin to prevent deep-vein thrombosis after hip replacement arthroplasty. *Lancet* 2:795-797, 1974.

11. Morris G.K., Henry A.P.J., Preston B.K.: Prevention of deep-vein thrombosis by low-dose heparin in patients undergoing total hip replacement. *Lancet* 2:797-799, 1974.

12. Salzman E.W., Harris W.H.: Prevention of venous thromboembolism in orthopedic patients. *J. Bone Joint Surg.* 58a:903-913, 1976.

13. Day L.J.: The incidence of fatal pulmonary embolism in patients with hip fractures. Unpublished manuscript.

14. Urokinase Pulmonary Embolism Trial. *Circulation.* 47(suppl.2):1-108, 1973.

15. Menzoian J.O., Williams L.F.: Is pulmonary angiography essential for the diagnosis of acute pulmonary embolism? *Am. J. Surg.* 137:543-548, 1979.

16. Stein P.D., Willis P.W. III, Dalen J.E.: Importance of clinical assessment in selecting patients for pulmonary arteriography. *Am. J. Cardiol.* 43:669-671, 1979.

17. Bell W.R., Simon T.L.: Current status of pulmonary thromboembolic disease: Pathophysiology, diagnosis, prevention, and treatment. *Am. Heart J.* 103:239-262, 1982.

18. Cheely R., McCartney S.W., Perry I.R., et al.: The role of non-invasive tests versus pulmonary angiography in the diagnosis of pulmonary embolism. *Am. J. Med.* 70:17-22, 1981.

19. Kafer F.R.: Respiratory function in pulmonary thromboembolic disease. *Am. J. Med.* 47:94, 1969.

20. McIntyre K.M., Sasahara A.A., Sharma G.V.: Pulmonary thromboembolism: Current concepts. *Adv. Intern. Med.* 18:199-218, 1972.

21. Fletcher J.W., James A.E., Holman B.L.: Regional lung functioning in cancer. *Prog. Nucl. Med.* 3:135-148, 1973.

22. Kipper M.S., Moser K.M., Kartman K.E., et al.: Long-term follow-up of patients with suspected pulmonary embolism and a normal lung scan. *Chest* 82:411-415, 1982.

23. McNeil B.J.: A diagnostic strategy using ventilation-perfusion scans with pulmonary angiograms. *Am. Heart J.* 92:700, 1976.

24. McNeil B.J.: A diagnostic strategy using ventilation-perfusion studies in patients suspect for pulmonary embolism. *J. Nucl. Med.* 17:613-616, 1976.

25. Kelley M.J., Elliott L.P.: The radiologic evaluation of the patient with suspected pulmonary thromboembolic disease. *Med. Clin. North Am.* 59:3-36, 1974.

26. Moses D.C., Silver T.M., Bookstein J.T.: The complementary roles of chest radiography, lung scanning, and selective pulmonary angiography in the diagnosis of pulmonary embolism. *Circulation* 49:179-188, 1974.

27. Dalen J.E., Brooks H.L., Johnson L.W., et al.: Pulmonary angiography in acute pulmonary embolism: Indications, techniques and results in 367 patients. *Am. Heart J.* 81:175-185, 1971.

28. Novelline R.A., Baltarowich O.H., Athanasoulis C.A., et al.: The clinical course of patients with suspected pulmonary embolism and a negative pulmonary arteriogram. *Diagn. Radiol.* 126:561-567, 1978.

29. Bell W.R., Simon T.L.: A comparative analysis of pulmonary perfusion scans with pulmonary angiograms: From a national cooperative study. *Am. Heart J.* 92:700, 1976.

30. Salzman E.W., Deykin D., Shapiro R.M., et al.: Management of heparin therapy: Controlled prospective trial. *N. Engl. J. Med.* 292:1046-1050, 1975.

31. Haeger K.: Problems of acute deep vein thrombosis. *Angiology* 20:280-286, 1969.

32. Hull R., Hirsh J., Sackett D.L., et al.: Replacement of venography in suspected venous thrombosis by impedance plethysmography and ^{125}I fibrinogen leg scanning. *Ann. Intern. Med.* 94:12-15, 1981.

33. Johnson W.C.: Evaluation of newer techniques for diagnosis of venous thrombosis. *J. Surg. Res.* 16:473-481, 1974.

34. Kakkar V.V., Howe C.T., Flanc C., et al.: Natural history of postoperative deep vein thrombosis. *Lancet* 2:230-232, 1969.

35. Palko P.D., Nanson E.M., Fedoruk S.O.: The early detection of deep venous thrombosis using ^{131}I tagged fibrinogen. *Can. J. Surg.* 7:215-226, 1964.

36. Albrechtson U., Olsson C.G.: Thrombotic side-effects of lower limb phlebography. *Lancet* 1:723-724, 1976.

37. Athanasoulis C.A.: Phlebography for the diagnosis of deep leg vein thrombosis, in *Prophylactic Therapy of Deep Venous Thrombosis and Pulmonary Embolism.* DHEW publication No. (NIH) 62. Washington, D.C., DHEW, 1975, pp. 76-866.

38. Mullick S.C., Wheeler H.B., Songster G.F.: Diagnosis of deep venous thrombosis by measurement of electrical impedance. *Am. J. Surg.* 119:417-422, 1970.

39. Kakkar V.V.: The diagnosis of deep vein thrombosis using the ^{125}I fibrinogen test. *Arch. Surg.* 104:152-159, 1972.

40. Harris W.H., Salzman E.W., Athanasoulis C., et al.: Comparison of ^{125}I fibrinogen count scanning with phlebography for detection of venous thrombi after elective hip surgery. *N. Engl. J. Med.* 292:665-667, 1975.

41. Wheeler H.B., Anderson F.A., Cardullo P.A., et al.: Suspected deep vein thrombosis: Management by impedance plethysmography. *Arch. Surg.* 117:1206-1209, 1982.

42. Hull R., Hirsh J., Sackett D.L., et al.: Combined use of leg scanning and impedance plethysmography in suspected venous thrombosis. *N. Engl. J. Med.* 296:1497-1500, 1977.

43. Barritt D.W., Jordan S.C.: Anticoagulant drugs in the treatment of pulmonary embolism. *Lancet* 1:1309-1312, 1960.

44. Moser K.M.: Pulmonary embolism. *Am. Rev. Respir. Dis.* 115:829-852, 1977.

45. Zilliacus H.: On specific treatment of thrombosis and pulmonary embolism with anticoagulants, with particular reference to postthrombotic sequelae: Results of 5 years' treatment of thrombosis and pulmonary embolism at series of Swedish hospitals during years 1940–1945. *Acta Med. Scand.* 171(suppl.):1-221, 1946.

46. Johnson R., Charnley J.: Treatment of pulmonary embolism in total hip replacement. *Clin. Orthop.* 124:149-154, 1977.

47. Sabiston D.C., Durham N.D., Wagner H.N.: The pathophysiology of pulmonary embolism: Relationships to accurate diagnosis and choice of therapy. *J. Thorac. Cardiovasc. Surg.* 50:339-356, 1965.

48. Alpert J.S., Smith R., Carlson J., et al.: Mortality in patients treated for pulmonary embolism. *JAMA* 236:1477-1480, 1976.

49. Parasakos J.A., Adelstein S.J., Smith R.E., et al.: *N. Engl. J. Med.* Late prognosis of acute pulmonary embolism. 289:55-58, 1973.

50. Basu D., Gallus A., Hirsh J., et al.: A prospective study of the value of monitoring heparin treatment with the activated partial thromboplastin time. *N. Engl. J. Med.* 287:324-327, 1972.

51. Porter J., Hirshel J.: Drug related deaths among medical in-patients. *JAMA* 237:879-881, 1977.

52. Vieweg W.V.G., Piscatelli R.L., Houser J.J., et al.: Complications of intravenous administration of heparin in elderly women. *JAMA* 213:1303-1306, 1970.

53. Young M.R., Norris J.R.: Femoral neuropathy during anticoagulant therapy. *Neurology* 26:1173-1175, 1976.

54. Snyder M., Renauden J.: Intracranial hemorrhage associated with anticoagulation therapy. *Surg. Neurol.* 7:31-34, 1977.

55. Sadjadpour K.: Hazards of anticoagulation therapy shortly after lumbar puncture. *JAMA* 237:1692-1693, 1977.

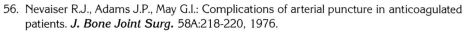

56. Nevaiser R.J., Adams J.P., May G.I.: Complications of arterial puncture in anticoagulated patients. *J. Bone Joint Surg.* 58A:218-220, 1976.
57. Babcock R.B., Dunper C.W., Scharfman W.B.: Heparin-induced immune thrombocytopenia. *N. Engl. J. Med.* 295:237-241, 1976.
58. Fratantoni J.E., Pollet R., Gralnick H.R.: Heparin-induced thrombocytopenia: Confirmation of diagnosis with in vitro methods. *Blood* 45:395-401, 1975.
59. Rhodes G.R., Dixon R.H., Silver D.: Heparin-induced thrombocytopenia with thrombotic and hemorrhagic manifestations. *Surg. Gynecol. Obstet.* 136:409-416, 1973.
60. Baird R.A., Convery F.R.: Arterial thromboembolism in patients receiving systemic heparin therapy. *J. Bone Joint Surg.* 59A:1061-1064, 1977.
61. Weismann R.E., Robin R.W.: Arterial embolism occurring during systemic heparin therapy. *Arch. Surg.* 76:219-227, 1958.
62. Meinhold J.M., Reale E.O., Miller W.A.: Audit of anticoagulant therapy of pulmonary embolus, deep vein thrombosis and thrombophlebitis. *Am. J. Hosp. Pharm.* 36:214-218, 1979.
63. Hattersley P.G., Mitsuyka J.C., King J.H.: Sources of error in heparin therapy of thromboembolic disease. *Arch. Intern. Med.* 140:1173-1175, 1980.
64. Rutkowski D.M., Burke W.S.: Advances in thrombolytic therapy. *Drug Intell. Clin. Pharm.* 16:115-121, 1982.
65. Sherry S.: Thrombolytic therapy of acute pulmonary embolism. *Drug Ther.* 8:72-80, 1983.
66. Gorlin R.: Fibrinolytic therapy in thromboembolic disease. *Hosp. Prac.* 17:146-160, 1982.
67. Bell W.R., Meek A.G.: Guidelines for the use of thrombolytic agents. *N. Engl. J. Med.* 301:1266-1270, 1979.
68. Ahlberg A., Nylander G., Robertson B., et al.: Dextran in prophylaxis of thrombosis in fractures of the hip. *Acta Chir. Scand. Suppl.* 387:83-85, 1968.
69. Clarke D.B.: Pulmonary embolectomy re-evaluated. *Ann. R. Coll. Surg. Engl.* 63:18-24, 1981.
70. Gorham L.W.: A study of pulmonary embolism. *Arch. Intern. Med.* 108:418-426, 1961.
71. Soloff L.A., Rodman T.: Acute pulmonary embolism: II. Clinical. *Am. Heart J.* 74:829-847, 1967.
72. Mattox K.L., Feldtman R.W., Beall A.C., et al.: Pulmonary embolectomy for acute massive pulmonary embolism. *Ann. Surg.* 195:726-731, 1982.
73. Menzoian J.O., LoGerfo F.W., Doyle J.E., et al.: Technical modifications in the placement of inferior vena caval filter devices. *Am. J. Surg.* 142:216-218, 1981.
74. Greenfield L.J., Peyton R., Crute S.: Greenfield vena cava filter experience. *Arch. Surg.* 116:1451-1456, 1981.
75. Silver D., Sabiston D.C.: The role of vena caval interruption in the management of pulmonary embolism. *Surgery* 77:1-10, 1975.
76. Stewart J.R., Peyton J.W.R., Crute S.L., et al.: History and physical examination in acute pulmonary embolism in patients without preexisting cardiac or pulmonary disease. *Am. J. Cardiol.* 47:218-223, 1981.
77. Donaldson M.C., Wirthlin L.S., Donaldson G.A.: Thirty-year experience with surgical interruption of the inferior vena cava for prevention of pulmonary embolism. *Ann. Surg.* 191:367-372, 1980.
78. Moskovitz P.A., Ellenberg S.S., Feffer H.L., et al.: Low-dose heparin for prevention of venous thromboembolism in total hip replacement and surgical repair of hip fractures. *J. Bone Joint Surg.* 60A:1065-1070, 1978.
79. Gallus A.S., Hirsh J., Tuttle R.J., et al.: Small subcutaneous doses of heparin in prevention of venous thrombosis. *N. Engl. J. Med.* 288:545-551, 1973.
80. Williams, J.W., Eikman E.A., Greenberg S.H., et al.: Failure of low dose heparin to prevent pulmonary embolism after hip surgery or above the knee amputation. *Ann. Surg.* 188:468-474, 1978.
81. Sharnoff J.G., Rosen R.I., Sadler A.H., et al.: Prevention of fatal pulmonary thromboembolism of heparin prophylaxis after surgery for hip fractures. *J. Bone Joint Surg.* 58A:913-918, 1976.

82. Harris W.H., Salzman E.W., Athanasoulis C.: Comparison of warfarin, low-molecular-weight dextran, aspirin, and subcutaneous heparin in prevention of venous thromboembolism following total hip replacement. *J. Bone Joint Surg.* 65A:1552-1562, 1974.

83. Johnson R., Green J.R., Charnley J.: Pulmonary embolism and its prophylaxis following Charnley total hip replacement. *Clin. Orthop.* 127:123-132, 1977.

84. Prevention of fatal postoperative pulmonary embolism by low doses of heparin: An international multicentre trial. *Lancet* 2:45-50, 1975.

85. Pachter H.L., Riles T.S.: Low dose heparin: Bleeding and wound complications in the surgical patient. *Ann. Surg.* 186:669-674, 1977.

86. Wessler S., Gitel S.N.: Low-dose heparin: is the risk worth the benefit? *Am. Heart J.* 98:94-101, 1979.

87. Bergqvist E., Bergquist D., Bronge A., et al.: An evaluation of early thrombosis prophylaxis following fracture of the femoral neck. *Acta Chir. Scand.* 138:689-693, 1972.

88. Fredin H.O., Nillius S.A., Bergqvist D.: Prophylaxis of deep vein thrombosis in patients with fracture of the femoral neck. *Acta Orthop. Scand.* 53:413-417, 1982.

89. Morris G.K., Mitchell J.R.A.: Warfarin sodium in prevention of deep venous thrombosis and pulmonary embolism in patients with fractured neck of femur. *Lancet* 2:869-872, 1976.

90. Zekert F., Kohn F., Vormittag E.: Prophylaxis of Thromboembolic Diseases in Traumatologic Patients, in *Proceedings of the 4th International Congress on Thrombosis and Haemostasis.* Vienna, 1973, p. 281.

91. Snook G.A., Chrisman O.D., Wilson T.C.: Thromboembolism after surgical treatment of hip fractures. *Clin. Orthop.* 155:21-24, 1981.

92. Harris W.H., Salzman L.W., Athanasoulis C.A., et al.: Aspirin prophylaxis of venous thromboembolism after total hip replacement. *N. Engl. J. Med.* 297:1246, 1977.

93. Ryde M., Eriksson H., Tangen O.: Comparison of the inhibition of activated factor S (Xa) and thrombin by heparin and polysulphated xylan (PZ68) in man, in Mediterranean League Against Thromboembolic Disease: *6th International Congress on Thrombosis.* Abstract No. 248, 1980.

94. Cotton L.T., Roberts V.C.: The prevention of deep vein thrombosis, with particular reference to mechanical methods of prevention. *Surgery* 81:228-235, 1977.

95. Roberts V.C., Cotton L.T.: Prevention of postoperative deep vein thrombosis in patients with malignant disease. *Br. Med. J.* 1:358-360, 1974.

96. Smith R.C., Elton R.A., Orr J.D., et al.: Dextran and intermittent pneumatic compression in prevention of postoperative deep vein thrombosis: Multiunit trial. *Br. Med. J.* 1:952-954, 1978.

97. Sabri S., Robert V.C., Colton L.T.: Prevention of early postoperative deep vein thrombosis by intermittent compression of the leg during surgery. *Br. Med. J.* iv:394-396, 1971.

98. Hills N.H., Pflug J.J., Jeyasingh K., et al.: Prevention of deep vein thrombosis by intermittent pneumatic compression of the calf. *Br. Med. J.* 1:131-135, 1972.

99. Rosengarten D.G., Laird J., Jeyasingh K.: The failure of compression stockings (tubigrip) to prevent deep venous thrombosis after operation. *Br. J. Surg.* 57:296-299, 1970.

100. Allan A., Williams J.T., Bolton J.P., et al.: The use of graduated compression stockings in the prevention of post-operative deep vein thrombosis. *Br. J. Surg.* 70:172-174, 1983.

Chapter 26

Delayed Union, Nonunion, and Malunion of Hip Fractures

Marvin H. Meyers, M.D.

Delayed union and nonunion of fractures occur more frequently at the femoral neck than at the intertrochanteric or subtrochanteric levels. The reported incidence is 10%–35% following displaced subcapital or transcervical fractures. There is a decreased incidence at the basilar neck level. Nonunion is infrequent at the intertrochanteric and subtrochanteric levels.

Although definitions of delayed union and nonunion are open to interpretation, the following is probably acceptable to most surgeons. Delayed union is present when a reasonable interval has passed between the time of the injury and the average time to union of a particular fracture, and there is still no radiographic or clinical evidence of osseous union. The potential still exists for union. Nonunion is present when all of the reparative processes necessary for healing have ceased and bone continuity has not been restored at the fracture site. One author[1] considered untreated femoral neck fractures to be nonunions 3 weeks following injury, another used 6 weeks as the criterion.[2] Many others believe untreated fractures of the femoral neck to be nonunions 3 months after injury.[3-6] Probably, fractures treated or untreated without clinical or roentgenologic evidence of union at 6 months are truly nonunions. Usually the patient complains of pain on stress with tenderness at the fracture site. X-ray films frequently demonstrate sclerosis of the fracture surfaces. There may or may not be increasing deformity on serial x-ray examinations. Bone atrophy on both sides of the fracture is present. There may be some callus around the fracture site, except at the level of the femoral neck, where external callus cannot develop, and a lucent interval in the callus.

There is controversy concerning the treatment of delayed union and nonunion of intracapsular fractures. Most authors agree that internal fixation, bone grafting, and osteotomy is the favored procedure for nonunions at the intertrochanteric and subtrochanteric levels. In general, any method that converts an ununited fracture to a soundly united one is preferable to artificial replacement, from both physiologic and functional viewpoints. Fracture union with a viable head will allow normal hip function.

Some authors advise against closed reduction and internal fixation of displaced femoral neck fractures which are older than 3 weeks. Others are opposed to open reduction and internal fixation of femoral neck fractures after 10 days.[7, 8]

343

FACTORS RESPONSIBLE FOR NONUNION

Several factors bear on the healing of hip fractures and the selection of a treatment method when delayed union or nonunion is evident. These are described below.

Age

Henderson, in 1940, opposed the use of a bone graft to treat ununited femoral neck fractures in patients under the age of 50.[5] However, if the patient is vigorous and likely to return to work or to remain active, an attempt at gaining osseous union with a bone graft with or without an osteotomy is justified, regardless of age. Some patients may be candidates for bone graft procedures up to 65 years of age or older. Several reports support this view.[9, 10] On the other hand, the elderly patient with a hip fracture is frequently in poor health, and osteoporosis is common, which makes fracture fixation difficult. Therefore, replacement arthroplasty may at times be preferable in the elderly.

Type of Fracture

There is a striking increase in the incidence of nonunion with displaced intracapsular fractures. Undisplaced or minimally displaced fracture which are fixed in situ rarely go on to nonunion.

The degree of posterior neck comminution probably is an important factor influencing the rate of nonunion. It is difficult to reduce the fracture and maintain reduction when there is severe comminution of the posterior neck. Bone grafting procedures are necessary.

The type of fracture probably has little influence on the cause of nonunion following fractures at the intertrochanteric and subtrochanteric levels.

Accuracy of Reduction

Anatomical reduction has little if any effect on the rate of osseous union of hip fractures except for intracapsular fractures. Anatomical reduction is difficult to achieve when the posterior aspect of the femoral neck is severely comminuted. It is difficult to assess rotational malposition after closed reduction of the fracture. Anatomical reduction can only be ascertained on direct visualization when the capsule is opened.

Vascular damage of the head fragment influences the rate of healing of intracapsular fractures and is related to the degree of fracture displacement. The more accurate the reduction, the better the prospects for revascularization of the head fragment.

A valgus reduction of an intracapsular or intertrochanteric fracture is more likely to heal since there is more of a compression force than a shearing force at the fracture line (see Fig 26–4,B).[11]

Treatment Method

Nonunion is frequently the result of delay or neglect in the surgical treatment of intracapsular fractures. Early closed reduction and internal fixation is the treatment of choice for displaced hip fractures. Unless fixation is rigid the incidence of nonunion will be high. Undisplaced fractures may be treated by immobilization without surgery. However, other factors bear on the selection of internal fixation for undisplaced fractures (see chapter 1).

Sliding nail plate devices, the Zickel nail, and occasionally a solid nail plate for intertrochanteric and subtrochanteric fractures have advocates. In terms of results, all seem to work well. There is little to choose between them. Bulky single nails like the Smith-Peterson triflanged nail do not seem to be as effective in achieving rigid stability of intracapsular fractures. The same can be said of sliding nail plates. Multiple pins placed in the optimal position provide the best fixation. Care must be taken that the threaded portions of pins do not bridge the fracture line. Otherwise, impaction may be inhibited, leading to delayed union or nonunion.

Impaction of the Fragments

Maximal impaction of fracture fragments reduces the fracture gap between the major fragments, permitting the optimal structural situation for bone healing. The wider the gap, the greater the potential for delayed union or nonunion. Impaction is essential for union of intracapsular fractures. In some reports nail plates have been noted to cause separation of intertrochanteric fracture fragments. Months after treatment, weight-bearing can cause metal fatigue, with breakage of the nail. Fracture of the metal is soon followed by impaction and osseous union in many cases.

Senn in 1883 stated that "The only cause for nonunion in the case of an intracapsular fracture is to be found in our inability to maintain coaptation and immobilization of the fragments during the time required for bone union to take place."[12] Coaptation of the fragments and rigid fixation are essential for good osseous union to occur.

Avascular Necrosis

Osseous union can take place in the presence of an avascular femoral head. However, viability of the femoral head may be an important factor in determining whether osseous union occurs. Banks reported that new bone is present at the intracapsular fracture line 10 days after fracture.[13] The repair process was present on both sides of the fracture only if the femoral head was viable.[13] It is apparent that union will take longer and may be in jeopardy if the femoral head is avascular. There is documentation that healing does occur in a significant number of cases with an avascular head.[14, 15]

Early Weight-Bearing After Internal Fixation

Early weight-bearing can cause collapse at the fracture site, with shortening, migration of the internal fixation device, and motion at the fracture site. Whether or not these consequences are seen depends in part on the vertical pattern of the fracture site.[11] Since it is not possible to obtain rigid fixation in the elderly patient with osteoporosis, motion at the fracture probably is present with increased stress. Motion is detrimental to healing of intracapsular fractures.

Recently there has been a move toward early mobilization and weight-bearing as a desirable goal in fracture treatment. However, since hip fractures are more prevalent in the elderly, they are better treated with internal fixation of the fracture and early mobilization without weight-bearing because of the soft bones and the difficulty in obtaining rigid fixation. Until there is some radiographic evidence that osseous union is progressing, weight-bearing is a risk.

DIAGNOSIS

As mentioned earlier, there is disagreement about what constitutes nonunion in hip fractures. It is safe to declare a nonunion when the fracture is ununited at 6 months. If there is no evidence of new bone bridging the fracture site at 3 months, one may make the interim diagnosis of delayed union. Pain at the fracture site on weight-bearing several months after injury is strongly suggestive of delayed union or nonunion. Marked absorption or sclerosis of contiguous fracture surfaces suggests nonunion. There may be times when the surgeon cannot decide whether there is nonunion of a hip fracture. Tomograms are useful in establishing the diagnosis (Fig 26–1). Occasionally, push-pull films are helpful in diagnosis.

Progressively increasing radiolucency around metallic devices (the windshield-wiper sign) is strongly suggestive of nonunion (see Fig 26–1,A).

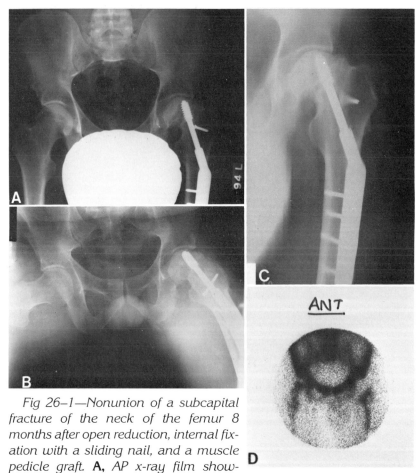

Fig 26–1—Nonunion of a subcapital fracture of the neck of the femur 8 months after open reduction, internal fixation with a sliding nail, and a muscle pedicle graft. **A,** *AP x-ray film showing varus deformity. Note "windshield-wiper" sign. Osseous union is questionable.* **B,** *lateral x-ray film does not show evidence of nonunion.* **C,** *tomogram showing radiolucent line at fracture site, evidence of a nonunion.* **D,** *technetium 99m sulfur colloid scan showing no activity in the femoral head.*

Bone scans can be helpful in establishing a diagnosis of nonunion. A technetium 99m MDP bone scan will show increased uptake at the fracture line in a healing fracture. A pseudarthrosis will have a radiolucent area in the center of the fracture. Frequently there will be increased uptake on both sides of the radiolucency.

TREATMENT

There are several treatment options for delayed union and nonunion of hip fractures. Renailing the fracture (Fig 26–2), or renailing with osteotomy when there is a deformity, have advocates (Fig 26–3). The procedures frequently require augmentation with a bone graft. Replacement arthroplasty is a popular operation for the ununited hip fracture in the elderly.

The Girdlestone procedure is reserved for some patients with infected nonunion and for severely debilitated individuals with severe pain as a consequence of the nonunion.

Renailing

Renailing as the principal treatment for ununited hip fractures without addition of a bone graft is rarely justified. However, occasionally renailing in conjunction with a valgus osteotomy will be successful. The latter should not be the procedure of choice without augmentation with a bone graft when nonunion is established. However, it may be an acceptable alternative for delayed union.

Renailing should be considered soon after the initial operation as a measure to prevent nonunion if reduction is lost, impaction cannot be maintained, or the fixation shifts.

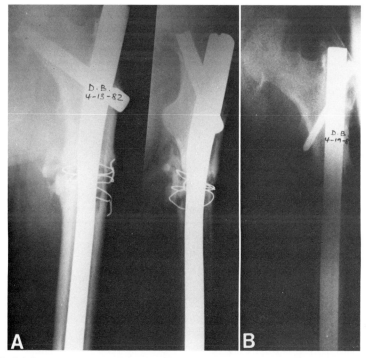

*Fig 26–2—**A,** nonunion of the subtrochanteric fracture after Zickel nailing. **B,** fracture renailed with interlocking nail and augmented with iliac bone graft.*

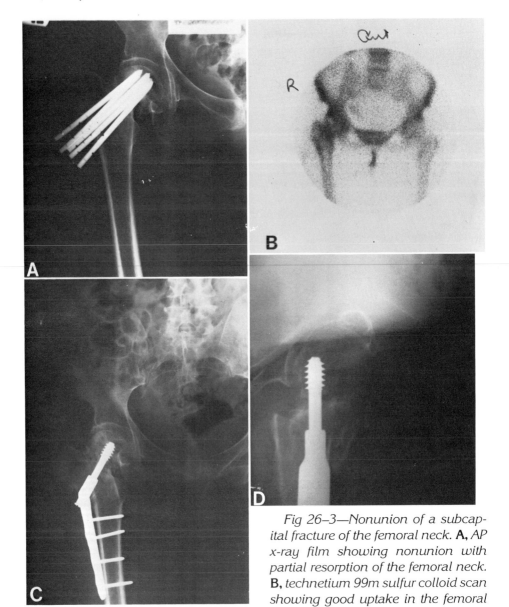

*Fig 26–3—Nonunion of a subcapital fracture of the femoral neck. **A,** AP x-ray film showing nonunion with partial resorption of the femoral neck. **B,** technetium 99m sulfur colloid scan showing good uptake in the femoral head. **C,** AP x-ray film after subtrochanteric osteotomy and internal fixation with a sliding nail. Note valgus position of the head fragment. **D,** lateral x-ray film after osteotomy and internal fixation.*

Osteotomy

Valgus osteotomy can eliminate shearing stress at the fracture site and introduce a compression force that facilitates osseous union. Pauwels reported significant increases in the rate of nonunion of intracapsular hip fractures as the angle of inclination of the fracture approached 70° (see Fig 4–1).[11]

Valgus osteotomy at the subtrochanteric level, in addition to renailing with or without a bone graft, has been particularly effective in treating nonunion of the femoral neck in the presence of a viable head and in treating intertrochanteric fractures that have migrated into a varus position (Figs 26–3 and 26–4).

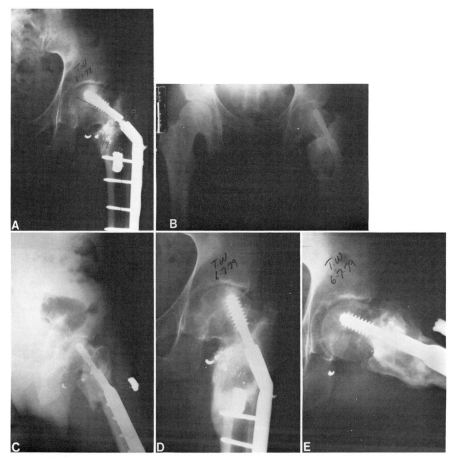

Fig 26–4—Nonunion of an intertrochanteric fracture of the hip. **A,** *AP x-ray film showing nonunion and broken nail.* **B,** *AP x-ray film after subtrochanteric osteotomy and renailing. Note valgus position of the proximal fragment.* **C,** *lateral x-ray film obtained postoperatively.* **D,** *AP x-ray film obtained 10 months after osteotomy and renailing, showing union of fracture and osteotomy.* **E,** *lateral x-ray film obtained 10 months after osteotomy and renailing.*

The operative procedure is done through a lateral approach. An incision is made over the lateral aspect of the thigh, beginning over the greater trochanter and proceeding distally for approximately 15 cm. The incision is developed through the subcutaneous tissue. The vastus lateralis muscle is severed at its origin at the base of the greater trochanter and elevated from the lateral aspect of the femur. Previous metal fixation devices are removed. A 140°–150° angle sliding nail is then inserted into the center of the head or the inferior half close to the subchondral surface. This is done without disturbing the area of delayed union or nonunion (Fig 26–5,A).

A dome osteotomy is then performed about 1–2 cm below the lesser trochanter (see Fig 26–5,A). Drill holes are made in a curvilinear pattern on the anterior surface of the femur. These are connected with an osteotome, creating a fracture at this level. The distal portion of the femur is then rotated laterally until it meets the side plate of the sliding nail (Fig 26–5,B). It is necessary to remove a small portion of the lateral cortex on the distal fragment to allow for the necessary rotation of the distal fragment (see Fig 26–5,A). Screws are then inserted through the nail plate into the distal fragment, securing the fixation.

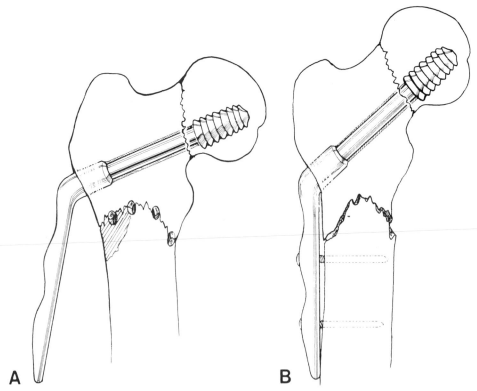

A   B

*Fig 26–5—Subtrochanteric osteotomy and nailing procedure for nonunion with deformity. **A** shows an ununited femoral neck fracture. The nonunion line is vertical. The nail is placed in the head and neck at the desired level. A dome pattern is outlined with drill holes and the osteotomy is then completed by connecting the drill holes with an osteotome. The shaded area on the superior, lateral aspect of the distal fragment must be removed to allow coaptation of the osteotomy fragments after rotation. **B,** final valgus position of the fragments with nail in place. Note fracture line in the compression mode.*

Postoperatively, the patient can be ambulatory on crutches or a walker without weight-bearing for several weeks. Usually partial weight-bearing can be resumed within 6 weeks. In addition to renailing and osteotomy, various bone grafting techniques, iliac bone grafts, fibular bone grafts, and the muscle pedicle graft may be utilized to stimulate osseous union. Intertrochanteric osteotomy and nail fixation without a bone graft for nonunion of the femoral neck when there is a viable head has been advocated by Kostuik.[9]

Dooly and Hopper recently reported satisfactory results in the treatment of fractures of the hip, both intracapsular and extracapsular, with internal fixation and a fibular bone graft.[15] In a few cases osteotomy was added to the procedure, although the authors concluded this was not necessary for a satisfactory result.

Hemiarthroplasty

Hemiarthroplasty is a procedure easily performed by skilled orthopedic surgeons, and many believe that the problem of the "unsolved fracture" has been solved by the use of this technique. Most reports in the literature describe failures in more than one third of all fresh fractures treated by hemiarthroplasty. Hemiarthroplasty has been carried over to the treatment of delayed union and nonunion of hip fractures. It must be reemphasized that the patient with a viable femoral head and osseous union of a hip fracture will have a superior result, compared to the result achieved with arthroplasty. The unacceptable failure rate with hemiarthroplasty should challenge the complacent attitude of many surgeons toward the solution of this particularly difficult fracture and should encourage a more aggressive approach to securing union and preserving the femoral head.

Total Hip Replacement

Total hip replacement is the treatment of choice in the elderly patient with nonunion of a femoral neck fracture. Occasionally total hip arthroplasty is required in ununited intertrochanteric fractures. Special devices must be used to obtain satisfactory arthroplasty at this level.

Girdlestone Operation

The Girdlestone procedure is occasionally necessary to control severe pain in the extremely debilitated patient. It is a viable procedure for the chronically infected nonunion.

Electrical Stimulation

Electrical stimulation may have a place in the treatment of delayed union or nonunion of hip fractures. The noninvasive techniques are preferred. However, electrical stimulation will not correct deformities. Osteotomy to correct the deformity requires an invasive procedure, and therefore bone grafting, and internal fixation is preferred to enhance the possibility of achieving osseous union.

Personal Preference for Treatment

I prefer renailing and subtrochanteric osteotomy augmented by an iliac bone graft for delayed union or nonunion of intracapsular fractures when the head is viable. A muscle pedicle bone graft is added to the procedure in selected patients when the head is nonviable. Arthroplasty, either hemi or total, is utilized to treat nonunion in the debilitated patient and the patient with a short life expectancy or serious disease that will not permit him or her to participate in the postoperative rehabilitation program. A cemented bipolar device is preferred when hemiarthroplasty is selected for treatment of a nonunion or delayed union. As more experience is gained with cementless replacements, now evolving, the need for cement in young patients will diminish. However, cement will still have a place in hemiarthroplasty for the older osteoporotic patient with a wide intramedullary canal.

Iliac bone grafting and renailing is the preferred treatment for delayed union or nonunion of the basal neck and intertrochanteric area. Osteotomy, internal fixation, and an iliac bone graft is the treatment of choice when a deformity is present.

Nonunion of subtrochanteric fractures is treated by renailing with a sliding nail plate or Zickel nail plus iliac bone grafting.

MALUNION

Malunion is a frequent complication of hip fractures. In the elderly patient this may be a result of failure to seek early medical attention after injury, or it may be a complication of surgical treatment. The general condition of the patient may not permit treatment for several weeks, and the soft bones in older patients makes it difficult to obtain firm fixation of the fracture fragments, allowing subsequent shifting of the pieces and union in malposition. Poor surgical technique is an additional factor resulting in malunion. Malunion in children was discussed in chapter 11.

The deformity is usually one of external rotation, coxa vara, and shortening. An internal rather than external rotatory deformity sometimes follows malreduction during open reduction and internal fixation. In untreated cases the rotatory deformity is almost always in external rotation. Shortening of more than 2.5 cm may require surgical lengthening of the femur, although in the very old patient who is minimally or moderately active, satisfactory function is possible, with a deficiency of as much as 5 cm, using a heel and sole lift.

Malunion Following Intracapsular Fractures

The position of malunion is almost always in varus and external rotation, with shortening rarely exceeding 2.5 cm. The decrease in length is due to the varus position and in part to partial absorption of the fracture surfaces prior to union.

Some disability accompanies the deformity. The patient usually limps and may have mild pain. Some form of external support may be necessary to permit ambulation. Surgical correction of the malunion and leg length discrepancy depends on the age, complaints, and needs of the patient. Most elderly patients can function at an acceptable level with the deformity. Others may have sufficient pain to require corrective surgery for relief. Patients older than 60 years are better served with an arthroplasty, either hemi or total. An osteotomy should be considered in the younger patient. In my experience either a wedge or a dome osteotomy (see Fig 26–5) is the procedure of choice to correct varus angulation or rotation. The change from varus angulation to normal or valgus angulation will restore some length, possibly as much as 2.0 cm, leaving a 0.5-cm discrepancy or less. That is an acceptable length.

Cervicotrochanteric Malunion

Coxa vara, external rotation of the distal fragment, and shortening occurs at this level. Shortening may reach as much as 5 cm. Severe disability in the older patient requires surgical correction of the varus angulation and malrotation by osteotomy and internal fixation with an angled nail plate. Correction of shortening of more than 2.5 cm necessitates a major procedure with skeletal traction or one of the various external devices such as the Wagner apparatus. Most elderly patients will not tolerate the leg-lengthening procedure, so osteotomy and internal fixation without an attempt at correction of the leg-length discrepancy ordinarily suffices. Younger patients may be considered for the osteotomy, internal fixation, and leg-lengthening procedure.

The wedge or dome osteotomy and correction of leg length with a Wagner device is my preference.

Tenotomy of tight hip adductors may be necessary to facilitate correction of the deformity after osteotomy.

Trochanteric Malunion

Malunion with internal or external rotation, coxa vara, and shortening of 2.5 cm or less can be corrected by a subtrochanteric wedge or dome osteotomy. The osteotomy can be done with an opening or closing wedge. I prefer the dome osteotomy. Occasionally an open wedge osteotomy is selected to provide some correction of shortening. Internal fixation with a nail plate is used to maintain stability.

Extreme shortening of 5 cm or more is present in some cases and the surgeon will have to consider the patient's age, functional status, and complaints in making a decision whether to add a lengthening procedure to the operation or to accept the leg-length discrepancy.

Tenotomy of the hip adductors may be necessary in some cases.

Subtrochanteric Malunion

In most cases dome osteotomy and internal fixation will provide a satisfactory solution to the problem.

REFERENCES

1. King T.: The closed operation for intracapsular fracture of the neck of the femur: Final result in recent and old cases. *Br. J. Surg.* 26:721, 1938-1939.
2. Reich R.S.: Ununited fracture of the neck of the femur treated by high oblique osteotomy. *J. Bone Joint Surg.* 23:141-158, 1941.
3. Bonfiglio M., Bordenstein M.B.: Treatment by bone grafting of aseptic necrosis of the femoral head and nonunion of the femoral neck (Phemister technique). *J. Bone Joint Surg.* 40A:1329-1346, 1968.
4. Caladruccio R.A.: Comparison of specimens from nonunion of neck of the femur with fresh fractures and avascular necrosis specimens. *J. Bone Joint Surg.* 45A:1471, 1963.
5. Henderson M.S.: Ununited fracture of the neck of the femur treated by the aid of the bone graft. *J. Bone Joint Surg.* 22:97-106, 1940.
6. Sherman M.S., Phemister M.D.: The pathology of untreated fractures of the neck of the femur. *J. Bone Joint Surg.* 29:19-40, 1947.
7. Coventry M.B.: Indications for prosthetic replacement. *Instr. Course Lect.* 16:292, 1959.
8. Eftekhar N.S.: Status of femoral head replacement in treating fracture of femoral neck. *Orthop. Rev.* 2:19-30, 1973.
9. Kostuik J.P.: Intertrochanteric osteotomy in non-union of femoral neck fractures. *Can. J. Surg.* 11:499-505, 1968.
10. Meyers M.H., Harvey J.P. Jr., Moore T.M.: Delayed treatment of subcapital and transcervical fractures of the neck of the femur with internal fixation and a muscle pedicle bone graft. *Orthop. Clin. North Am.* 5:743-756, 1974.
11. Pauwels F.: Der Schenkelhadsbruch: Ein mechanisches Problem. Grundlagen des Heilungsvorganges Prognose und kausale Therapie. *Beilag. Z. Orthop. Chirurg.*, 1935.
12. Senn N.: Fractures of the neck of the femur with special reference to bony union after intracapsular fracture. *Trans. Am. Surg. Assoc.* 1:333-441, 1883.
13. Banks H.H.: Tissue response at the fracture site in femoral neck fractures. *Clin. Orthop.* 61:116-128, 1968.
14. Banks H.H.: Non-union in fractures of the femoral neck. *Orthop. Clin. North Am.* 5:865-885, 1974.
15. Dooley B.J., Hooper J.: Fibular bone grafting for nonunion of fracture of the neck of the femur. *Aust. NZ J. Surg.* 52:134-140, 1982.

Chapter 27

Malignant Pathologic Fractures About the Hip Joint

Kevin D. Harrington, M.D.

The incidence of pathologic fractures about the hip joint has increased markedly in the past two decades as aggressive palliative treatment of established metastatic malignancies by means of hormonal manipulation, chemotherapy, and radiotherapy, has resulted in markedly extended patient survival. The mean survival for patients following a first long bone pathologic fracture improved from 7.2 months in 1966 to 18.8 months in 1982.[1-5] When pathologic fractures are analyzed by origin of the primary malignancy, those patients with pathologic fractures from metastatic carcinoma of the breast, the most common metastatic lesion in bone, had a mean survival of 22.6 months.[1] Patients with pathologic fractures secondary to primary tumors in the prostate and kidneys had mean survival times of 29.3 and 11.8 months, respectively. In contrast, patients with lung primaries still have a mean survival of less than 4 months.[1]

The reasonable anticipation of prolonged survival in selected patients engendered new enthusiasm among orthopedic surgeons for undertaking extensive reconstructive procedures necessitated by metastatic bone destruction about major weight-bearing joints. Approximately three quarters of malignant pathologic fractures requiring operative fixation occur about the hip joint.[1] With respect to operative and reparative techniques, these may be subdivided into fractures of the femoral neck, intertrochanteric and subtrochanteric fractures, combined fractures of the proximal femur, and fractures of the acetabulum. In addition, it is appropriate to consider prophylactic fixation of destructive lesions in the acetabulum or the proximal femur, where the risk of fracture is high.

FEMORAL NECK FRACTURES

Fractures involving the femoral neck are rarely amenable to internal fixation because ordinarily there is insufficient bone remaining in the proximal femur to allow adequate fixation of the fracture fragments by any technique. Consequently, prosthetic replacement is the treatment of choice in more than 90% of cases.

Important technical principles of prosthetic replacement include the following: (1) reestablishment of rigid contact between the prosthesis and the distal femoral neck, with interposed methylmethacrylate used only when absolutely necessary; (2) the use of a long-stemmed prosthesis, ideally 10–12 inches long, both to enhance intramedullary fixation and prophylactically to reinforce the femoral shaft, frequently also involved by tumor; (3) restoration of femoral length, both to minimize leg length discrepancy and to ensure hip joint stability. Failure to adhere to these principles will result in the type of complication illustrated in Figure 27–1,A.

The operative procedure is performed with the patient in the lateral decubitus position and using a Moore or modified Gibson posterolateral approach to the hip joint. Transection of the greater trochanter is rarely necessary. The femoral canal is rasped and curretted and the tumor debulked as thoroughly as possible to enhance the efficacy of postoperative irradiation.[6] After the femoral canal has been prepared the prosthesis is fitted into place and the hip reduced. The correct seating of the prosthesis within the shaft is checked by direct vision to evaluate both limb length and joint stability. If the reduced hip is unstable and dislocates easily, usual causes include inappropriate rotation of the prosthesis, impingement between bony prominences secondary to limb deformity, and, most commonly, inadequate restoration of femoral length. If limb length must be recreated, this can be performed easily using a custom-made prosthesis or by interposing methylmethacrylate between the apron of the prosthesis and the structurally adequate remaining femoral cortex. The latter alternative, assuming a long-stemmed prosthesis is used, has given results equal to those achieved with the custom-made prosthesis.[1] The methylmethacrylate can be molded about the flanged upper stem of the prosthesis by wrapping a malleable hard rubber dam around and above the proximal part of the femur to hold the acrylic in a form approximating the proximal femoral cortex (Figs 27–1,B and C).

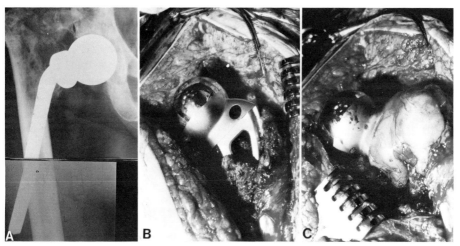

*Fig 27–1—***A,** *pathologic fracture due to primary carcinoma of the breast. Prosthetic replacement of the proximal femur failed because the bone in the cortex of the medial femoral neck did not support the prosthesis and was displaced. The distal prosthetic stem also penetrated through the tumor-infiltrated femoral shaft. (From Parrish F.F., Murray J.A.: Surgical treatment for secondary neoplastic fractures: A retrospective study of ninety-six patients. J. Bone Joint Surg. 52A:665-686, 1970. Reproduced by permission.)* **B,** *operative view during prosthetic replacement of the left proximal femur. Tumor and structurally weak bone have been resected, and a Moore prosthesis has been inserted. The prosthesis is unstable because there is no contact between the remaining bone and the apron of the prosthesis.* **C,** *methylmethacrylate has been poured into the medullary canal and built up around the upper stem of the prosthesis, thereby reestablishing structural continuity.*

The production of heat great enough to burn surrounding tissues has never been reported, although when large volumes of acrylic cement are used, the bed must be irrigated with cool saline during the later stages of polymerization.

Before the prosthesis is cemented in place, the hip joint is relocated and the limb distracted to an appropriate length so that the surgeon can determine under direct vision the amount of methylmethacrylate that must be built up under the apron of the prosthesis and the femoral shaft to obtain the appropriate limb length.

An attempt is made to fill the entire femoral medullary canal with methylmethacrylate. Occasionally a 0.5-cm hole can be drilled percutaneously through the distal femoral cortex and a vacuum created in the medullary canal, using suction, to enhance filling of the distal femoral canal with cement. The use of low-viscosity acrylic cement injected under pressure through a long nozzle syringe enhances this filling.

Attempting to reconstitute the missing cortical bone by bone grafting is futile because such a graft is rarely incorporated unless at least 1 year has elapsed since the completion of local radiotherapy.[7] Similarly, attempts to transplant the greater trochanter distally in an effort to improve joint stability are inadvisable, as the osteotomized trochanter often does not heal at the new site of its attachment owing to the effects of radiation therapy.

If, after placement of a prosthesis, the stem has perforated a weakened area in the femoral shaft (see Fig 27–1,A), the prosthesis should be removed and replaced with one having a longer stem. The perforation must be exposed under direct vision to ensure that all residual acrylic from the original prosthesis has been removed and that the new longer stem has passed the weakened area of bone without reperforating the cortex. Moreover, the cement can be injected into the distal femur more effectively through the perforation than through the more proximal femoral canal.

Lytic lesions of the femoral diaphysis that develop some time after the insertion of the proximal prosthesis can be stabilized by inserting an intermedullary Kuntscher nail retrograde through the femoral interchondylar notch (by a knee arthrotomy).[7] The fixation can be reinforced by methylmethacrylate, also injected retrograde. However, such a potential complication is better anticipated at the time of the original prosthetic placement by using a long-stemmed prosthesis and reinforcing the entire femoral shaft.

Prophylactic antibiotic irrigation is used intraoperatively, and systemic cephalosporins are administered prophylactically immediately preoperatively and for 48 hours postoperatively.

INTERTROCHANTERIC FRACTURES

Fractures across the intertrochanteric femur are the most common pathologic fractures secondary to metastatic malignancy. Lytic changes within the greater trochanter are common in patients with metastatic bone disease, approaching a 50% incidence in patients dying of cancer.[2, 8] When a trochanteric lytic focus becomes associated with similar lytic destruction of the lesser trochanter or medial cortex, the two areas may become connected by a fracture through relatively intact cortical and cancellous bone between. Because of the loss of cortical continuity medially, the proximal head neck fragment tends to angle into a varus position (Fig 27–2,A).

Conventional fracture fixation (by a nail plate device with its fulcrum of stress *lateral* to the fracture site) usually is doomed to eventual failure unless reconstruction of the *medial* cortical stability is achieved as well (Figs 27–2,B and C).[4, 8] It must be reiterated that most such fractures are irradiated, and that failure of bony union following irradiation is the rule rather than the exception.[6, 9, 10] Therefore, even the

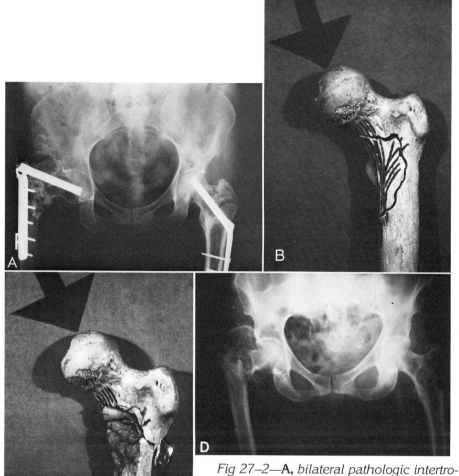

*Fig 27–2—**A,** bilateral pathologic intertro-chanteric fracture due to primary carcinoma of the breast. An attempt at internal fixation of the right hip fracture using a conventional nail and plate device resulted in severe varus malalignment and a nonunion of the fracture. The nail plate device failed because the fracture reduction-fixation had inadequate support along the medial cortex. (From Parrish F.F., Murray J.A.: Surgical treatment for secondary neoplastic fractures: A retrospective study of ninety-six patients. **J. Bone Joint Surg.** 52A:665-686, 1970. Reproduced by permission.) **B,** cadavar femur demonstrating an area of bone deficit where bone is typically destroyed by metastatic tumor. The primary compressive trabeculae along the medial neck cortex have been disrupted. Conventional fixation of the ensuing fracture would fail to correct this structural defect, and normal stresses of weight-bearing or muscle pull across the hip would favor angulation of the proximal fragment into varus. **C,** the structural defect has been filled with methylmethacrylate, which has the single asset of great compressive strength (15,000 psi), preventing varus angulation of the fracture. **D,** AP view of the pelvis of a woman, aged 72 years, with metastatic melanoma. There is a pathologic fracture through the base of the right femoral neck with extensive destruction of cortical bone proximally and distally. Prophylactic internal fixation of the left proximal femur is indicated because of destruction of most of the trochanteric cortical and cancellous bone by tumor lysis.*

strongest nail plate device will fail eventually if continual motion at the fracture site is not prevented.

Intermedullary fixation devices, such as the Zickel nail,[11] may be considered, but rarely with an intertrochanteric fracture is there sufficiently strong bone remaining in the proximal fragment to ensure adequate fixation. In instances of extremely advanced tumor lysis at the intertrochanteric fracture site (Fig 27–2,D) replacement of the proximal shaft by a specialized prosthesis may be required. However, whenever salvage of the femoral head by fracture fixation is possible, that technique is preferable to the use of a large custom-made prosthesis with its increased risk of infection, dislocation, loosening, and metal failure.

Ideally, medial cortical stability should be reconstituted using methylmethacrylate. This acrylic possesses excellent resistance to compression loads and, when combined with the excellent torque and shear strength inherent in the compression hip screw, affords secure and lasting fixation (see Fig 27–2,C).[1, 7, 12-14]

The technique for fixation begins with a closed reduction of the fracture on a standard fracture table and using image intensification for control. A conventional lateral approach is used and the vastus lateralis is elevated to expose the greater trochanter and femoral shaft distal to it. A 1.5-cm window is created in the lateral cortex just distal to the greater trochanter. With a rongeur and curet, the structurally inadequate bone and gross tumor tissue are removed as thoroughly as possible in order to debulk the tumor mass and to afford space for methylmethacrylate to fill the ensuing defect. In the conventional manner, a smooth Steinmann pin is inserted through the window into the femoral head and neck and its position confirmed as central within the head by both anteroposterior and lateral roentgenographic views. The corkscrew portion of a compression hip screw is then inserted over the Steinmann pin as far proximally into the femoral neck as possible.

A side plate of appropriate length (usually a five-hole side plate) is inserted over the proximal hip screw, with care taken to ensure that no impediments exist to positioning the plate against the lateral femoral cortex. Plate positioning should be practiced several times so that no delay will occur in placement once the acrylic cement has been injected within the medullary canal.

The methylmethacrylate is injected in liquid form as far proximally as possible around the shaft of the compression screw, and distally to a point well below the level of the destroyed medial cortex. With counterpressure exerted against the soft tissues of the medial side to minimize extrusion of the soft cement outside the medullary canal, the cement is digitally packed into the medial cortical defect. The side plate is then reapplied and clamped into place until polymerization of the cement is complete. It is inadvisable to drill holes for screw fixation of the side plate until the cement is quite hard, because prior to polymerization of the methylmethacrylate the drill bit will tend to bind in the adhesive cement mass and break. In contrast, solid acrylic cement can be drilled and tapped in the same manner as cortical bone.

SUBTROCHANTERIC FRACTURES

The highest incidence of fixation failure has occurred with subtrochanteric fractures, whether or not methylmethacrylate is used as an adjunct to such fixation. It appears that this is primarily because such fractures, unlike those of the intertrochanteric region, often involve extensive destruction of cortical bone circumferentially, and often over an extended length of the proximal femoral shaft (Fig 27–3). In such instances even intermedullary acrylic offers little restoration of medial cortical stability against weight-bearing varus stress.

Subtrochanteric fractures are not amenable to fixation with a nail plate device, even if augmented by acrylic cement. The torque and shear forces on the relatively weak side plate at the subtrochanteric level eventually lead to metal failure (see Fig 27–3,A). In addition, subtrochanteric fractures frequently occur in conjunction with metastatic lesions elsewhere in the femoral shaft. Prophylactic fixation of the entire shaft before the institution of radiotherapy is advisable in such instances.

Consideration of these factors warrants intermedullary fixation of subtrochanteric fractures using a device that not only reinforces the femoral shaft, but also reinforces the proximal intertrochanteric region and femoral neck as well. The Zickel nail is ideal for this purpose (Fig 27–3,B).[11]

For insertion of a Zickel nail, the patient is positioned on a standard operating table in the lateral decubitus position and with the affected leg draped free. An incision is made over the greater trochanter and the femoral cortex is penetrated at the superomedial aspect of the greater trochanter. Care should be taken not to penetrate the neck medial to the trochanteric sulcus for fear of further weakening bone that is probably already affected by tumor lysis. The intramedullary canal is reamed ante-

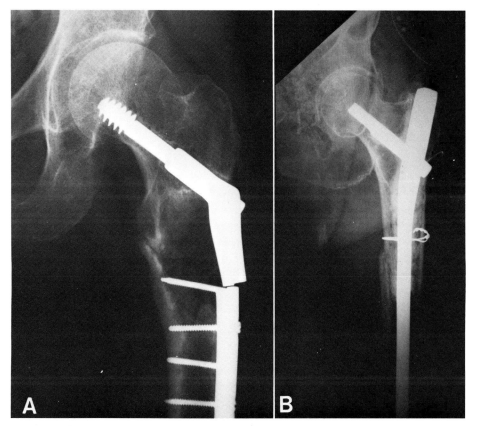

*Fig 27–3—**A,** solitary myeloma with extensive circumferential cortical bone loss. An attempt at fixation with a compression hip screw and methylmethacrylate failed because of insufficient bone stalk. An intramedullary device such as a Zickel nail would have been a better choice, with methylmethacrylate augmentation to minimize the risk of shortening. **B,** subtrochanteric fracture of the right femur secondary to extensive cortical bone destruction from metastatic carcinoma of the breast. The fracture has been internally fixed with a Zickel nail augmented by radiolucent methylmethacrylate.*

grade, up to 15 mm in the diaphysis and 17 mm in the intertrochanteric region, if possible.

If there is an extensive loss of cortical bone, the fracture site itself is exposed and curetted so that the defect may be filled with methylmethacrylate to prevent telescoping of the major bony fragments.

Prior to insertion of the cement, the Zickel nail should be inserted antegrade until its tip is visible at the fracture site when viewed from below. The lytic focus and the distal femoral canal are filled with methylmethacrylate and the Zickel nail is driven across the soft mass prior to its polymerization. It is not necessary to fill the proximal canal with methylmethacrylate because the bulk of the Zickel nail at its upper end together with the proximal fixation nail prevents rotation of the proximal fragment. The canal should be filled with cement distally, however, because the Zickel nail tapers at its lower end and prevention of rotation is thereby minimized.

When a subtrochanteric pathologic fracture has been internally fixed by a nail plate device which then failed, removal of the hardware is appropriate rather than attempting to reinforce the failed fixation by the application of additional side plates. If intermedullary methylmethacrylate was used at the time of the original (failed) fixation, the cement may be removed by exposing the fracture site and morselizing the acrylic with a small, straight osteotome and rongeur. Use of a high-speed power burr is inadvisable under these circumstances because the burr easily penetrates the weakened femoral cortex above and below the actual fracture.

FRACTURES OF THE ACETABULUM

Pathologic fractures involving the acetabulum occur because of destructive osteolysis of the acetabular rim, superior dome, medial wall, or a combination of these areas. Although open reduction and fixation of such a fracture may appear advisable on occasion, the reader should be cautioned that the extent of bony lysis always is greater than can be appreciated on roentgenograms and that efforts to reinforce such fixation by bone grafting are fruitless in the face of local irradiation.[9, 15] Consequently, the basic mode of reconstruction for such fractures should be total hip arthroplasty whenever possible. However, specialized techniques are required to ensure that the prosthetic acetabular component does not loosen or migrate but remains securely fixed to the remaining intact periacetabular ilial bone stock (Fig 27–4,A). The simple expedient of replacing the tumor-destroyed periacetabular bone with methylmethacrylate (Fig 27–4,B) is inappropriate. It leads to rapid loosening of the acetabular component because the acrylic has poor resistance to shear stresses and because there has been no reconstitution of weight-bearing support from the acetabulum across the medial ilium and sacroiliac joint and into the sacrum.

The most frequent complication occurring in periacetabular lytic lesions is due to failure to appreciate the extent of bone destruction or the risk of fracture before instituting prophylactic radiotherapy. During the early stages of radiation, a temporary but sometimes pronounced hyperemic softening occurs in the periace-tabular bone, particularly along the medial wall. This often results in a secondary protrusio deformity of the medial wall (Fig 27–4,C). This effect must be taken into account when reconstructive techniques are assessed. Moreover, in addition to its effect in temporarily weakening bone, local radiotherapy also effectively blocks bone healing in most instances, thereby negating the possibility of using bone graft or osteotomies to reinforce fixation of the prosthetic acetabular component.

The reconstruction must be fashioned so that subsequent weight-bearing stresses will be transmitted from the acetabular component into some area of strong bone capable of withstanding weight-bearing load and thereby capable of preventing migration of the prosthesis. To accomplish this aim, the condition of the acetabulum should be rated in one of the following classes, and reconstruction pursued accordingly:

Class I: Lateral cortices and superior and medial walls are all structurally intact (Fig 27–4,D).

Class II: Medial wall deficiency (see Fig 27–4,C).

Class III: Lateral cortices and superior walls are deficient (Fig 27–4,E).

Class I

Patients with class I fractures of the acetabulum, although often showing extensive invasion of bone by metastases, have sufficient unaffected periacetabular bone that conventional fixation of the acetabular component will result in no higher than usual an incidence of loosening or migration. If the extent of medial wall or acetabular rib involvement is in question, a computerized tomographic scan of the hip often is helpful in assessing the extent of tumor lysis. On occasion a technetium bone scan will reveal extensive tumor invasion of the affected hemipelvis, although plain roentgenograms may not suggest major destruction of the weight-bearing dome or medial wall. In such instances it would not be inappropriate to assign the fracture to class III for reconstructive purposes.

In most instances of prosthetic loosening following reconstruction for class I lesions of the acetabulum, there has been extensive and/or progressive superior or medial wall destruction. In the unusual event of acetabular component loosening and bony destruction definitely of class I severity only, revision of the hip arthroplasty should be performed, following the principles widely espoused for revision of any conventional total hip arthroplasty.

Class II

Patients with class II fracture of the acetabulum have in common a loss of structural continuity of the medial acetabular wall. However, the superior wall, the roof of the acetabulum, and the lateral cortices of the ilium, ischium, and pubis adjacent to the acetabulum (acetabular rim) are structurally intact.

Conventional seating and fixation of an acetabular component under these circumstances is associated with a high incidence of medial migration and loosening. As illustrated in Figure 27–4,A, the use of mesh reinforcement along the medial wall cannot be considered a deterrent to such migration.

The Oh-Harris protrusio shell (see Fig 27–5,D) is employed in order to transmit the stresses of weight-bearing on the acetabular component completely away from the deficient medial acetabular wall and onto the intact rim of the acetabulum. Mesh may be placed along the medial wall in some instances as well, but only in an effort to minimize cement extrusion into the pelvis.

Class III

Patients with class III fracture of the acetabulum have in common a loss of structural continuity not only of the medial acetabular wall, but also of the superior acetabular roof and acetabular rim as well (see Fig 27–4,E). In most instances there is extensive lysis of the ischium and/or pubis, making the inferior acetabular rim functionally nonexistent. Effective fixation of the acetabular prosthetic component in

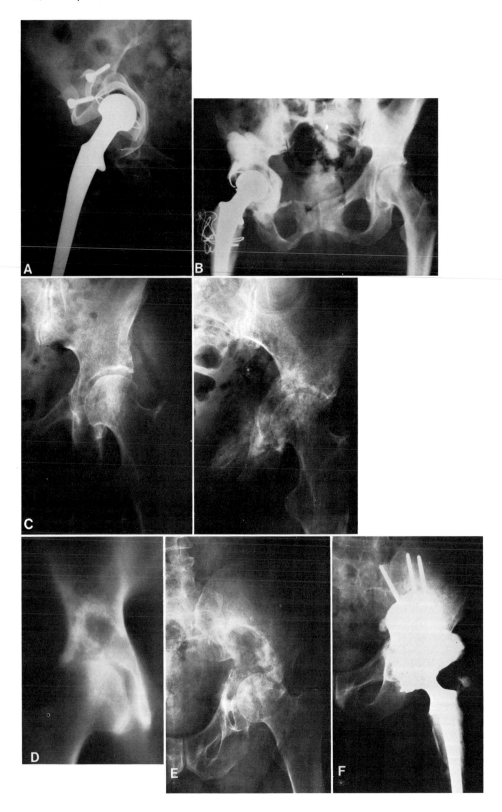

its normal location would be impossible even using the Oh-Harris protrusio ring because fixation of the acetabular component depends on transmission of the weight-bearing load onto structurally intact bone of the ilium and sacrum well superior to the area of tumor lysis.

The reconstruction of a hip joint for a class III lesion is an extremely challenging undertaking. At operation, gross tumor tissue and bone fragments should be removed until structurally intact bone can be palpated superiorly. This usually results in the creation of a large cavity within the supra-acetabular ilium as well as exposure of an extensive defect of the medial wall (Figs 27–5,A–C). Once all tumor tissue and destroyed bone have been removed, the importance of transmitting acetabular weight-bearing into the intact bone of the upper ilium and sacrum is more apparent.

Large-threaded Steinmann pins are drilled from the upper reaches of the defect into the good bone of the superior ilium, particularly along the medial rim of the ilium and across the sacroiliac joint into the lateral sacrum. An attempt is made to curve the flexible pins during the drilling, thereby allowing them to follow the concavity of the intermedullary space of the ilium (Figs 27–4,F and 27–5,C–E). In most instances positioning the pins so that their longitudinal axis follows the normal weight-bearing stress lines of the ilium and across the sacroiliac joint into the sacrum is preferable.

Once the threaded pins are in place, their distal ends should be cut off so as just barely to avoid interference with the normal positioning of the protrusio ring and of the acetabular prosthetic component. It is often difficult to position the pro-

---

*Fig 27–4—**A,** AP view of the right hip in a patient undergoing hip replacement for a pathologic fracture of the medial acetabular wall. The surgeon attempted to achieve fixation of the acetabular component by a combination of mesh and methylmethacrylate. Medial and superior migration of the component has occurred. **B,** an attempt was made to bridge an area of extensive bone loss using methylmethacrylate alone for fixation of the acetabular component. Predictably, loosening of the acetabular component occurred soon after weight-bearing began, with eventual migration superomedially. **C,** AP view of the left hip of a woman, aged 52 years, with metastatic carcinoma of the rectum. A lytic infiltration of the medial acetabular wall with a minimally displaced fracture is apparent. Six weeks later, after the completion of local irradiation (4,000 rad), there was more extensive lysis and softening of the bone, with displacement of the femoral head. Protrusio has resulted from softening of the bone caused by a combination of tumor lysis and postirradiation hyperemia. **D,** AP tomogram of the right hip of a 40-year-old patient with metastatic cylindroma of the submaxillary gland. The patient complained of severe pain in the right hip on weight-bearing. Conventional AP x-ray films revealed blastic changes in the supra-acetabular ilium but no evidence of destruction of the weight-bearing dome of the acetabulum. **E,** AP view of the left hip of a man, aged 51 years, with metastatic carcinoma of the adrenal cortex. Extensive lytic destruction of the supra-acetabular bone is apparent, with migration of the femoral head proximally. **F,** 18 months after resection of the destroyed bone and tumor and hip replacement, the acetabular component remains securely fixed to the pelvis by a combination of threaded Steinmann pins, wire mesh, a protrusio shell, and methylmethacrylate. The lucent halo above the cement mass was apparent from the time of surgery. Lack of apparent loosening of the fixation pins attests to the stability of fixation.*

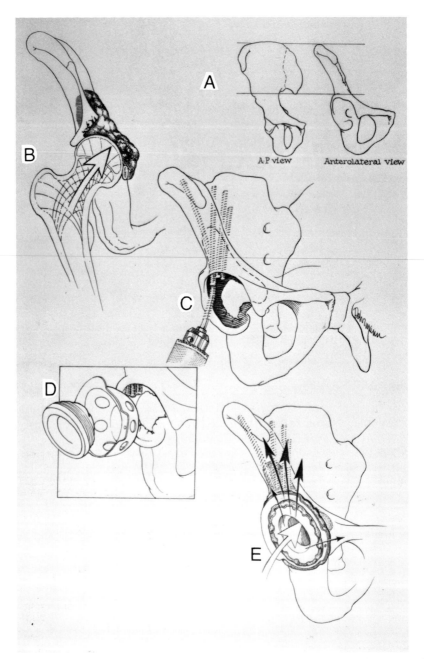

*Fig 27–5—**A,** anterolateral view of the pelvis demonstrating the thinness of the ilium superior to the acetabulum. **B,** tumor has destroyed the superior and medial acetabular bone, leaving minimal intact cortex for fixation of the acetabulum component. **C,** after tumor tissue is resected, large threaded Steinmann pins can be driven from the periacetabular cavity into the structurally sound bone of the superior ilium and across the sacroiliac joint. **D,** acetabular component as it sits in the protrusio shell. **E,** the combination of acetabular cup, protrusio shell, and Steinmann pins incorporated into methylmethacrylate effectively transmits weight-bearing stresses onto the strong bone of the ilial wing and sacrum.*

trusio ring in the presence of the Steinmann pins and it may be necessary to use a vice-grip pliers to twist the pins and force them deeper into the upper ilial bone. The pins should not be bent away from the protrusio component, because such a maneuver tends to loosen the fixation across the sacroiliac joint.

The superacetabular cavity and acetabulum itself are packed with methylmethacrylate and the components are cemented in place to form a biomechanical continuum between the prosthetic acetabulum, protrusio ring, Steinmann rings, and intact bone superiorly.[15]

Class III fractures result from aggressive metastatic foci which frequently are highly vascular lesions. The typical primary tumors resulting in such lesions are myeloma, lymphoma, or carcinoma of the lung, kidney, thyroid, or colon. When a sharp, sclerotic, reactive rim is apparent roentgenographically (see Fig 27–4,E), it is likely that the host bone has reacted to the destructive tumor focus and that that focus is not highly vascular. However, when extensive reticulated osteolysis exists and extends irregularly and vaguely into the iliac wing (see Fig 27–4,C), consideration should be given to preoperative arteriographic evaluation of the area for assessment

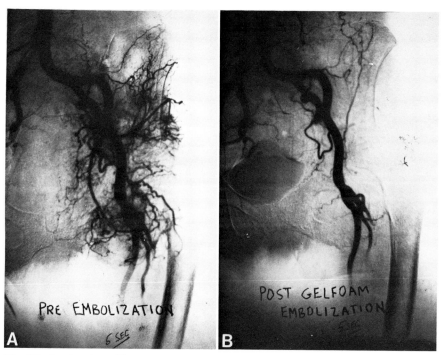

*Fig 27–6—**A,** class III metastatic carcinoma of the colon has caused extensive destruction of the medial, inferior, and superior acetabular walls. After a full course of radiotherapy, the femoral head migrated medially and superiorly through bones weakened by a combination of tumor osteolysis and hyperemia after irradiation. An x-ray film demonstrating diffuse and poorly circumscribed tumor osteolysis, particularly when secondary to metastatic carcinoma of the colon, strongly suggests a highly vascular lesion. Aortogram demonstrates hypervascularity of the metastatic focus with tumor vessels, all emanating from the hypergastric artery. **B,** aortographic appearance after selective embolization of the hypogastric artery with Gelfoam. Joint reconstruction using threaded Steinmann pins and methylmethacrylate then was accomplished with minimal blood loss.*

of its vascularity and for possible embolization of the tumor bed to minimize operative blood loss.[7]

When the arteriogram demonstrates excessive vascularity (Fig 27–6,A) one should embolize the major arterial trunk from which the tumor vessels arose. Strips of Gelfoam (2 × 20 mm) are cut and then morselized with sterile saline to make a syrup of a consistency that can just be forced through the catheter by injection. The Gelfoam effectively occludes the tumor vessels (Fig 27–6,B), thus devascularizing the operative site sufficiently to minimize blood replacement requirements. It is not essential to follow this arteriographic devascularization with immediate surgery. Delays of 24–48 hours do not result in any increased incidence of infection secondary to tumor necrosis.

When an excessively vascular lesion has not been anticipated or controlled preoperatively, blood loss at the time of operation may occur. In the majority of instances this bleeding is from tumor vessels within bone that cannot be controlled by electrocautery. Synthetic clotting substrates [Gelfoam or tribomoethanol (Avetine)] also are minimally effective. The otherwise uncontrollable hemorrhage from within the confines of such a bony tumor focus can be controlled effectively by packing the site with methylmethacrylate in its doughy prepolymerized state. As the acrylic polymerizes it expands, compressing the bleeding surfaces. In addition, the heat of polymerization may assist in cauterizing exposed tumor vessels. After 15 minutes the solid methylmethacrylate may be removed piecemeal using a small straight osteotome, exposing a dry bony bed. Reconstruction can then proceed in a blood-free field.

It should be noted that this procedure is not an appropriate alternative to preoperative embolization. Before methylmethacrylate can control hemorrhage effectively, most or all of the gross tumor tissue present must be removed. Blood loss during this procedure may be extreme, and by the time effective packing of the lesion with cement can be performed, the technique may become a lifesaving procedure to abate exsanguination.

PROPHYLACTIC FIXATION OF IMPENDING FRACTURES

In patients presenting with metastatic tumor foci in bone which are recognized before the development of a fracture, pain and progression of the lesion can usually be reversed by radiotherapy. This is the treatment of choice unless the bone is likely to fracture. However, the initial response of bone to radiation, particularly during the second week of therapy, is hyperemia at the periphery of the tumor focus with temporary softening of adjacent bone and an increased risk of spontaneous fracture. This is particularly true when the lesion is primarily lytic, but a similar phenomenon has been observed with primarily blastic lesions as well. Radiotherapists have become increasingly concerned that cancer patients will suffer a fracture during the course of radiation therapy, and consequently have become more adamant in demanding prophylatic fixation of impending fractures before radiation is instituted.[6, 9]

Neither a bone scan nor a roentgenogram alone of the affected area can be relied on to indicate completely the extent of tumor involvement or the risk of impending fracture. However, well-accepted criteria do exist and are reliable in most instances in predicting the likelihood of a fracture through a lytic metastatic focus. Femoral lesions which are primarily lytic, which are 2.5 cm or larger in the femur, or which involve destruction of 50% or more of the femoral cortex circumferentially are highly susceptible to fracture.[6, 16] Fidler and others demonstrated conclusively that a long bone lesion involving 50% of the cortex had at least a 50% chance of spontaneous fracture if not prophylactically reinforced.[17, 18] The most common indication for prophylactic fixation, however, is the persistence of pain with weight-bearing even in the face of effective radiation therapy.

Blind intramedullary nail fixation of impending long bone fractures is inadvisable if more than 75% of the cortex has been destroyed. All too often, with the progression of the lytic lesion, a telescoping fracture of the bone will occur despite such fixation, resulting in an unacceptable protrusion of the nail proximally. The only means of preventing this is to approach the potential fracture site directly, debulk the gross tumor tissue and destroyed bone by curettage, and pack the defect with methylmethacrylate while internally fixing the remaining bone with an intramedullary nail. The nail will resist shear and torque stresses and the cement will prevent telescoping.

Once prophylactic fixation of the affected long bone has been achieved, radiotherapy may be completed without risk of complications by fracture. There is good evidence that radiotherapy is neither adversely affected by the presence of acrylic cement nor interferes with the stability of such fixation.[3, 19, 20]

POSTOPERATIVE CARE

Patients are encouraged to be out of bed on the second or third postoperative day and to begin ambulation with full weight-bearing as soon as possible with the assistance of a trained physical therapist.

Patients who have not already received a full course of local irradiation to the tumor focus should have this initiated beginning 2–3 weeks postoperatively. As noted, there is no evidence that the presence of methylmethacrylate interferes with the efficacy of local irradiation, although a local ionization effect has been demonstrated at the site of a metal implant.[20] No clinical effects from this phenomenon have been recognized.[3]

Most pathologic fractures must be approached on an individualized basis depending on the extent of bone destruction, the location of the fracture, and the general condition of the patient. Treatment calls for some ingenuity on the part of the surgeon, and rigid standardization of technique is impossible. Nevertheless, the use of acrylic for fixation is not difficult technically and is well within the grasp of the orthopedic surgeon skilled in more conventional fracture management. Because acrylic fixation affords immediate fracture stability, almost all patients are able to resume walking and enjoy good relief of pain.

REFERENCES

1. Harrington K.D., Sim F.H., Enis J.E., et al.: Methylmethacrylate as an adjunct in the internal fixation of pathological fractures. *J. Bone Joint Surg.* 58A:1047-1055, 1976.
2. Marcove R.C., Yang D.J.: Survival times after treatment of pathological fractures. *Cancer* 20:2514, 1967.
3. Murray J.A., Bruels M.D., Lindberg R.D.: Irradiation of polymethylmethacrylate: In vitro gamma radiation effect. *J. Bone Joint Surg.* 56A:311-312, 1974.
4. Parrish F.F., Murray J.A.: Surgical treatment for secondary neoplastic fractures: A retrospective study of ninety-six patients. *J. Bone Joint Surg.* 52A:665-686, 1970.
5. Perez C.A., Bradfield J.S., Morgan H.C.: Management of pathologic fracture. *Cancer* 79:684-693, 1972.
6. Blake D.D.: Radiation treatment of metastatic bone disease. *Clin. Orthop.* 73:89, 1970.
7. Harrington K.D.: *The Management of Malignant Pathological Fractures.* American Academy of Orthopaedic Surgeons, *Instructional Course Lectures,* vol. 26. St. Louis, C.V. Mosby Co., 1977, pp. 147-162.

8. Coran A.G., Banks H.H., Aliapoulios M.A., et al.: The management of pathologic fractures in patients with metastatic carcinoma of the breast. *Surg. Gynecol. Obstet.* 126:1225, 1968.

9. Bonarigo B.C., Rubin P.: Nonunion of pathologic fracture after radiation therapy. *Radiology* 88:889, 1967.

10. Galasko C.W.B.: Pathological fractures secondary to metastatic cancer. *J. Coll. Surg. Edinb.* 19:351-362, 1974.

11. Zickel R.E., Mouradian W.H.: Intramedullary fixation of pathological fractures and lesions of the subtrochanteric region of the femur. *J. Bone Joint Surg.* 58A:1061-1066, 1976.

12. Charnley J.: *Acrylic Cement in Orthopaedic Surgery.* Baltimore, Williams & Wilkins Co., 1970.

13. Harrington K.D.: The use of methylmethacrylate as an adjunct in the internal fixation of unstable comminuted intertrochanteric fractures in osteoporotic patients. *J. Bone Joint Surg.* 57A:744, 1975.

14. Sloof T.J.: The influence of acrylic cement. *Acta Orthop. Scand.* 42:465, 1971.

15. Harrington K.D.: The management of acetabular insufficiency secondary to metastatic malignant disease. *J. Bone Joint Surg.* 63A:653-664, 1981.

16. Beals R.K., Lawton G.D., Snell W.E.: Prophylactic internal fixation of the femur in metastatic breast cancer. *Cancer* 28:1350, 1971.

17. Fidler M.: Prophylactic internal fixation of secondary neoplastic deposits in long bones. *Br. Med. J.* 1:341, 1973.

18. Rubin P., Green J.: *Solitary Metastases.* Springfield, Ill., Charles C Thomas, Publisher, 1968, pp. 143-167.

19. Bremner R.A., Jelliffee A.M.: The management of pathological fracture of the major long bones from metastatic cancer. *J. Bone Joint Surg.* 40:652-659, 1958.

20. Eftekhar N.S., Thurston C.W.: Effect of irradiation on acrylic cement with special reference to fixation of pathological fractures. *J. Biomech.* 8:53-56, 1975.

Chapter 28

Management of Infections Following Fracture of the Hip

Michael J. Patzakis, M.D.

Sepsis following postoperative treatment of hip fractures requires prompt diagnosis, accurate assessment of the extent of the infection, prompt emergency surgical treatment, and institution of appropriate systemic antibiotic therapy. Not only can sepsis be life-threatening, the socioeconomic impact is great because of the frequent necessity for prolonged and repeated hospitalizations. The end result may be impaired function and increased morbidity because of interference with the osteogenic process, destruction of the hip joint itself, or the performance of resectional arthroplasty as a salvage procedure. For these reasons it is imperative that the operating surgeon have a rational approach to the management of the infected hip fracture.

DIAGNOSIS AND ASSESSMENT OF INFECTION

The cardinal feature in the treatment of postoperative infection of hip fractures is prompt diagnosis. Clinical signs of infection such as postoperative fever, persistent pain, swelling, erythema, edema of the wound, and drainage should all make one suspect the likelihood of infection. Laboratory aids and diagnostic tools include (1) the complete blood cell count and erythrocyte sedimentation rate, (2) blood cultures, (3) Gram stain and culture of wound drainage, (4) aspiration of the operative site, (5) roentgenography, (6) sinography, (7) abscessography, (8) arthrography, and (9) bone scanning. Although the laboratory aids are helpful in increasing the index of suspicion for infection, the diagnosis is based on identification of the organism on Gram stain or culture of material drained from the wound and/or aspirated from the fracture site or hip joint. Because the cultures generally take 24–72 hours to grow, the Gram stain is an important factor in starting specific antibiotic therapy as well as undertaking prompt surgical treatment.

Joint space narrowing on x-ray films in the postoperative hip patient should be considered to be caused by infection until proved otherwise. Joint space narrowing develops later in the postoperative period, generally after several weeks have elapsed. In patients that have a draining wound or sinus, a sinogram obtained using radiopaque contrast material delineates the extent of the infection and aids in determining whether the infection is superficial or deep, thus allowing one to assess the extent of the infection. For patients whose wounds are not actively draining but in whom frank

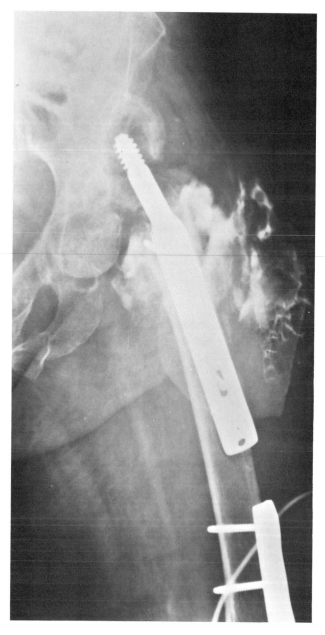

*Fig 28–1—
Abscessogram in a 69-
year-old woman with an
infected intracapsular
fracture. The
compression screw has
cut out of the femoral
head.*

pus is encountered when the fracture site is aspirated, the injection of radiopaque contrast material will help delineate the extent of the abscess cavity (Fig 28–1).

In patients with intracapsular fractures, it is imperative that the joint be aspirated and arthrography performed to document the location of the aspiration (Figures 28–2 and 28–3). Often, if no fluid is obtained when the hip joint is aspirated, one may misinterpret the aspiration findings and believe that sepsis of the joint is not present when in fact the needle did not enter the joint space. In addition, if purulent material is encountered, the arthrogram may show capsular ruptures and document the extent of infection at that time. Technetium 99 methylene diphosphonate and especially gallium 67 scans are more useful in late infections; radio-

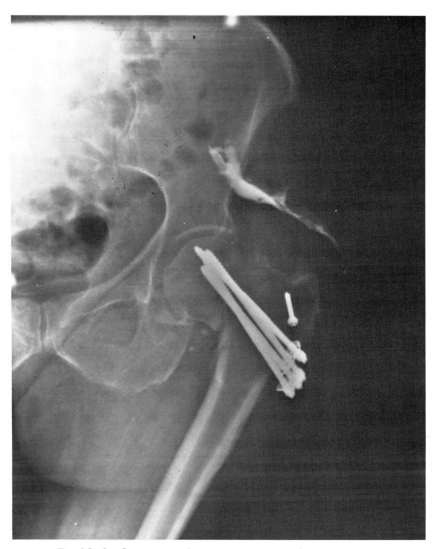

Fig 28–2—Sinogram showing extracapsular sinus tract.

actively tagged indium blood cells are also useful in diagnosis and they help in assessing less obvious infections that may be present.

SURGICAL TREATMENT

Once the diagnosis of infection is made, all patients must undergo formal irrigation and debridement of the wound in the operating suite, with excision of all necrotic bone and soft tissue. The objective is to convert a contaminated infected wound to a clean surgical wound. Copious amounts of irrigating fluid should be utilized. We use 10 L of irrigating fluid, usually 8 L of normal saline and 2 L of antibiotic solution containing 50,000 units of bacitracin and 1 million units of polymyxin per liter of normal saline.

For purposes of treatment, infected hip fractures can be grouped into extracapsular and intracapsular fractures. With respect to infected extracapsular fracture

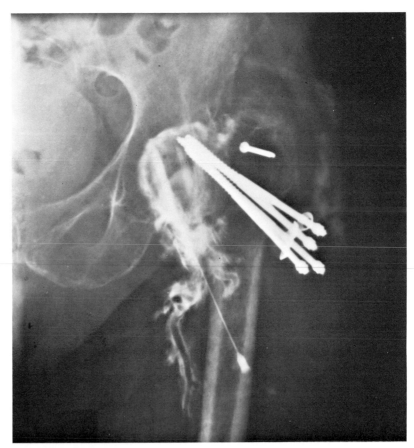

Fig 28–3—Aspiration of the hip joint with arthrogram. Some contrast material has been inadvertently injected into the femoral artery sheath.

of the hip, once the extent of the infection has been assessed in the acute postoperative period following internal fixation, the patient should be taken to surgery and the wound should be extensively debrided. If the internal fixation device is providing stability it should not be removed. If it is not providing stability, it should be removed and the fracture stabilized with another internal fixation device or with skeletal traction. Figures 28–4 and 28–5 are roentgenograms of a patient who was transferred to our institution following an extracapsular fracture for an injury sustained in an automobile-train collision. The patient was febrile and had clinical evidence of a hip infection. An abscessogram was obtained (see Fig 28–4) and the patient was taken to surgery, where formal irrigation and debridement were performed and the internal fixation device, a Jewett nail, at the time thought not to be providing adequate stability, was removed and replaced with a Richard compression screw. The wound was closed over tubes and the bone subsequently united without further evidence of infection.

Figures 28–6 through 28–8 are roentgenograms of a patient in whom, because of medical problems, surgery on the intertrochanteric fracture was delayed. A metastatic hematogenous infection of the fracture site subsequently developed and the patient was taken to surgery, where the wound was debrided and irrigated and left open and the fracture was treated in traction. The wounds healed by secondary intention, and subsequently the intertrochanteric hip fracture also healed.

When postoperative infection develops after the fracture has united, the internal fixation device should be removed at the time of surgical drainage and debridement as it is no longer necessary, and the foreign body may become a nidus for continuing infection. Patients with infected intracapsular fractures inadvertently have pyarthrosis. If the fracture has displaced and there is destruction of the joint as well as of the femoral head, and the head is not salvageable, it is advisable to remove all of the internal fixation devices as well as the necrotic femoral head and convert the fracture to a resectional arthroplasty (Girdlestone procedure).

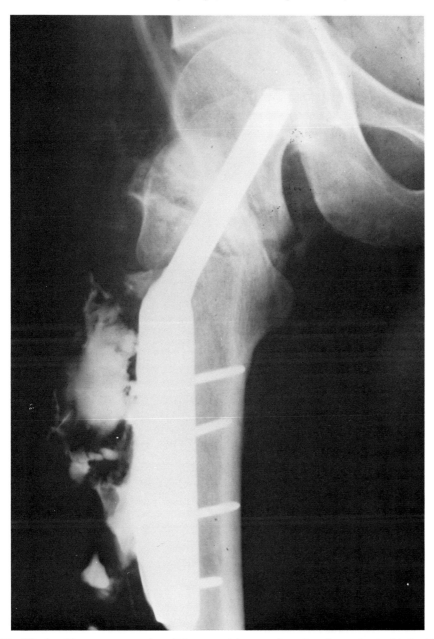

Fig 28–4—Abscessogram in a 54-year-old man showing the extent of infection. Fracture is displaced.

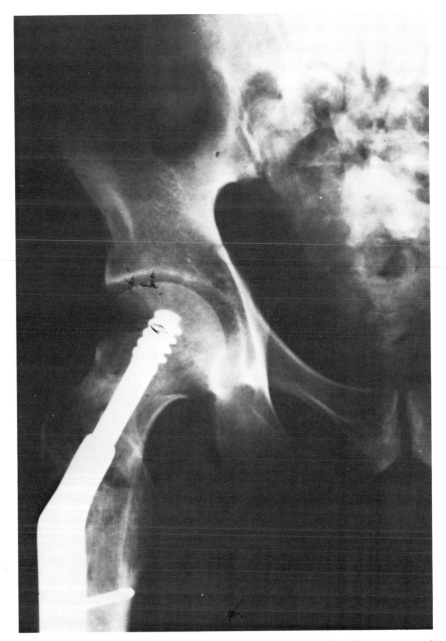

Fig 28–5—Same patient as in Figure 28–4. Jewett nail has been removed and fracture reduced and fixed with a compression screw blade plate.

Following extensive irrigation and debridement of the wound, patients are placed in skeletal traction. Because many patients with hip fractures are elderly, they often cannot tolerate 6 weeks of skeletal traction, as was recommended by Girdlestone in his original article.[1] Therefore, we have treated the majority of our patients with 3 weeks of traction and have seen no additional shortening using this protocol as opposed to 6 weeks of traction. Similar conclusions were reported by Parr et al.[2] in their series: they found no correlation between the length of time the patient was held in traction postoperatively and the ultimate shortening or loss of function.

Figures 28–9 and 28–10 are roentgenograms of a 62-year-old woman who was treated with a muscle pedicle graft and multiple pin fixation. A postoperative infection developed with loss of reduction, and the head was nonviable. A Girdlestone arthroplasty procedure was performed, followed by 3 weeks of traction. A roentgenogram obtained 10 months after surgery is shown in Figure 28–10.

Figures 28–11 through 28–13 are roentgenograms of a 73-year-old woman who had been treated with a Moore prosthesis for a transcervical fracture of the femur. The fracture subsequently dislocated and a deep wound infection ensued that necessitated removal of the implant. In patients who because of medical problems or pressures sores cannot tolerate continuous traction, we use intermittent traction, and if it is imperative to have the patient out of bed, we use an abduction thigh brace or pillow to keep the hip abducted and the proximal femoral shaft from putting pressure on the soft tissues, which would cause wound breakdown.

Resection of the head and neck of the femur is a salvage procedure used for control of the infected hip fracture when there is both joint and femoral head

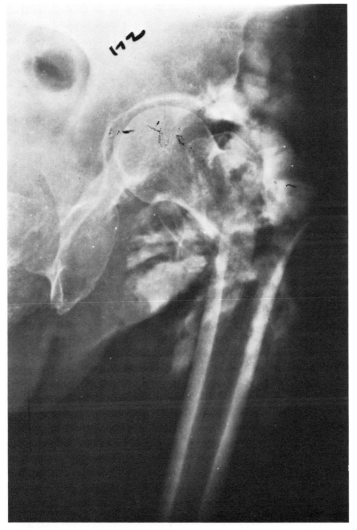

Fig 28–6—Abscessogram of a 57-year-old woman with hematogenous seeding of an intertrochanteric fracture.

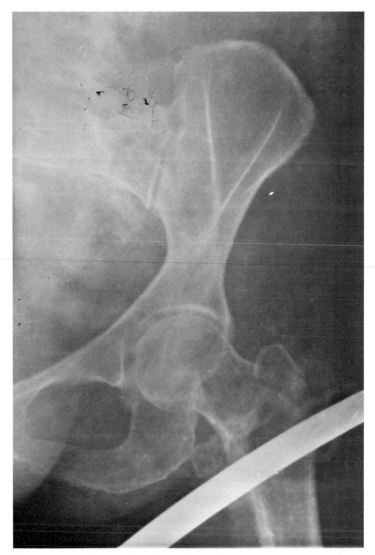

Fig 28–7—Same patient as in Figure 28–6. Fracture was treated in traction.

destruction. This procedure was first described in 1849 after White[3] resected the hip joint of a 9-year-old boy with septic arthritis. Girdlestone[1,4] reported using the procedure to treat tuberculosis of the hip in 1928, and again in 1943 to treat acute pyogenic arthritis of the hip.

Parr, Croft, and Enneking[2] in 1971 reported control of infection in 11 of 12 patients. From a functional standpoint, reports in the literature[5,6] suggest that Girdlestone resection arthroplasties provide a poor functional result and are generally painful. In selected patients the Girdlestone resectional arthroplasty can later be converted to a total hip arthroplasty. Figure 28–14, A and B are roentgenograms of a 52-year-old woman in whom a Girdlestone resectional arthroplasty was converted to a total hip arthroplasty after more than 12 months of no clinical reactivation of a staphylococcal infection, confirmed by laboratory tests and repeated aspirations. Nine years after total hip conversion she continued to function without any signs of reactivation of the previous infection.

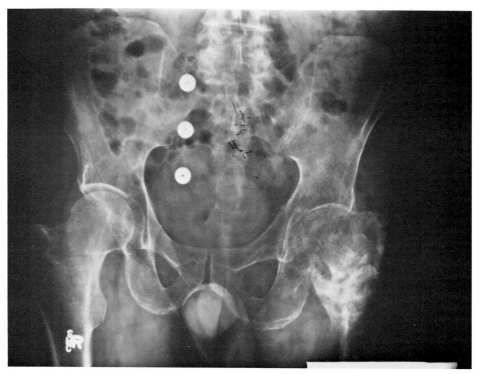

Fig 28–8—Same patient as in Figure 28–6. Fracture at 3 months is on its way to union.

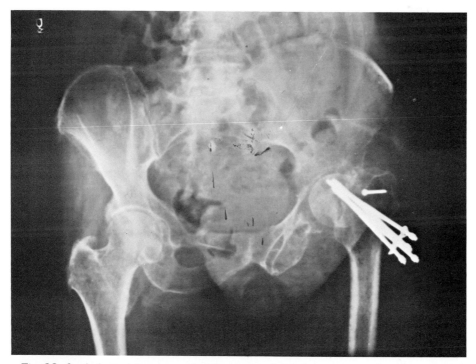

Fig 28–9—Infected transcervical fracture of the femur treated with a muscle pedicle graft and multiple pin fixation.

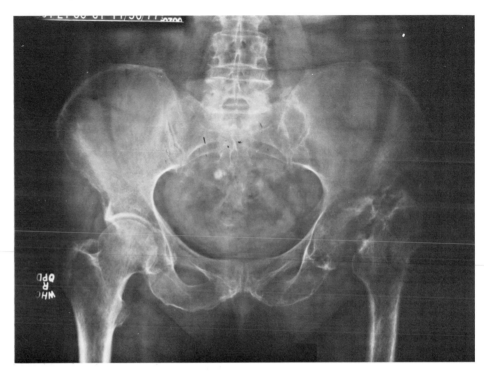

Fig 28–10—Same patient as in Figure 28–9. Hip appearance 10 months after
Girdlestone arthroplasty.

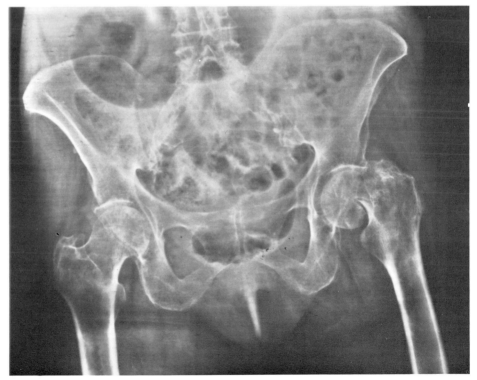

Fig 28–11—73-year-old woman with a left transcervical femur fracture.

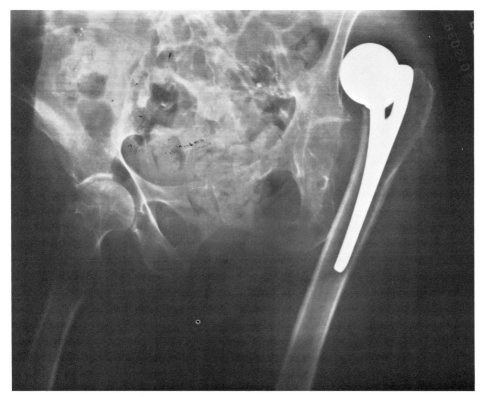

Fig 28–12—Same patient as in Figure 28–11. Left hip is dislocated.

SURGICAL PROCEDURE FOR RESECTIONAL ARTHROPLASTY

If an incision was made previously, we attempt to incorporate lateral scars into the present incision. We use a posterolateral incision extending along the lateral aspect of the femoral shaft to the greater trochanter and then proceeding posteriorly toward the posterosuperior iliac spine. The incision is then carried down through the skin and subcutaneous tissue and the fascia tensor. The fascia lata is incised along its plane and the fascia of the gluteus maximus is cut and the muscle split. The gluteus medius and minimus muscles are retracted anteriorly and the external rotators are identified and incised. The piriform tendon lies just superior to the capsule. Once this tendon is incised, the capsule can be identified. The capsule is then excised and the hip joint and fracture site are exposed. Internal fixation devices are removed. All necrotic bone, including the femoral head, is removed, and all necrotic tissues, including synovium, are excised. The excision should be as complete as possible, leaving raw surfaces of vascular cancellous bone with beveled smooth surfaces.[7] The wound is irrigated with copious amounts of irrigating solution and hemostasis is effected so that the wound is dry prior to closure. The surgeon should feel that the wound has been converted to a clean surgical wound.

If the wound is not clean and there is extensive abscess present, the wound should be packed open. If the wound is closed, the wound should be closed either over closed suction irrigation or Hemovac drains. In our early series we used closed suction irrigation, but recently we have used just closed Hemovac drains for 48 hours. The reason for using drainage rather than suction irrigation is to avoid the possibility of contamination by hydrophilic organisms, primarily gram-negative ones that we

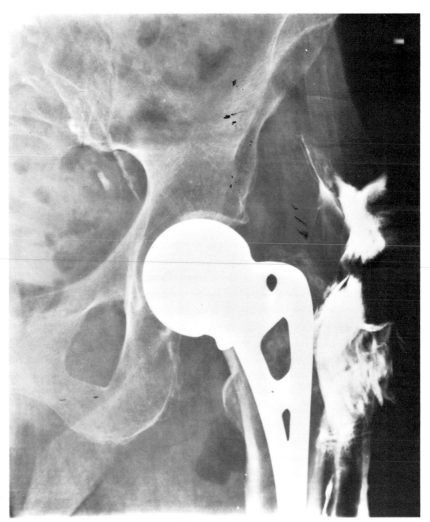

Fig 28–13—Same patient as in Figure 28–11. Abscessogram shows extent of deep infection. Prosthesis was subsequently removed.

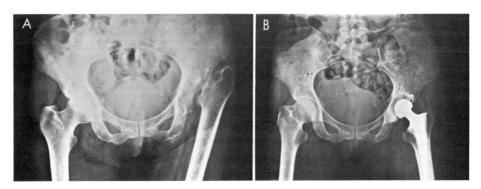

Fig 28–14—**A,** AP x-ray of pelvis before surgery of a 52-year-old woman who had Girdlestone arthoplasty several years ago. **B,** 9 years after total hip replacement there was no evidence of infection.

and others have reported in the literature.[8-10] For closed suction irrigation we have used an antibiotic solution containing 50,000 units of bacitracin and 1 million units of polymyxin per liter of fluid, in the amount of 2 L of fluid a day for 48 hours. On the third day, both the ingress and egress tubes are hooked up to Emerson suction pumps, and after 24 hours of suction, both tubes are removed. It is imperative that both tubes be placed on suction drainage for at least 24–48 hours after the ingress irrigating solution has been stopped, in order to decompress the dead space as well as remove all fluid and hematoma present. Otherwise an abscess cavity will remain and the likelihood of success will be diminished.

Wounds that are left open may either be allowed to granulate by secondary intention or may be converted to closed wounds by delayed closure in 7–10 days. Prior to secondary closure a quantitative wound culture should be done and there should be fewer than 10^{-5} organisms present; otherwise the wound should not be closed secondarily. At the time of delayed closure the entire wound must be excised so that all contaminated tissue is removed. This is a major step contributing to the success of delayed closure. At surgery the entire wound should be excised and debrided, thereby converting it to clean healthy tissue prior to closure.

ANTIBIOTIC THERAPY

Antibiotic therapy is instituted based on the Gram stain, culture results, and sensitivity reports. The usual dosages for antibiotics are listed in Table 28–1. In patients that have *Pseudomonas* infections a combination of an aminoglycoside such as tobramycin or gentamicin and a synthetic penicillin such as piperacillin gives the best response to treatment. Antibiotic toxicity should be monitored, and it is imperative that an infectious disease consultant help manage the patient and observe for antibiotic side effects. The length of antibiotic therapy reported in the literature varies but is usually 3–6 weeks. We have found that 3 weeks of intravenous antibiotic therapy is adequate and additional therapy should be based on clinical need. In our experience, when failures occur, it is usually not because of the length of antibiotic therapy, but because the wound was not converted to a clean wound and debridement was not thorough. A surgeon must constantly monitor the wound, and decisions for redebridement should be made as early as possible after the first debridement in order to prevent the morbidity and antibiotic toxicity consequent on prolonged an-

TABLE 28–1.—Commonly Given Antibiotics and Usual Dosages

Antibiotic	Dosage
Synthetic penicillins Methicillin Oxacillin	1–2 gm q4h IV, or 100–200 mg/kg/24 hours
Penicillin	10–20 million units/24 hours, IV
Cephalosporins	1–2 gm q4h IV, or 100–150 mg/kg/24 hours
Cefamandole	12 gm, maximum
Keflin	18 gm, maximum
Cefadyl	18 gm, maximum
Piperacillin	Usual dosage, 3 gm q4–6h IV, or 200–300 gm/kg/24 hours
Vancomycin	500 mg q6–8h IV
Clindamycin	600 mg q6h IV, maximum 2.4 gm/day

tibiotic therapy. Patients that are on aminoglycoside therapy should have peak and trough serum levels assessed in order to ascertain whether they are receiving adequate and safe therapeutic dosages.

REFERENCES

1. Girdlestone G.R.: Arthrodesis and other operations for tuberculosis of the hip, in *The Robert Jones Birthday Volume.* London, 1928, p. 347.
2. Parr P.L., Croft C., Enneking W.F.: Resection of the head and neck of the femur with and without angulation osteotomy. *J. Bone Joint Surg.* 53A:935-944, 1971.
3. Obituary of Anthony White. *Lancet* 1:324-325, 1849.
4. Girdlestone G.R.: Acute pyogenic arthritis of the hip: An operation giving free access and effective drainage. *Lancet* 1:419-421, 1943.
5. Bittar E.S., Petty W.: Girdlestone arthroplasty for infected total hip arthroplasty. *Clin. Orthop.* 170:84, 1982.
6. Clegg J.: The results of pseudoarthrosis after removal of an infected total hip prosthesis. *J. Bone Joint Surg.* 59B:298, 301, 1977.
7. Taylor R.G.: Pseudoarthrosis of the hip and foot joint. *J. Bone Joint Surg.* 32B:161-165, 1950.
8. Kelly P.J., Martin W.J., Conventry M.B.: Chronic osteomyelitis: Treatment with closed irrigation and suction. *JAMA* 213:1843-1848, 1970.
9. Leddy J.P., Grantham S.A., Stinchfield F.E.: Hip mold arthroplasty and postoperative infection. *J. Bone Joint Surg.* 53A:37-46, 1971.
10. Patzakis M.J., Dorr L.D., Moore T.M., et al.: The early management of open joint injuries. *J. Bone Joint Surg.* 56A:532-541, 1974.

Index